INTEGRATIVE THERAPIES
FOR
FIBROMYALGIA,
CHRONIC FATIGUE SYNDROME,
AND
MYOFASCIAL PAIN

"This integrative holistic approach to these conditions is what is needed throughout medicine today. Empowering us to become part of our own health and healing process is such a powerful approach to these conditions or any others. I applaud the authors, and hope they inspire others to follow their lead."

BILL DOUGLAS, AUTHOR OF
THE COMPLETE IDIOT'S GUIDE TO T'AI CHI & QIGONG

INTEGRATIVE THERAPIES
FOR
FIBROMYALGIA, CHRONIC FATIGUE SYNDROME,
AND
MYOFASCIAL PAIN

The Mind-Body Connection

CELESTE COOPER, R.N.,
AND JEFFREY MILLER, Ph.D.

Healing Arts Press
Rochester, Vermont • Toronto, Canada

Healing Arts Press
One Park Street
Rochester, Vermont 05767
www.HealingArtsPress.com

Healing Arts Press is a division of Inner Traditions International

Note to the reader: This book is intended as an informational guide. The remedies, approaches, and techniques described herein are meant to supplement, and not to be a substitute for, professional medical care or treatment. They should not be used to treat a serious ailment without prior consultation with a qualified health care professional.

Library of Congress Cataloging-in-Publication Data
Cooper, Celeste.
  Integrative therapies for fibromyalgia, chronic fatigue syndrome, and myofascial pain : the mind-body connection / Celeste Cooper and Jeffrey Miller.
    p. cm.
  Includes bibliographical references and index.
  ISBN 978-1-59477-323-5 (pbk.)
  1. Fibromyalgia—Alternative treatment. 2. Chronic fatigue syndrome—Alternative treatment. 3. Myofascial pain syndromes—Alternative treatment. I. Miller, Jeffrey. II. Title.
  RC927.3.I58 2010
  616.7'42—dc22

                                                            2009044469

Printed and bound in the United States by P. A. Hutchison

10 9 8 7 6 5 4 3 2 1

Text design by Jon Desautels and layout by Priscilla Baker
This book was typeset in Garamond Premier Pro, with Helvetica Neue and Gill Sans used as display typefaces

Trigger point art on pages 41 and 43 is reprinted from Clair Davies's book *The Trigger Point Therapy Workbook,* 2nd ed. (Oakland, Calif: New Harbinger Publications, 2004), pages 21 and 37. Used by permission of Amber Davies.

Excerpt on page 143 from Carol Eustice reprinted by permission of Carol Eustice, Arthritis .about.com.

"The Sickening Six" on page 191 reprinted from *Arthritis Survival* by Robert S. Ivker and Todd Nelson, copyright © 2001 by Robert S. Ivker. Used by permission of Jeremy P. Tarcher, an imprint of Penguin Group (USA) Inc.

Excerpts on pages 302 and 304 from *Driving Your Own Karma* by Swami Beyondananda (Steve Bhaerman) reprinted by permission of Inner Traditions International, Rochester, Vermont, www.InnerTraditions.com.

To send correspondence to the authors of this book, mail a first-class letter to the authors c/o Inner Traditions • Bear & Company, One Park Street, Rochester, VT 05767, and we will forward the communication.

Contents

Foreword

Managing one invisible and often misunderstood chronic illness is a challenge. Functioning well with three of them can seem overwhelming. Fibromyalgia, chronic fatigue immunodysfunction, and chronic myofascial pain can wear you down if you aren't prepared. The general support systems that automatically kick in for people who have more obvious or better-known illnesses are absent. Life doesn't end when you get these illnesses, but it does change and a new life begins. It's up to you to determine the quality of that life. These conditions require many changes if you are to successfully navigate the often-treacherous currents in the river of life. One of the most important changes is that of your own attitude toward life and to the illness that complicates it.

Integrative Therapies for Fibromyalgia, Chronic Fatigue Syndrome, and Myofascial Pain: The Mind-Body Connection is a good guidebook to facilitate this positive change.

DEVIN J. STARLANYL

Devin J. Starlanyl is former director of the Fibromyalgia and Chronic Myofascial Pain Institute and is the author, with Mary Ellen Copeland, of *Fibromyalgia and Chronic Myofascial Pain: A Survival Manual* and *The Fibromyalgia Advocate*.

Preface

The writing of this book started as an exercise for mental health. Toward the end of a twenty-year nursing career in critical care, emergency nursing, and education, my musculoskeletal symptoms had become severe. I had spent approximately six years juggling chronic pain, family, and work. I cut back my work from full time to part time and tried changing the focus of my career. Because of my disorders, I found that the work I loved so much was no longer possible. My story is typical.

I was fortunate to find a neurologist knowledgeable in myofascial pain before the full implications were realized. He was actually able to see the twitch response on my back when he gave me trigger point injections and taught me about this telltale response of trigger points to injections and pressure. He also suggested alternative treatments.

However, before I was diagnosed with fibromyalgia (FM), I suffered through more than five years of unrelenting, unforgiving symptoms of body-wide pain, fatigue, and flu-like symptoms.

As happens to so many of us, I was also the target of remarks that threatened my self-esteem. When I was finally diagnosed with fibromyalgia (FM), an additional, separate disorder from chronic myofascial pain, I had reached a point of desperation and despair over my feelings of loss. Being a "type A" personality, I couldn't accept lack of control.

My psychotherapist was able to help me address my reactions to others and to the health care community of which I had once been a part. That therapist is now my friend and coauthor of this book.

After my diagnosis, I knew I needed to learn as much as I could about these disorders. It was through people like Devin Starlanyl, Dr. I. Jon Russell, and Clair Davies, as well as the Fibromyalgia Network, The Forum, and my support group members that I discovered why birds flock together. You will see references throughout the book recognizing these people for what they have done for so many others and for me.

I was disheartened by the ignorance regarding fibromyalgia (FM), chronic fatigue immunodysfunction (CFID), and chronic myofascial pain (CMP) in the medical community. To my dismay there were many who did not know the difference between the tender points of FM and the trigger points of CMP, or between the fatigue associated with FM and the overwhelming, life-altering fatigue of CFID. Among them were some health care providers and specialists who professed that they knew about fibromyalgia, chronic fatigue, and chronic myofascial pain.

Understanding the differences and the similarities of these three disorders, and knowing how to respond to others in an informative way will contribute to making you the star player in your own show.

Acknowledgments

I believe God is responsible for certain people crossing another's life path. Some believe it is destiny. For me (Celeste), this is an acknowledgement of God's undying love. He never promised me that life would have no trials and tribulations. He did, however, promise to be there to help me through. Without Him, I would be nothing; without Him, none of these people would have been there for me.

First, I want to thank my mother for always encouraging me to be the best I could be, and for teaching me by example that nothing worth having comes without sacrifice.

To my sis, what can I say? You build me up. You give me confidence in myself.

I thank my husband for picking up when I could no longer handle the job. I know my illnesses have affected your life as well. Because of these unrelenting illnesses and their unpredictability, there is little left of me, and writing uses most of that. May God bless you for sacrificing so that I might continue to help others.

I thank my friends—the ones I have left—for hanging in there with me. Thank you for being there when I didn't think I could make it through another day; for listening when I needed to talk, even though I'm sure you didn't want to hear it again; for understanding when I couldn't repay a favor; and for accepting me as I am.

All my FMily members are so very important to me. It is essential to have a strong support system to make it through the trials of chronic illness. Being able to talk to people who understand exactly what it is like for you brings comfort. Thank you for being there.

Thank you to the person who coined the term FMily, Devin Starlanyl. You have been everything and more to me and your contribution to this book has been invaluable. You picked me up and dusted me off as a new writer. Few would make the personal sacrifices you made to help me be the best I could be. You are all that a mentor should be. You guided me so that I could grow and you corrected me so my readers would have the best information. You did more than just coin the term; you became part of my FMily.

Thanks also to Sondra Cooper, human resource specialist, and Josh Joseph Sonsiadek, chiropractic physician and biochemist, for your helpful contributions to the book.

I cannot conclude these acknowledgments without recognizing all those at Inner Traditions/Healing Arts Press who have morphed my dream into reality. First and foremost, thank you Laura, my project editor, for all your care for not only the book, but for me as well. Your unending dedication and personal concern will forever remain in my heart. Abigail, my copy editor, thank you for your meticulous attention to detail, even though there were times when I wished you weren't quite so good at your job. I only mean that lovingly; it is because of the questions you asked and the overwhelming time I know you spent researching that I know you have been truly vested in our book. To all the people at Inner Traditions who had a hand in the publication of this book, I have some experience working with others, and I can tell you, you are all number one, without exception. The pleasure in working with all of you is truly mine. What more could a writer possibly ask for?

This book is dedicated to all of those, both in the present and in the past, who have been instrumental in my life and believed in me—I will meet you again one day.

CELESTE COOPER

I would like to thank my parents for their unwavering support. My thanks to the professors who turned the lamp on for me, Jay Haley, Milton Erickson, B. F. Skinner, Roger Ulrich, Hilary Karp, Duane Hartley, and Bill Jesse. My family deserves an award for putting up with Daddy's writing schedule; much love to Marji, Corina, and Wilson. Most special thanks to my best teachers who graciously drive to my office and take their hour teaching me about their conditions as they grow and improve, and to Celeste for kicking me where and when it was needed and proving me "write." My work here is respectfully dedicated to my late brother, Bob, a brilliant educator shining bright too briefly.

JEFFREY MILLER

Introduction

We hope you find this book informational, motivational, interactive, and integral to your health care treatment plan. We encourage you to share what you discover with your family, friends, and health care providers.

For people who suffer chronic disorders, advocating is more than just therapeutic. In my case, it has been essential for my mental health. Because of the need for research, fueling this type of work has been a means of using my talents to help others in ways that support our cause. One of my main obstacles to writing is "brain fog," or cognitive deficit. It was the need to address my feelings of isolation and psychological despair that caused me to begin writing this book. What started as therapy has come into reality due to encouragement, help, and correction by my dear friend and coauthor, Dr. Jeffrey Miller. Through his help I have been able to produce my portion of this book.

Fibromyalgia (FM) and chronic myofascial pain (CMP) are thought by many, including some health care providers, to be interchangeable. Nothing could be further from the truth. However, they do often coexist in the same patient, which makes accurate diagnosis difficult at best. It is important to know if a patient has one or both disorders so that the correct treatment plan can be developed. As a patient with both, I can tell you that some treatments for FM may actually aggravate the symptoms of CMP, and vice versa. Some treatments, such as those discussed in chapter 4, may be beneficial for both.

Fibromyalgia and chronic fatigue immunodysfunction (CFID) are often lumped together as the same disorder. Both involve fatigue, which is the primary symptom of CFID, but the two disorders are dissimilar and have different diagnostic criteria, noted in chapter 1. The two conditions are similar in that both are thought to be caused by a disruption in the central nervous system, but they are dissimilar in the actual pathway of disruption. The treatments for FM and CFID, however, are similar, with a few differences.

It is not uncommon for the same patient to have a combination of any two or all three conditions. Since they have common treatment modalities, as well as conflicting therapeutic interventions, it is important to include all three in one book.

Understanding the three disorders will empower you. Chapter 1 will help you to identify the different symptoms of fibromyalgia, chronic fatigue immunodysfunction, and chronic myofascial pain; distinguish which warning signs apply to you; and determine what information is important to share with your doctor. Whatever your conclusions, it is important to learn what aggravates or alleviates your symptoms, and how to relate your findings to those who will be helping with your care. Whether you actually have all three conditions, a combination of two, or only one, the topics discussed in this book will be applicable.

Learning to deal with the psychological issues that can and do evolve with chronic pain disorders like these can have a profound impact on your relationships and on the way you feel emotionally, physically, and spiritually. All too often there is fear of sharing underlying concerns, and the value of mental health is not recognized. This book will help you to address your apprehension without fear of consequence.

We feel spiritual health is just as important as mental and physical health. Jeff, my co-author, is Buddhist by faith and his spirituality defines his total being. I rely on my spiritual base as a Christian; my spirituality has played an integral part in learning who I am as a whole person, and in how I deal with chronic illness. We both believe that one aspect of health relies on spiritual fulfillment, and that religious beliefs are a way to meet that need. Perpetual enrichment of spirit is as vital to total well-being as food is necessary for sustaining the body. We hope our book will help you to understand what a difference it can make to be mentally clear and nourished in body, mind, and spirit.

No matter how much we think we are in control of what is happening to us and around us, we are not prepared for a crisis. Chapter 6 will give you some tips for dealing with a catastrophe or calamity.

There is no reason for you to feel alone, isolated, or without resources. From the front cover to the back, this book is packed with helpful tools for dealing with pain, exhaustion, fatigue, health care providers, family, friends, coworkers, self-esteem, depression, anxiety, stress, and medical and legal red tape. Last, but not least, we hope the information on advocacy and dealing with the health care system will empower you and give you a sense of control.

This book is specifically dedicated to providing you with the means to find the support you need.

1

Fibromyalgia Pain, Chronic Fatigue Immunodysfunction, and Chronic Myofascial Pain from Trigger Points

In order to address and identify personal needs we must first be able to define what they are and how they affect our lives. This chapter is devoted to promoting a better understanding of fibromyalgia (FM), chronic fatigue immunodysfunction (CFID), and chronic myofascial pain (CMP).

By reviewing the definition, history, demographics, etiology, genetic or gender predisposition, diagnostic criteria, symptoms, and prognosis, you should be able to identify certain characteristics of each disorder. You will receive enough information to complete the interactive exercise at the end of each section. By the end of the chapter you will see how the disorders share certain symptoms, but are differentiated by others.

Our greatest desire is for you to realize you are not alone. We are learning together and by sharing our knowledge, we can make a difference in combating these disabling illnesses.

New studies, theories, and discoveries will continue after the publication of this book, and the resource section includes the best tools available at the time of publication for locating current and breaking information. There are many helpful links at TheseThree.com, which are updated periodically.

Throughout this book fibromyalgia is referred to as FM, chronic fatigue immunodysfunction is referred to as CFID, and chronic myofascial pain is referred to as CMP. All three of these disabling disorders are considered chronic illnesses and can be a devastating disruption to your lifestyle, psyche, and general well-being.

COMMONLY USED ABBREVIATIONS

FM: fibromyalgia or fibromyalgia syndrome (FMS)

CFID: chronic fatigue immunodysfunction syndrome
Also known as:
chronic fatigue syndrome (CFS)
and myalgic encephalomyelitis (ME)

CMP: chronic myofascial pain
Also known as:
myofascial pain syndrome/disease (MPS)

It's important to have a clear understanding of what is known to us now and what remains to be discovered. We hope that having a clearer understanding will help you to identify symptoms related to your disorder(s) and to set goals for enhancing your quality of life. As you journey through the words, paragraphs, and pages of this book, keep in mind that the guidelines and interactive exercises are intended to augment or complement medical care and treatments, not replace them.

During your journey take time at each summary exercise to reflect on the section of road you have just traveled. Brain fog and concentration may be a huge obstacle, but it is important to read the chapters in order, because the information in each one builds on the previous chapter. Don't get discouraged if you start to feel fatigue; just come back to it when you feel "on top" of things, and you'll be glad you did. This is a self-help book that depends on your reactions and interactions; it is about you and for you. Have a great journey.

All About Fibromyalgia

It's Not All in a Name

The term fibromyalgia gives the impression it is a muscle disorder. After reading the rest of this chapter, you will know that this is inaccurate. Research suggests it is a disorder of the central nervous system that affects the muscles and the relay system of brain messaging.

It's difficult to find correct terminology for each of the three disorders discussed in this book. Although that may seem trivial to some, the name of a disorder can have a tremendous impact on the way it is perceived and treated. Someday, through scientific discovery and advocacy by patients and the health care community, we will get away from ambiguous terms.

---

fibro: from the word fibrous, meaning "composed of fibers"; an elongated threadlike structure (in this case pertaining to fibers, fascia, tendons, and ligaments).

muscle fibers: having the power to contract and produce movement; fibers responsible for locomotion and performing vital body functions.

algia: pain.

myalgia: muscle pain.

allodynia: "other pain"; pain from stimuli that are not normally painful.

pain: a feeling of distress, suffering, or agony caused by stimulation to specific nerve endings. Usually a protective mechanism that alerts the sufferer to early tissue damage somewhere in the body.

pain threshold: the level that must be reached for a stimulus to be recognized as painful.

Definition

Fibromyalgia is defined as follows, according to American College of Rheumatology (ACR) criteria:

From patient history: widespread aching lasting more than three months
From examination: local tenderness at eleven of eighteen specific sites

Please keep in mind that the ACR criteria, while still used for diagnosis, may lead to underdiagnosis in many people, both women and men. More importantly, FM is a disorder characterized by widespread pain, abnormal pain processing, sleep disturbance, fatigue, and sometimes psychological distress. People with fibromyalgia may also have other symptoms, such as morning stiffness, tingling or numbness in hands and feet, headaches (including migraines), irritable bowel syndrome, problems with thinking and memory (sometimes called "fibro fog"), painful menstrual periods, and other pain syndromes.[1] It is a chronic, noninflammatory disorder characterized by widespread allodynia, fatigue, and multiple tender points. Although it's not a life threatening or progressive illness, symptoms can intensify or diminish without warning.

History

Fibromyalgia is not a new syndrome or disorder. It has been officially recognized by the health care industry for the past two decades, and has been known to exist for more than a hundred years. Symptoms of what we know today as FM were first described in the seventeen hundreds, and the disorder was first observed and documented by British surgeon William Balfour in 1816. In 1904 the same collection of symptoms was recognized by another British fibromyalgia pioneer, Sir William Gowers, who described chronic soft tissue syndromes as fibromyocitis.[2]

When Dr. Gowers identified this same collection of symptoms, he described it as "a disorder affecting women of blameless habits and abstentious clergymen," and treated these patients with exercise instead of aspirin.[3] This treatment suggests that as early as the nineteen hundreds Dr. Gowers did not consider this disorder inflammatory by nature, even though many of his colleagues of those days thought it was. He was a true pioneer in understanding the symptoms of fibromyalgia.

Later in the nineteen hundreds the term *fibrositis* appeared in North American rheumatology textbooks. In the 1940s fibromyalgia was thought to be associated with depression and stress, and later, in 1975, Harvey Moldofsky and Hugh Smythe, both Canadian medical doctors, noted sleep abnormalities and fatigue in patients with diffuse musculoskeletal tender points. They also believed that fatigue could occur due to a disruption in an individual's normal circadian rhythm, regardless of normal sleep duration.[4] Even today, there are those who believe FM may be secondary to psychological stress or disordered sleep. Today evidence includes the physiological upset, regardless of what the aggravating factor might be. Still, by the very name itself—fibrositis—it seems the medical community back in

1904 believed the disorder to be inflammatory in nature. Conventional medical practitioners would have considered it foolhardy for someone to follow Dr. Gower's theories and delay proper treatment.

Finally, in 1981 a connection was made between fibromyocitis and the non-inflammatory systemic symptoms. This led to adoption of the term "fibromyalgia" to identify the syndrome variously described as fibromyocitis, muscular rheumatism, tension myalgia, psychogenic rheumatism, tension rheumatism, neurasthenia, and fibrositis.[5]

EARLIER TERMS FOR FIBROMYALGIA

fibromyocitis

muscular rheumatism

tension myalgia

psychogenic rheumatism

tension rheumatism

neurasthenia

fibrositis

Twenty years ago, fibromyalgia as we now understand it was unrecognized, but the continued symptoms of diffuse muscle pain and fatigue suffered by people with FM led them on a quest for help. Today, it can no longer be denied. History has changed the future for those of us who suffer from this disabling disorder.

Demographics (Age, Gender, and Genetic Predisposition)

The predisposition to FM comes from multiple factors. Often identified as triggers are virus, trauma (accidental or surgical), chemical exposure, abuse (emotional or physical), a prior debilitating illness, or any of these in combination.

According to the Centers for Disease Control and Prevention (CDC), approximately 2 percent of the U.S. population has FM, and the ratio of women to men is 7:1.[6] While the onset of the syndrome can occur at any age and affect either gender, it predominately affects females between puberty and menopause and knows no boundaries related to economic, social, or racial status.

Likewise, the severity of symptoms cannot be correlated to any particular factor. FM is mostly discussed as a female disorder, but in a study done in Israel in 2000, men affected by FM reported more severe symptoms than women and showed decreased functional status.[7] This study suggests that it may be important to include males in proportionate numbers in all studies.

Fibromyalgia is the third most prevalent rheumatologic disorder in the United States,[8] and may often co-occur (up to 25-65 percent) with other rheumatic conditions, such as rheumatoid arthritis (RA), systemic lupus erythematosus (SLE), and ankylosing spondylitis (AS).[9] Despite these staggering statistics, physicians are given little or no training regarding identification or treatment of any conditions that cause muscle dysfunction.

Diagnostic criteria for fibromyalgia were finally established in the late twentieth century. In 1990 the American College of Rheumatology published what is now considered official diagnostic criteria for fibromyalgia. The criteria were originally to be used for a scientific study on FM and were not intended to be the *standard* for diagnosis of the illness. However, in 1993 the World Health Organization officially recognized the syndrome—fibromyalgia—and adopted the ACR criteria, which are recognized by leading authorities today.

The average FM patient visits more than five physicians or health care practitioners and spends thousands of dollars before a diagnosis is made. Does this sound like your experience? You will read many articles on how much fibromyalgia costs the health care system, articles that often seem to blame patients for rising health care costs. All illnesses cost health care dollars, and we are no more to blame for our symptoms than the health care community is to blame for not finding the cause. Rising health care costs are not due to FM any more than cancer, heart disease, arthritis, or any number of conditions for which patients seek help. The medical system's survival depends on illness. Shouldn't we blame exorbitant intermediary costs, the insurance and pharmaceutical industries, greed for profit, and the cost of technology?

Patient care delivery today has been affected by the cost of the technology that we as consumers have come to expect and the demand for doctors to see more patients in less time. To an older health care consumer like me, it seems as if these new health care systems are nothing less than big business. The compassion that once fueled a desire to help people with disease and illness has been squeezed out of health care like the last bit of toothpaste from its tube. The days of compassionate nurses and religious orders caring for the infirm are long gone. That is not to say nurses no longer care, but they are allowed little time to care for their patients, and they become frustrated, too. The point is that today's health care delivery does not have the same meaning it did in the days of Florence Nightingale. We've come a long way and developed far superior technology, but what is it costing us? In this day of large health care conglomerates, few health care providers have time to give the "special touch."

Unfortunately, the captains at the helm don't see "compassionate moments" as an important factor in patient outcomes.

The lack of education for health care providers and an untimely diagnosis can be devastating to the patient and to the health care community in general. The cost of making repeated doctor visits for the same complaints and waiting for up to five years to receive a diagnosis could be avoided if doctors and the medical community were more aware of the latest research, and diagnostic criteria. This atrocity can only be remedied by educating practicing physicians, advocating for increased awareness, and securing funding for research. This book includes entire subsections addressing our dilemma.

Objective Data

In addition to lack of knowledge by medical practitioners, a major obstacle in diagnosing FM has been the lack of objective physical findings. The diagnostic exam in which the doctor palpates the eighteen tender points characteristic of FM relies solely on the patient's report of pain when pressed in these areas. Routine test results appear normal, so the physician must rely heavily on the patient's ability to give an accurate history. Increasingly, researchers give credibility to the physiological and biological symptoms of fibromyalgia.

objective findings: conclusions made by the examining practitioner through observation of conditions that can be seen, heard, or felt.

Although functional imaging is used only in research, the results document the physiological disruption that occurs in FM. Thanks to the due diligence of investigators who use this new technology to determine and provide objective data, we now have validation for the presence of pain and the dysfunction associated with it.

Diagnostic Criteria

Unlike other disease processes, the symptoms of fibromyalgia affect all four quadrants of the body equally. In other words, tender points are found on both sides of the upper body (above the waist) and both sides of the lower body (below the waist). If there is a tender point in the left elbow, there will be another tender point in the same spot on the right elbow. Painful tender points are consistent and are considered chronic because they persist for a period of at least three months.

According to the ACR criteria, tender points are assessed by applying pressure (four kg/cm^2) to specific points on the body.[10] This would be enough pressure to make the examiner's fingernail blanch (turn pale) when pressure is applied. The patient may experience other tender points, but it is generally believed that these specific model sites are more exquisitely tender to the FM patient. Another distinguishing characteristic is that FM pain does not radiate to other parts of the body. Careful examination technique should be used since the exam alone can actually perpetuate a flare in the fibromyalgia patient, causing undue distress. If the practitioner finds eleven of the eighteen tender points identified by the ACR model that fit the pattern previously described, the patient is diagnosed with fibromyalgia.

Tender Points by Description

Front—Upper Body

- Mid-anterior cervical—on the neck, just below where the head meets the neck, just above the collar bone.
- Second rib—just below the collar bone approximately three finger widths down.

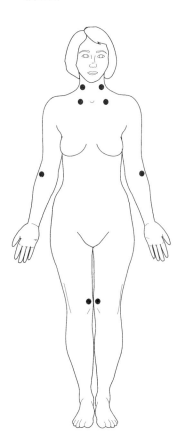 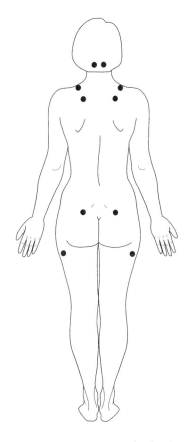

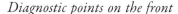

Diagnostic points on the front   *Diagnostic points on the back*

- Lateral epicondyle of humerus—inner elbow on the same side as the thumb.

Front—Lower Body

- Knee—on the inner side of the knee where you can feel a fat pad.

Back—Upper Body

- Occiput—on each side of the spine where the head and neck meet.
- Inferior neck—on the upper line of the shoulder, slightly less than halfway from the shoulder to the neck.
- Suprascapular—along the upper margins of the shoulder blade, three finger widths on a diagonal plane toward the spine.

Back—Lower Body

- Sacrolateral—on the upper buttock close to the "dimple" area, approximately one-half the distance to the spine from the hip.
- Posterior greater trochanter—just below the fold of the buttocks, close to the outside edge of the thigh.

Symptoms

Fibromyalgia symptoms may vary from person to person, day to day, and/or minute to minute. They also fluctuate in severity. Many people equate the symptoms of fibromyalgia and chronic fatigue immunodysfunction to those of the flu. If you do not have FM or CFID, imagine what it would be like to wake up every day feeling this ill. Identifying what triggers a flare is essential in learning to keep these occurrences to a minimum.

symptom: an indication of disease perceived by the patient.

subjective findings: symptoms that can be perceived only by the subject, you, and not by the examiner. The examiner must rely on you to report these problems.

Common Symptoms

- Pain (often severe and disabling)
- Widespread body aches and soreness
- Morning stiffness

- Tender points
- Non-restorative sleep (even with eight hours of sleep)
- Malaise—lack of zest or energy, fatigue

Associated Symptoms

Other symptoms that may accompany FM are listed below. This list has been compiled from National Institutes of Health, Centers for Disease Control, Mayo Clinic, National Fibromyalgia Association, and FM Network News.

CAUTION

The other symptoms could be attributed to a separate problem. Do not automatically attribute them to FM. If you have them, discuss them with your doctor; additional diagnostic tests may be needed. Be sure to ask if your doctor is also familiar with chronic fatigue immunodysfunction and chronic myofascial pain.

- Anxiety and/or depression
- Bladder difficulties (pain, urinary frequency and/or urgency, burning, difficulty urinating)
- Bowel habits altered (irritable bowel syndrome, diarrhea, constipation, painful cramping, bloating, gas, other related symptoms)
- Chemical sensitivity
- Chest wall pain
- Cognitive disturbances (inability to remember or stay focused—brain fog, or fibro fog—short-term memory problems)
- Cold intolerance (feeling cold when others do not)
- Dizziness
- Dry eyes and mouth
- Gynecological disturbances or premenstrual syndrome (PMS)
- Headaches, severe and chronic, including migraine
- Impaired coordination
- Irritability or mood changes
- Jaw pain
- Paresthesias, unexplained (numbness or tingling, particularly in the arms or legs)
- Photophobia (sensitivity to light)

- Raynaud's syndrome
- Restless leg syndrome (RLS) and/or periodic limb movement (PLM)
- Ringing in the ears (tinnitus)
- Sensitivity to odors
- Sensitivity to noise
- Skin sensitivities, mottling, and rashes
- Subjective swelling (an unobservable feeling of being swollen)
- Visual problems

Some symptoms may be due to myofascial trigger points (TrPs) associated with chronic myofascial pain, for instance, bladder difficulties, altered bowel habits, chest wall pain, gynecological disturbances, chronic severe headaches, pain that isn't in the joint but feels as if it is, RLS, PLM, and subjective swelling. Many of the symptoms can be explained by trigger points. Paresthesias—unexplained numbness or tingling, particularly in the arms or legs—is usually caused by nerve entrapment and can be due to untreated trigger points. Again, FM patients, CFID patients, and CMP patients should be studied separately or closely screened for coexistence of two or all three of the disorders.

Chest wall movement is decreased in many FM patients, which could be due to underlying undiagnosed chronic myofascial pain (CMP) or because it aggravates chest wall tenderness. Lack of chest wall motion can do two things: intensify pain and cause a lack of oxygen. Our bodies require oxygen in order to be healthy. The benefits of deep breathing will be discussed later. If you have both FM and CMP, trigger points cause the pain of CMP, and FM intensifies it. If you have both CFID and CMP, trigger point treatment produces byproducts that can bring on, or intensify, symptoms of CFID.

Following is my personal testimony, which I'm providing for you because I believe it is validating for all of us to write our experiences in a journal. Once validation is made, you can let it go. There still will be difficult times, but I have learned that journaling helps me to better manage my illnesses.

Learning how to express our feelings, focus on positives, and communicate needs helps us in immeasurable ways. To eliminate even one symptom temporarily can make a difference in total emotional, physical, spiritual, and mental well-being.

——————   *Personal Testimony*   ——————

I am so tired. However, as I resign myself to bed each night I strive to embrace sleep that may or may not come. If I do slumber, I am too often awakened with the feeling that my extremities have been amputated with the ax of a grim reaper. My thrashing about and kicking brings unwelcome remarks from a spouse who swears I am physically abusing him in retaliation for his snoring.

When I get the nerve (literally) to get my feet on the floor, I seldom feel them. When I do, they feel like a ripe tomato that will rupture with weight. Every muscle seems to work against the other, and I pray not to topple until the feeling of the needles in the bottom of my feet passes, pleading that it will pass and the morning hours turn the day into one that is more acceptable. I examine everything I do or do not put into my mouth, from diet to medications, for fear in a few hours my head will feel like I am on a whirlybird, death-drop ride that won't stop. I toil to embrace my body's alarm system. What do I do now?

Weakly, I wonder if I will be up shortly with the abdominal flu-like pain of irritable bowel and an odor that nauseates me and awakens my husband. Then I ask . . . why would my partner not grieve the loss of the person he once knew?

I experience bladder pain with burning, urgency, and frequency, only to be told, "You have a condition that is aggravated by the medications you are on to treat your other problems. And once again, there is no cure; we don't know what causes it."

I scrutinize my clothing, down to my bra, because if it is too constricting I hurt to the bottom of my soul from pressure on places I didn't know existed until FM, CFID, and CMP. Should my shirt button because I can't lift my arms, or not button because my hands won't work?

I am a 50-something woman in an 80-something body. My bones are brittle and I can no longer hold my urine because of pelvic floor trigger points that twitch faster than an electrical current.

Others look at me as if I have lost my mind because I am dressed for the Artic when we are experiencing a midwestern heat wave.

When I do try to exercise, every step makes me feel as if my left leg has been put in a vise, then dumped into a blender; and when I proceed in a drunken walk, I end up with bruises that forbid the stylish clothes of my peers without unwelcome comments. These symptoms are aggravated by chronic hip bursitis, piriformis syndrome, or some sympathetic nerve disorder yet to be determined.

When I try to tell the doctor that the "newest" medication I'm on is not producing the results we expected, I hear, "I don't know why; studies show this medication works for most people." This leaves me feeling not trusted and somehow responsible for my pain.

Music I once loved now seems to be convoluted and loud to my ears only. Why is this? Why does something others enjoy so much make my thoughts even more disjointed than they already are? And did I mention the incessant eye twitch that challenges the speed of light? All this leaves me with the choice of being agitated, anxious, or in pain, versus being rude and difficult to be around.

When I drop things—because my hands are more like rags than the helpmates they are intended to be—those around me respond with, "You should be paying closer attention"; once again, I thought I was.

Fatigue and exhaustion have ruined relationships. I have had to accept that when I feel the need to hang on to my sanity, apart from my support group, others cannot truly understand that this is not "an excuse," but just one more thing that is out of control.

When I am "out to lunch" in an FM fugue state, friends and family may say, "Why weren't you listening?" They are unaware that such comments leave me feeling guilty and inadequate. They don't understand and I must accept that.

Then there are some who say they want to understand, but seem to change the subject when I feel the need to share my experience of FM.

Sharing my invisible conditions with family, friends, and even health care providers makes me feel like a whiner. So I withhold the complaints thinking this will somehow improve the way others perceive me, only to be told, "You are looking good, you must be better." To say how I really feel, well . . .

When I hear FM is a "wastebasket diagnosis," I ponder . . . a wastebasket would be a wonderful place to put all the uncaring, critical opinions of others who threaten our sense of self-worth with their seemingly unkind words.

What do we do with all our untold thoughts, feelings, and physical pain? If only . . .

ETIOLOGY OF FIBROMYALGIA

A scientific **hypothesis** must be formed and backed by scientific data in order to secure funding for research. This is why theories must be derived from solid information. Let me say here, I am not a researcher or a scientist. Some of the information in the etiology sections of FM, CFID, and CMP is very detailed and scientifically oriented. Please do not be intimidated if you don't understand it. I do have a medical background, yet much of the research reported here is out of my league. Where I have made interpretations of the studies, I have done so as I understand them. But my knowledge base on some of the information is very limited.

As with many disorders that are not clearly understood, the information is new to the investigator too. Research is about proving a certain theory or hypothesis; some researchers get the expected results and some don't. When they do, they know they are heading down the right road, and when they don't, the unexpected results offer up the opportunity for developing a new hypothesis. Researchers keep working hard at getting the answers. I apologize if I have misinterpreted any of the studies.

All three of these disorders could have some element related to the central **nervous system** (see p. 19). The brain is an awesome and very complex organ. We are learning more and more every day, but we are just chipping away at the tip of the iceberg. We are truly pioneers in this gateway to enlightenment. The one thing I hope you take away from the etiology sections is that the history of scientific study has led us to a better understanding of what might cause these disorders. We aren't there yet, but we must not become discouraged and drop the ball. These scientists are trailblazers and should be recognized for all their hard work. They should be acknowledged by us and by those who care for us.

Sometimes described as an "orphan" disorder, FM is much like an unclaimed waif. Finding its closest molecular relative will determine its scientific classification.

Fibromyalgia is a chronic pain condition of unknown origin; however, scientists have identified multiple abnormalities, including autonomic, peripheral, and central nervous system permutations. The brain has difficulty processing information, and the central nervous system is easily excited by input it receives from the **peripheral nervous system**. The pain of FM is the result of peripheral stimulation and central sensitization. Glial cell activation (to be discussed later) may play a role in the initiation and perpetuation of this sensitized state.[11] A better understanding of these important neurochemical interactions may provide relevant insights into future effective therapies. Following is a brief overview of

---

etiology: the scientific study of a disorder's origin.

hypothesis: a supposition that appears to explain a group of phenomena and is assumed as a basis of reasoning and experimentation. A theoretical assumption is created for the purpose of investigation.

nervous system: the organ system that, along with the endocrine system, helps the body adjust to internal reactions and environmental conditions. It consists of the central nervous system and the peripheral nervous system.

some theories involved in research over the past two decades.

Structural

Structure malformations may be predisposing factors to the symptoms associated with FM, CFID, and CMP. However, correcting the structural problem, when possible, will not cure FM or CFID.

Structural changes brought about by contracted muscles due to trigger points (TrPs) found in chronic myofascial pain are profound and can play a significant role for someone who has fibromyalgia/chronic myofascial pain complex (FM/CMP).[12] It is even more significant in Stage II CMP, when there is central sensitization. Stage II CMP will be defined at length in a contributing chapter (by Devin Starlanyl) in the upcoming *Myofascial Trigger Point Manual,* 3rd edition, by Dr. David Simons, a textbook for physicians.[13]

It is important to know about different conditions or symptoms that can coexist or mimic any of the three disorders, FM, CFID, and CMP. They will be discussed at length in chapter 2.

Genetic

Although the cause is unknown, (which is why FM is classified as a syndrome rather than a disease), there is some evidence suggesting it is an inherited disorder.[14] Incidental findings regarding children and parents with similar histories of pain-related problems have led to studies regarding a possible genetic connection. In a more recent review of literature on genetic and familial factors regarding certain syndromes, particularly fibromyalgia, evidence suggests that serotonin and dopamine-related genes may play a role.[15] Although it is useful to understand the possible relationship between heredity and FM, genetic influence is not something we can treat, at least for now.

Immunity

A certain subset of patients with what is referred to by scientists as "immune-mediated demyelinating polyneuropathy" has responded favorably to treatment with intravenous immunoglobulin (IVIg).[16] This suggests a disruption in the immune system may exist in some patients. It may be that these particular patients have both FM and CFID, which would illustrate the importance of accurately screening study participants.

Muscle Hypoxia and Growth Hormone Deficiency

Deductive reasoning suggests that if a person experiences pain when pressure is applied to soft tissue, or experiences muscle pain (myalgia), weakness, and stiffness, there is a problem

---

peripheral nervous system: the voluntary (somatic) and the autonomic nervous systems:

- **voluntary nervous system:** somatic. Consists of motor and sensory nerves, controls skeletal muscles, and carries messages to the brain. It is responsible for helping you carry out tasks, such as taking a drink from a glass (motor, efferent), or

reflexively removing your hand from a hot burner (sensory, afferent).

- **autonomic nervous system (ANS):** consists of the sympathetic and parasympathetic nervous systems. It operates without conscious control (see p. 22).

hypoxia: low oxygen level resulting in diminished oxygen nurturance to the body.

in the muscle itself. This is not necessarily the case.

Muscle biopsy studies have been conducted since 1957. Many of these studies reported pathological abnormalities, meaning the tissue was not the same as tissue from a normal individual. A study by Dr. Muhammad Yunus at the University of Illinois in 1986 finally laid this issue to rest by showing the muscle tissue to be no different from that of pain-free subjects.[17]

Muscle pain and fatigue in FM may be due to microcirculation abnormalities.[18] Theoretically this would mean that the shortage of energy normally provided by oxygen to the muscle causes improper functioning. Robert Bennett, M.D., at the University of Oregon, has analyzed the relationship of disrupted stage-4 sleep to muscle damage. Growth hormone (GH), which is essential to muscle tissue repair and health, is released during stage-4 sleep, but FM patients never reach or stay at this level, making the hormone unavailable.[19] Research continues to show many FM patients have GH deficiency.[20] This may account for slow wound healing in some FM patients.

Research is being conducted regarding treatment with growth hormone to determine its future effectiveness in treatment of FM symptoms in a certain subset of patients.[21] The drawback for now is that this therapy is being used in clinical trials, suggesting more investigation is needed. It is unlikely that this will be the last we hear regarding GH and its affects on FM in this subset of patients.

Sleep Anomalies

Drs. Moldofsky and Smythe first began studying the relationship of sleep to pain in FM. In 1975 they published results of a study that used an EEG (electroencephalograph) to measure brain wave patterns. They found that patients exhibiting what we know today as FM symptoms were deficient in stage-4 sleep. In 1977 they did a study on healthy subjects and found that when deprived of stage-4 sleep for three nights, subjects began to complain of tenderness, pain, and stomach upset.[22] This might suggest that if you correct the sleep problem, FM could be eradicated; however, not all people with sleep apnea or other primary sleep problems affecting stage-4 sleep have FM. Most leading authorities today agree that FM is a disorder involving the central nervous system, and is not the result of a sleep anomaly.[23]

Although sleep disruption can be linked to depression, fatigue, gastrointestinal upset, and other symptoms experienced by FM patients, correcting sleep problems with medication does not significantly improve the overall well-being of many FM sufferers.[24]

However, treatment of the sleep anomaly related to FM and CFID is imperative. Lack of sleep or disrupted sleep can manifest in agitation, disordered thought, and amplification of any stimulus.[25] Providing rest for the brain and body will help you control at least one of your aggravating factors. Studies exploring non-restorative sleep problems associated with FM are in progress.

HPA Axis

The hypothalamic-pituitary-adrenal (HPA) axis is one of the body's major stress response systems and may be altered in FM. The hypothalamus is a small gland in the brain that, simply stated, "receives input from the body." It then relays this input to the pituitary, or "master gland." The pituitary is the size of pea and sits in a small recess at the base of the brain. The "master" regulates many other **endocrine glands** by coordinating hormone production in the way that a conductor coordinates the individual musicians in a symphony orchestra. When the pituitary is alerted by the hypothalamus that the body is experiencing some sort of stress, it sends the message on to the adrenal glands, which sit on top of the kidneys. The adrenal glands produce adrenaline and many other chemicals that the body uses for its fight-or-flight response. The balance among these is called the HPA axis. The symphony of the hypothalamus, pituitary, and adrenals is normally perfectly orchestrated, and any disruption—any "player" that forgets a note, strums the wrong string, or misses a cue—can change the way the body responds. The abnormalities in FM patients are consistent with loss of HPA axis resiliency.[26] Reduced adrenal reactivity has been noted in FM patients, particularly lowered cortisol release, even though free cortisol is unaltered, suggesting we somehow adapt to the reduced cortisol.[27] Cortisol has been dubbed the "stress hormone" because the levels rise during the body's fight-or-flight response. High levels of cortisol, in turn, trigger the relaxation response, which helps to body return to normal. Because release of cortisol is low in some FM patients, it may not trigger the relaxation response that should follow, meaning the "stress state" never lets up. This is why it is particularly important for FM patients to participate in the relaxation therapies discussed later.

Central Nervous System

Fibromyalgia is a disorder that causes pain amplification. Many believe this pain intensification is the result of **central nervous system (CNS)** neurotransmitter feedback loop deregulation. This suggests that the message of "relieve pain now" is blocked and can't get through; or that the dispatch is intercepted somewhere in the system. Repeated studies using functional magnetic resonance imaging (fMRI) show these same results.[28, 29]

Two key chemicals play an important role in neurotransmission: substance P and serotonin. The disruption of these two chemicals can have a profound effect on pain perception.

---

endocrine gland: a gland that regulates bodily functions by secreting hormones that are delivered directly into the blood. Each of the endocrine glands has a specific function; however, they all rely on other glands in the system for maintenance of normal hormonal balance in the body.

central nervous system (CNS): consists of the brain and spinal cord. It contains neurons and glia. Neurons command the message retrieval and emissions, and secrete certain neurotransmitters. Glia, also called glial cells, provide support and nutrition, maintain homeostasis, form myelin (to protect nerves found in the CNS), and participate in signal transmission. Glia are now believed to also secrete certain neurotransmitters. Spinal extensions of the CNS—nerve roots—affect skeletal muscles and organs in the body.

Substance P, which has been found in increased amounts in FM patients, is a peptide substance in spinal fluid (fluid that circulates in the central nervous system); its job is to regulate pain information.[30] Serotonin, a neurotransmitter produced by tryptophan, an **essential amino acid,** is stored in the central nervous system; its role is to reduce the intensity of the pain signal and help with sleep regulation and mood. Some researchers believe that FM patients are low in serotonin, and thus, have a decreased capacity for pain relief modulation. Neurotransmitters are a complex lot, and their deregulation can affect any number of symptoms, including those associated with fibromyalgia.[31]

It is believed that **central pain** processing is altered in patients with fibromyalgia because of altered serotonin metabolism, especially changes in the functioning of the 5-HT3 receptor. Tropisetron and other selective 5-HT3 receptor antagonists show promise in the treatment of FM.[32] Serotonin is being studied using the **functional MRI (fMRI).** The brain is a magnificent thing and complete understanding of how it works is elusive to even the sagest of investigators, so don't labor over these studies, just know that there are people out there who are doing their best to help.

One school of thought holds that serotonin in patients with FM is being filtered out by the blood brain barrier, a membrane that is supposed to block substances that could damage the brain, but may also filter out necessary substances like serotonin.[33]

Recent work with single photon emission computed tomography (PET) imaging of the brain has revealed that regional blood flow to areas in the brain is decreased in patients with FM and other disorders associated with chronic pain, when compared to healthy controls.[34] The functional MRI supports the hypothesis that FM is caused by the brain's cortical, or subcortical, augmentation of pain processing.

A study conducted by Baraniuk, Whalen, Cunningham, and Clauw at the Chronic Pain and Fatigue Research Center at Georgetown University found that "central nervous system opioid dysfunction may contribute to pain in fibromyalgia."[35]

I suspect a disruption of chemical messaging in the central nervous system. This might explain why so many of us also have one or more overlapping, unexplained clinical conditions. CFID, irritable bowel syndrome, temporomandibular disorder, and the multiple chemical sensitivities that often coexist in FM patients.[36]

FM literature links a wind-up phenomenon to a possible central sensitization abnormality. Brain images confirm central nervous system changes picked up on the brain scan

---

essential amino acid: an amino acid that is not produced by the body, making it essential to the human diet. Some sources, meat, cheese, eggs, fish and poultry.

central pain: pain associated with a lesion (disruption) of the central nervous system.

functional MRI (fMRI): a type of MRI that measures brain function by using magnetic imaging to register the quick, tiny, metabolic changes in an active part of the brain. Among other things, it is being used to see how a person's brain interprets pain. A painful stimulus is applied to the patient, and the brain's response is mapped.

that are consistent with painful stimulation to the patient.[37] Central pain processing, the way the brain processes the message of pain being sent from outside the brain or spinal cord, is more sensitive to stimuli in the FM patient. The central nervous system is in a state of hyperexcitability and there is increased wind-up after sensations have been induced.[38] We seem to be suspended in space, swirling and twirling without reason or awareness. Do you ever feel as if you just can't take one more thing on your plate without exploding? This is the way your central nervous system feels when you have FM. Just one more stimulus that by itself would amount to nothing causes your central nervous system chemicals to be off and running, spinning like the wheels of a bike with no brakes. This central sensitized state is perpetuated by many peripheral events, but for many of us there is one specific, always present culprit. That culprit is CMP. Chronic myofascial pain from trigger points keeps the already sensitive state of the FM patient constantly bombarded with new painful stimuli, perpetuating the symptoms of FM.

Trigger points, or TrPs, are the most common loci of peripheral sensitization (meaning outside the nervous system).[39] This relentless source of peripheral stimulation adds fuel to the fire of an overexcited state of the brain (central sensitization) that is constantly maintained in FM. This easily explains why those of us with both FM and CMP have such a difficult time dealing with symptoms. We think we are getting a handle on the body-wide pain of FM, and then we sneeze, pick up something heavy, ignore our needs, get cold, or just live, and those trigger points we thought were gone are suddenly back. They were merely dormant, waiting for the opportunity to pop back up and start the cycle all over.

Glial Cells

In addition to central nervous system chemical disruption, a type of central nervous system cell may play a role—the glial cell. Glial cells are one of two types of cells found in the CNS, and there are many different kinds of glial cells. They provide support and nutrition, maintain balance (**homeostasis**), form myelin (to protect the nerves found in the CNS), and participate in signal transmission. Some types of glial cells are created by inflammation and injury to tissue, which in turn releases cytokines from nerve cells to the surrounding area. There is growing evidence suggesting that peripheral pain mediators—predominantly immune and glial cells—are important mediators of persistent pain states and can act at several locations.[40] In conditions such as FM, the glia, which normally are quiet, are activated and produce a longer than normal release of "pro-inflammatory **cytokines**."[41] This can happen during pathological pain[42] and can affect the release of neurotransmitters, such as substance P.

---

homeostasis: a tendency of biological systems to maintain stability by continually adjusting to conditions that are optimal for survival.

cytokines: small, secreted proteins that mediate and regulate immunity, inflammation, and the formation of blood cell components.

One study investigated the role of cytokines and adhesion molecules involved in directing immune cells. The study revealed a slight disturbance in FM patients, suggesting an enhanced adhesion and recruitment of leukocytes to inflammatory sites.[43]

Some believe glial cells can produce cytokines without nerve injury or some other stressor, which means that inflammation may not need to occur. The possible correlation of cytokines to FM are being studied aggressively. "Drugs that attack the chemical substances released by glial cells are predicted to be powerful remedies for people in pain."[44]

Autonomic Nervous System

The autonomic nervous system (ANS) is made up of the **sympathetic and parasympathetic nervous systems**. Heart rate variability present in some FM patients indicates a disruption in the ANS.[45] This disruption may be in the feedback loop of the ANS among target organs, structures, and the central nervous system (CNS), and may cause inappropriate information (neurotransmitters) to be released or blocked along the information loop.[46] This theory may not replace the HPA theory, but actually support it and help explain hypo-reactive sympathetic difficulties, neuro-

hormonal abnormalities, and inappropriate reactions in the sympathetic nervous system of FM patients.[47] It's like a broken piston; the cylinder misfires and gasoline doesn't circulate through the system, resulting in sputtering, coughing, and sometimes loss of locomotion.

Symptoms such as enhanced pain sensitivity, increased muscle tension, numbness and tingling sensations, non-restorative sleep, brain fog, migraine, odor sensitivity, sensitivity to light and noise, visual disturbances, dry eyes and mouth, gastrointestinal problems, urinary disorders, exhaustion, low blood pressure, dizziness or faintness, shortness of breath, Raynaud's symptoms, anxiety, and cold intolerance may be the result of disruption in the feedback loop between the autonomic and the central nervous system.

Conclusion

The relationship of adenosine phosphate and altered glucose metabolism in red blood cells, low insulin-like growth factor, elevated serum hyaluronic acid level, disordered regulation of cortisol, high circulating levels of nitric oxide (NO),[48] thyroid resistance,[49] and the role of gastrointestinal proteins[50] are also being studied.

The one thing universally agreed upon is that abnormal widespread pain sensitivity is a

sympathetic nervous system: responds to danger with an excitatory effect and initiates the fight or flight response. It discharges stimulating secretions, like adrenalin and cortisol, at nerve junctions. These secretions are then discharged into the blood to help start muscle action quickly. An example of a sympathetic response is an increase in heart rate and respiration, shunting of blood from the digestive tract, and constriction of blood vessels to give the body the extra energy it needs at times of stress, that can

range from doing exercise to being physically or emotionally distressed.

parasympathetic nervous system: prevents the body's responses to sympathetic stimulation from accelerating to extremes, and influences organs toward restoration and energy conservation. Secretions are discharged to slow heart and lung activity, restore digestive function, and limit the constriction of blood vessels. This acts as a damper unless the challenge demands a prolonged effort.

distinctive trait of FM. Persistent peripheral stimulation can lead to changes in the central nervous system causing central sensitization and pain. It seems that once this central sensitization is established, it takes very little peripheral input to maintain a chronic pain state.[51] Regardless of varying theories, the end result points to alterations in CNS function. Understanding these mechanisms and their relationship to central sensitization and clinical pain will provide new approaches for the prevention and treatment of fibromyalgia and other chronic pain syndromes.

Because of the close relationship with other syndromes and diseases, understanding the causes of fibromyalgia will not only help sufferers control pain to lead more productive lives, but may decrease the incidence of such syndromes and disorders as irritable bowel syndrome, irritable bladder, and migraines in otherwise healthy individuals not affected by FM.

Other Disorders

There are disorders that often coexist with, and aggravate, FM. There are also conditions that mimic FM. The important thing is that you understand the role other conditions play in the way you deal with FM. These will be discussed in chapter 2.

Your doctor can help you see how any coexisting conditions may affect you. It is essential to note any coexisting conditions for proper treatment, for two very important reasons: The first is to eliminate the possibility that your symptoms are from something other than FM (or CFID or CMP). The second is to identify the role another condition can play.

There are diseases with symptoms similar to FM (and CFID and CMP) that can be life threatening. Proper treatment should not be delayed because of a misdiagnosis. Please consult your physician regarding your complaints.

Prognosis

Although symptoms seem to accumulate over time, fibromyalgia is not a fatal or progressive disorder.

---

flare: a period of time in which symptoms are not under control, or worsen.

It is the tendency of the *fibromite* (a term those of us with FM use to describe ourselves in an online support group, the Fibrom-L community) to have a worsening of symptoms when they are left untreated. We are susceptible to a flare when we deviate in any way from our personally tailored, multidisciplinary treatment plan. This worsening of symptoms does not mean FM is progressing from one step to the next in the disease process. "Unpredictable" is the best way to describe the way symptoms occur.

It is literally a 24/7 job for all of us, and varies in difficulty from one patient to another. A lot depends upon how long it took before we were diagnosed and the number of symptoms and coexisting conditions that afflict us. The good news is that with proper treatment and identification of aggravating factors, symptoms can be eradicated for some, and at least controlled by the rest of us.

To be in control when everything seems out of control is quite an undertaking, but extremely rewarding.

The ultimate measure of a man is not where he stands in moments of comfort, but where he stands at times of challenge and controversy.

MARTIN LUTHER KING JR.

Summary Exercise: FM

Can you briefly describe the key points listed below?

- Definition of Fibromyalgia
- History and demographics
- Symptoms
- Personal testimony (a narrative of your own experience)
- Objective findings (those findings noticed by your examiner, such as bumping into walls, pulling away from painful stimulus, test results, or mottled skin)
- Subjective findings (those symptoms that only you, the subject, can feel)
- Etiology
- Genetics
- Prognosis
- What do you do if you experience a new, undiagnosed symptom?
- What did you learn about the effects of FM on your life?

Your Inventory of Symptoms

Which of the following symptoms do you have? (Check all that apply.)

Diagnostic Criteria

The first group of symptoms listed are integral to a diagnosis of fibromyalgia.

☐ Symptoms that affect all four quadrants of the body equally

☐ Pain that *does not* radiate to other parts of the body when a tender point is pressed

☐ Tender points on both sides of the upper body (above the waist)

☐ Tender points on both sides of the lower body (below the waist)

☐ Tender points that have persisted for a period of at least three months

Which tender points do you have? Eleven of the eighteen points must be tender for a diagnosis of fibromyalgia. (*Circle your tender points on the illustrations below.*)

Common Symptoms

☐ Pain (often severe and disabling)

☐ Widespread body aches and soreness

☐ Morning stiffness

☐ Tender points

☐ Non-restorative sleep (even when eight hours of sleep is achieved)

☐ Malaise—lack of zest or energy, fatigue

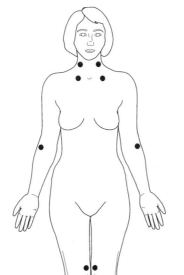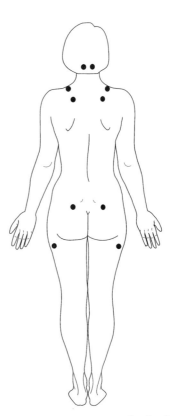

Diagnostic points on the front   *Diagnostic points on the back*

Other Symptoms That May Accompany FM

- ☐ Anxiety and/or depression
- ☐ Bladder difficulties (pain, urinary frequency or urgency, burning and/or difficulty urinating)
- ☐ Bowel habits altered (irritable bowel syndrome, diarrhea, constipation, cramping, bloating, gas, and other disturbances)
- ☐ Chemical sensitivity
- ☐ Chest wall pain
- ☐ Cognitive disturbances (inability to remember or stay focused—brain fog, or fibro fog; short-term memory problems)
- ☐ Cold intolerance (feeling cold when others are not)
- ☐ Dizziness
- ☐ Dry eyes and mouth
- ☐ Gynecological disturbances or premenstrual syndrome (PMS)
- ☐ Headaches, severe and chronic, including migraine
- ☐ Impaired coordination
- ☐ Irritability or mood changes
- ☐ Jaw pain
- ☐ Paresthesias, unexplained (numbness or tingling particularly in the arms or legs)
- ☐ Photophobia (sensitivity to light)
- ☐ Raynaud's syndrome
- ☐ Restless leg syndrome (RLS) and/or periodic limb movement (PLM)
- ☐ Ringing in the ears
- ☐ Sensitivity to odors
- ☐ Sensitivity to noise
- ☐ Skin sensitivities and rashes
- ☐ Subjective swelling (a feeling of being swollen that is not observed by the examiner)
- ☐ Visual problems

Chronic Fatigue Immunodysfunction— The Muster to Master

Chronic fatigue immunodysfunction (also known as chronic fatigue syndrome), its definition, how it is diagnosed, the population it affects, possible causes, and prognosis can be found in multiple references. This subsection of chapter 1 is a summary of the condition put together from various resources.

Definition

Chronic fatigue immunodysfunction (CFID) has been described as a debilitating condition that causes prolonged, severe fatigue not relieved by rest. This fatigue may be worsened by physical or mental activity, and lasts for six months or longer. A clinical diagnosis is made after other medical conditions are excluded. It is associated with four or more specific symptoms noted in the diagnostic criteria following in the text. "These symptoms must have persisted or recurred during six or more consecutive months of illness and must not have predated the fatigue."[52] CFID may be accompanied by multiple nonspecific symptoms.

In studies done by the Centers for Disease Control and Prevention (CDC) the most commonly reported CFID symptoms were sore throat, fever, muscle pain, and muscle weakness at the onset of the illness. As the illness progressed, reports of muscle pain and forgetfulness increased and the reporting of depression decreased.[53]

History

Some suggest chronic fatigue syndrome is a new illness, but Dr. Peter Rowe at Johns Hopkins Medicine, Baltimore, maintains the symptoms that define CFID have been around for many decades. It is recognized by several names in different parts of the world. In 1940, MacLean and Allen described a syndrome with coinciding symptoms present in a certain subset of patients afflicted today. Those patients have neurally mediated hypotension (NMH).[54]

Chronic fatigue syndrome (CFS) is also known as "myalgic encephalomyelitis" (ME) in the United Kingdom and Canada. Even older terms, such as "neuralgia" or "atypical polio," described the same symptoms. The term "chronic fatigue syndrome" was adopted in the late 1980s.

The determination as to what term best describes this condition is controversial and still under debate. Patients and researchers believe "chronic fatigue syndrome" is unacceptable and perhaps vilifies the disorder, in that it focuses on only one aspect of the syndrome and does not give a clear picture of symptoms. Similarly, approximately thirty years ago MS (multiple sclerosis) was inaccurately referred to as "hysterical paralysis," and most patients and researchers believe that such labeling places undue stress on patients.[55] These labels also have significant effects on relationships and the patient's ability to cope. The term "chronic fatigue" implies there is something we can do about it. We don't plan to be tired, we are not lazy, and most of us have been physically active in our lives prior to CFID. We have all heard comments like, "Just get up and go," "I get tired, too," "I don't use fatigue as an excuse to stay in bed," "I make myself get on with the day when I don't sleep well," "Why don't you get more rest?" If the disorder were called something like polyimmuneglobulinemia (PGE)—my own made-up term—people would be far less likely to blame the patient.

MOST COMMON TERMS

CFS: Chronic Fatigue Syndrome

CFID: Chronic Fatigue Immunodysfunction

ME: Myalgic Encephalomyelitis

Other Terms

Neuralgia

Atypical polio

Yuppie flu

Fatigue—chronic

Immune dysfunction syndrome

Epidemic neuromyasthenia

Post-viral fatigue syndrome

Demographics (Age, Genetics, Gender, Population, Incidence)

CFID seems to affect females predominantly, but not to the extent that FM does. Of the more than one million Americans with chronic fatigue syndrome, females are affected four times more frequently than males. There are more people in the United States suffering from CFID than from multiple sclerosis, lupus, lung cancer, or ovarian cancer, and it knows no socioeconomic boundaries.[56]

More recent studies suggest an equal or greater occurrence among adults than in adolescents, and CFID is less common in children.[57] However, because children have difficulty relating their symptoms or voicing their concerns, they are difficult to diagnose. Children who experience acute onset of flu-like or mononucleosis-like symptoms are more likely to describe their symptoms, because they are differentiated in their minds. Yet children who experience gradual onset usually do not initially perceive themselves as ill, because they have grown accustomed to their symptoms. Gradual onset CFID frequently leads to underdiagnosis in children. They may go on to experience "childhood migraine, Crohn's disease, atypical epilepsy, school phobia, attention deficit disorder, rheumatoid arthritis, chronic rheumatic fever, irritable bowel syndrome, and others."[58] We can anticipate further investigation of CFID and FM prevalence and repercussions in children.

The CDC says chronic fatigue syndrome affects more than one million people in the United States; however, it has also been reported in Europe, Australia, New Zealand, Canada, Iceland, Japan, Russia, and South Africa. Developing countries are most likely also affected by this disabling disorder, but the collection of this evidence is beyond their capabilities or they have other priorities, such as life-threatening disease, hunger, and lack of shelter.

Current CFID demographics may change with greater recognition of proper diagnostic tools and reporting methods.

Diagnostic Criteria

As with other disorders, such as rheumatoid arthritis, lupus, and hypertension, CFID is classified as a clinical condition rather than a disease because a direct cause cannot be identified.

The criteria for diagnosing chronic fatigue syndrome were set by the CDC. The assessment should include a complete physical exam; an in-depth medical history; a thorough investigation of environmental, viral, and chemical exposure issues; a mental status exam; lab tests; and other diagnostic tests. Chronic fatigue immunodysfunction is a diagnosis of exclusion, so other conditions that can mimic CFID *must* be ruled out before the diagnosis can be made. However, other clinical conditions, such as FM, multiple chemical sensitivity (MCS), and Gulf War syndrome (GWS) cannot be excluded until it is determined that they do not coexist with CFID.

Because fatigue can be present in so many illnesses, you should expect your physician to conduct tests that will help rule out other causes. These tests will evaluate for infections, autoimmune disorders, tumors, malignancies, muscle or nerve diseases, endocrine disorders (such as hypothyroidism), sleep apnea, narcolepsy, psychiatric or psychological illnesses, drug or alcohol dependency (or side effects), and other underlying conditions such as heart, kidney, or liver disease.

According to the 1994 revision of the 1988 CDC diagnostic criteria for CFID, there must be unexplained persistent or recurring chronic fatigue of new onset, not alleviated by rest, that significantly affects the person's activities of daily living, including occupational, educational, social, and personal activities. The symptoms must have persisted for at least six or more months and must not have predated the fatigue.[59]

Four or more of the following symptoms must be present in order to meet the criteria.

- Cognitive impairment, substantially reduced short-term memory, or loss of concentration (brain fog—difficulty processing information or finding words)
- Sore throat—nonexudative pharyngitis (unexplained inflammation without secretions)
- Lymph node tenderness
- Muscle pain (myalgia) that is persistent and reproducible on repeated examination
- Joint pain, multiple, without swelling or redness (arthralgias)
- Headaches of a new type, pattern, or severity
- Non-restorative sleep
- Post-exertional malaise (generalized ill feeling) lasting more than twenty-four hours

---

CAUTION

If another diffuse joint abnormality (arthropathy) is found and is associated with warmth or inflammation, then another cause of pain should be considered. It could involve an inflammatory process, such as arthritis.

(This, along with other similar disorders, is considered in chapter 2.)

Other Symptoms that May Accompany CFID

According to CDC, the following are commonly observed symptoms in addition to the eight primary defining symptoms of CFID.[60]

- Allergies or sensitivities to foods, alcohol, odors, chemicals, medications, or noise
- Brain fog (poor concentration, comprehension, word finding, reasoning, and memory)
- Chills and night sweats
- Chest pain

- Chronic cough
- Irritable bowel, abdominal pain, nausea, diarrhea, or bloating
- Irregular heartbeat
- Jaw pain
- Difficulty maintaining upright position (orthostatic instability, dizziness, balance problems, or fainting)
- Psychological problems (depression, irritability, mood swings, anxiety, or panic attacks)
- Shortness of breath
- Visual blurring, eye pain, or dry eyes
- Weight loss or gain

The CFID Association of America advocates for CFID in the community, with the government, and with health care professionals. They also provoke CFID research and provide education. Following are symptoms they have noted in addition to those listed by the CDC.[61]

- Alcohol intolerance
- Gynecological problems, including PMS and endometriosis
- Low-grade fever or low body temperature
- Muscle twitches
- Paresthesias—abnormal sensations (burning, numbness, or tingling)
- Ringing in the ears (tinnitus)
- Seizures
- Sensitivity to heat and/or cold
- SICCA-like symptoms (mucosal dryness, such as dry mouth and eyes)

CAUTION

Chest pain, bowel dysfunction, irregular heartbeat, jaw pain, balance problems, headaches, muscle pain, paresthesias, tinnitus, shortness of breath, SICCA-like symptoms, sore throat, and visual disturbances can also be caused by untreated trigger points found in chronic myofascial pain. If those are the only contributing symptoms, chronic myofascial pain should be excluded before a diagnosis of CFID is made.

Symptoms vary among individuals. They can linger for at least six months and often, for years. Treatment should be designed to help patients and their families adjust to living with this disabling chronic illness.

If any of these symptoms are new or you have not been diagnosed, please consult with your physician.

Chronic fatigue immunodysfunction is not always a stand-alone disorder. It is possible to have both FM and CFID, both CFID and CMP,[62] or even all three disorders. It is important to know if you have been correctly diagnosed with either FM or CFID, or both. You should also understand the importance of knowing if you have CFID and CMP, and after reading the next section on CMP, the picture should come into focus for you. This does not mean that the overlapping symptoms of CFID are attributed to FM or CMP, only that they could be; for your sake, it should be considered. This is why fibromyalgia pain, chronic fatigue immunodysfunction, and chronic myofascial pain from trigger points are grouped in this book.

ETIOLOGY OF CFID

Thus far, scientists have not determined a standard cause of CFID. Although triggers may contribute to the onset of CFID, they are not connected with any certainty to a particular cause.[63] No single genesis has been defined as typical of the syndrome.

Triggers

Some experts believe CFID is triggered by a particular event, for example toxic exposure to chemicals,[64] toxic mold exposure,[65] or viruses,[66] including, but not limited to, mononucleosis[67] and tick-borne diseases,[68] (one being Lyme disease). Some believe systemic mycoplasma infections can mimic Lyme symptoms, and should be considered in CFID and FM patients;[69] however, this does not mean mycoplasma causes CFID, only that it may be present in some of these patients. Others say that although a large subset of CFID patients show evidence of bacterial and/or viral infection(s), and patients with multiple infections do have more severe signs and symptoms, there is no correlation between the types of coinfection.[70] Emotional stress can trigger a cascade of symptoms; however, these immunological responses are not limited to CFID and may manifest in other types of illness.[71] It is important to keep in mind that there can be a difference between subsets of CFID patients in regards to those who are more susceptible to infection and those who are not.

There is no indication that chronic fatigue immunodysfunction is a contagious disorder, and reported outbreaks are difficult to prove or validate.[72] One might conclude from this that it's not transmitted via viruses or bacteria.

With all that said, it's difficult to know where to begin.

Central Mediation, Immunological Factors, and the Role of the HPA Axis

In a 2004 study done by Siemionow, Fang, Calabrese, Sahgal, and Yue at the Lerner Research Institute in Cleveland, Ohio, physical activity–induced **EEG** signal changes were found in CFID patients and may serve as physiological indicators for a more objective diagnosis. Specifically, what the study showed was "altered central nervous system signals in controlling voluntary muscle activities, especially when the activities induce fatigue."[73] In other words, there is objective validation of CFID; the patient's subjective input has been proven by scientific measures.

In the section on fibromyalgia we discussed the role of serotonin, one of the neurotransmitters in the central nervous system, in reducing the intensity of the pain signal and regulating sleep and mood. A **PET** study regarding the role of serotonin in relationship to symptoms of CFID showed a reduced density of serotonin transporters (5-HTTs) in the brain of CFID patients. This alteration of serotonin is believed to play a key role in the abnormal physiology of chronic fatigue syndrome.[74] If a patient has fewer "feel good trains" to transport "feel good chemicals," or the "feel good, be happy" rail car is empty, the result is increased pain.

Because of the increased incidence of allergy in chronic fatigue immunodysfunction, some feel CFID may be connected to immune system dysfunction. Certain biochemicals are released as part of the centrally mediated effort of the HPA axis—the hypothalamus, pituitary, and adrenals—in response to stress.[75] As you may recall from the previous section, disruption or dysfunction of the HPA axis can cause inflammation of pathways in the nervous system and trigger an unwarranted immune response. The hormone cortisol is released to suppress inflammation and activate cellular immunity, and some studies suggest a lower level of cortisol in CFID patients, a disturbance of central neurotransmitters, and a disturbance of the relationship between cortisol and central neurotransmitter function. However, these findings do not consistently correlate to CFID symptoms. There is reduced HPA function and enhanced 5-HT function on neuroendocrine challenge tests.[76] A study done in 2004 suggests that the HPA axis is altered in both FM and CFID when compared to controls; however, the alterations differ between FM and CFID,[77] and some researchers believe that an all-inclusive claim of dysfunction of the HPA axis is not represented in CFID patients. More research into the way other aspects of the neuroendocrine system relate to CFID is needed. The origin

---

EEG: electroencephalogram, the record produced by tracing electrical impulses of the brain.

PET scan: positron emission tomography. PET is a diagnostic technique that looks at the body on a cellular level. The patient receives an injection of a small amount of radioactive material, which is absorbed by the body as it travels through. Detection of tiny particles emitted from this radioactive substance measure cellular energy. These measurements interface with a computer to produce three-dimensional images of the patient's body that can be used to record cellular energy and evaluate a variety of diseases. PET has been used, among other things, to study FM, CFID, and memory disorders of an undetermined cause.

of CFID and FM may be similar in that both show a disruption in the HPA axis; however, the type or extent of disruption may be different. Causes could be from different factors. Researchers will continue to form hypotheses for research, but once more is understood regarding the brain's function, its pathways, and how its chemicals all talk to one another, we will be closer to understanding these and many other disorders thought to be governed by the central nervous system, and closer to more significant treatment.

Adrenal steroid abnormalities have also been suggested in relationship to CFID. It appears DHEA hormone levels are elevated in CFID and show a correlation with reported symptoms leading to disabilities. This is important because hydrocortisone therapy in these particular patients may help reduce DHEA levels and thereby reduce symptoms.[78]

In autoimmune disorders, tissue damage is present. The type of tissue damage typical of autoimmune disorders is not present in CFID patients. However, researchers report a similarity to autoimmune diseases in that there is a decrease in both the natural killer (NK) immune cells (the frontline against invasion) and T-cell activation markers (crucial to the immune system) in CFS patients.[79] Another promising study shows that patients with CFID have an "underlying detectable abnormality in their **immune** cells."[80]

Three other hypothetical causes have been posited, including deregulation of the 2-5A synthetase/RNase L pathway (part of the antiviral defense mechanism). There may be abnormal messaging that can initiate both intracellular hypomagnesaemia in skeletal muscles and transient hypoglycemia. Researchers think this might explain muscle weakness and the poor utilization of oxygen typically seen in CFID patients.

The second hypothesis under discussion is that the observed excessive nitric oxide (NO) production in a subset of CFID patients may be due to the activation of the protein kinase R enzyme. Elevated nitric oxide is known to induce blood vessel dilation, so this may help explain a drop in blood pressure following exercise, thus explaining the exercise intolerance reported by a certain subset of CFID patients to be discussed shortly.

The last of the three hypotheses debates the potential interrelationship of several types of infections frequently identified in CFID patients.[81]

Autonomic Nervous System

As in FM, dysautonomia, a disruption in the autonomic nervous system, cannot be ruled out as a possible origin of CFID. Autonomic dysfunction is strongly associated with fatigue in some CFID patients.[82] These findings may help explain autonomic dysfunctions, like neurally mediated hypotension (NMH) and abnormal heart rhythms. Some researchers believe patients with these symptoms should be targeted for intervention studies that would eventually lead to effective treatment for these particular symptoms.

---

immune: a process or condition characterized by the reaction to, and interaction with, substances that are interpreted by the body as being "not self."

neuro: having to do with the nervous system.
ology: the study of (something).

Other Factors that May Affect Chronic Fatigue

Neurally mediated hypotension has been reported in a significant number of CFID patients.[83] However, not all CFID patients have a hypotensive response (drop in blood pressure), nor do they have other accompanying symptoms of **NMH,** such as slow response to verbal stimuli, visual disturbances, or reports of lightheadedness with the three-stage, seventy-degree tilt test. Neurally mediated hypotension may not cause chronic fatigue immunodysfunction, but it does exist in a certain subset of CFID patients. Proper diagnosis of this particular patient population could provide the necessary treatment for their symptoms.

There could be specific oxidative modifications to muscles, according to an Italian study done in 2003.[84] They found a deregulation of basic cellular pumps and the way they regulate cellular activity across cellular membranes. When the pumps aren't functioning properly, allowing basic cellular metabolism and oxygen transmission and utilization, the body's "teeter-totter" gets "monkey wrenched," causing an upset in the way cellular metabolism helps the body regulate and maintain stability.

Laboratory findings that are part of the diagnostic criteria for another subset of patients with CFID include the ANA (antinuclear antibody), altered levels of immunoglobulins, and antibodies related to the Epstein-Barr virus.

The thyroid gland, located in the neck near the "Adam's apple," is responsible for storing iodine and metabolizing food and oxygen into energy for cellular activity. It produces a hormone called thyroxine (T4). Thyroxine is converted into another hormone, called T3. The levels of these hormones affect heart rate, body temperature, growth, energy, disposition, and other metabolic activities. Some patients may have normal levels of thyroid hormones, but as happens in reactive hypoglycemia, their peripheral tissue is resistant. Thyroid resistance is thought to have a possible connection to FM in certain patients, and according to Garrison and Breeding, this hypometabolism may also be present in CFID.[85]

Abnormalities have been observed on MRI and SPECT scans in CFID patients. Chronic fatigue immunodysfunction patients have exhibited marked difficulties in mental processing despite IQs within normal range. Sleep abnormalities, neuroendocrine dysfunction, and autonomic dysfunction can also be seen in CFID patients. There continues to be an immune activation that can lead to symptoms lasting for decades. This may be the result of secretion of pro-inflammatory cytokines and nitric oxide, with "resulting injury to the peripheral nervous system and chronic low level immune activation in the brain." Some laboratory results show increased neutrophil apoptosis, and microbiological studies show "many different post-viral fatigue states."[86] A neutrophil is a type of white blood cell that kills and digests waste and foreign matter. Apoptosis is programmed cell death.

Other Names for NMH: vaso-vagal hypotension, delayed orthostatic hypotension, postural orthostatic tachycardia syndrome, idiopathic hypovolemia

The neutrophil typically lives for about three days. An increase in neutrophil activity would be an abnormal finding.

Other studies indicate dysfunction in growth hormone (GH),[87] natural killer cells,[88] and IgM antibodies.[89] There has also been research and some discussion related to ciguatera toxin (also known as fish toxin) and CFID.[90]

All symptoms and potential explanations go back to the way the complex internal messaging system works—the contents of the envelope, how the mail is delivered, and the forwarding address. The necessity of keeping up with the latest scientific findings about any given disorder places an overwhelming educational burden on those who treat patients. Dedicated scientists are still looking for the one connection that will bring clarity—the "aha moment."

Literature review shows that even though chronic fatigue immunodysfunction has a common set of symptoms, it may be caused by various infectious or noninfectious factors, immunological responses, or some type of disruption in the central and/or autonomic nervous systems. Responses that occur at the cellular level may be influenced by hormonal responses. The etiology is still under investigation, so we must seek more information and thank those who have already contributed so much.

Late-breaking News on CFID Research

As this book moves into the production phase, scientists at the Whittemore-Peterson Institute for Neuro-Immune Disease in Reno, Nevada (www.wpinstitute.org), have made a groundbreaking discovery. They, in collaboration with the National Cancer Institute and the Cleveland Clinic, have found antibodies to the bloodborne retrovirus, XMRV, Xenotropic MuLV-Related Virus, in CFID patients. (This virus was originally discovered in prostate cancer tumors.) The original findings of a 67 percent positive correlation for CFID patients were published in the journal, *Science,* one of the world's leading journals of original scientific research, in the article titled "Detection of Infectious Retrovirus, XMRV, in the Blood Cells of CFS Patients." Additional study results reported indicate that in these further studies as many as 95 percent of CFS patients test positive for the retrovirus.

This discovery will catapult research on CFID and FM in a new direction. A small sampling of FM patients was tested for the virus, as well, and they too tested positive. However, it is possible that some members of this sample group had been originally misdiagnosed with FM when they actually had CFID. More research is needed to determine whether the virus is a causative factor or has only a casual link to CFID or other related neuro-immune disorders, and further research for demographics, possible treatments, and method of transmission is indicated. Current retrovirus treatment is toxic with many side effects, so a benefit/risk/morbidity analysis will be imperative. To date, testing for the virus has been done only as part of research, but it is expected to be available to the public eventually.

Honestly, I didn't think I would live long enough to experience all that this discovery means to us. Listen up, dear readers, no longer will CFID be a wastebasket diagnosis, nor will we be told that our symptoms are all in our heads. I feel certain that the CDC will recognize the need for a name change. Glory, Halleluiah.

idiopathic chronic fatigue: unexplained chronic fatigue that fails to meet the criteria for diagnosis of CFS.

Never doubt that a small group of thoughtful, committed citizens can change the world. Indeed, it is the only thing that ever has.

MARGARET MEAD

Prognosis

Chronic fatigue immunodysfunction is not considered a progressive illness. The symptoms seem to be more severe at the onset and typically stabilize, but they may be chronic, come and go, or improve. Some patients partially or fully recover, and others recover and then relapse.

According to the CDC, "the clinical course of CFID varies considerably. The percentage of patients who recover is unknown, and the definition of what should be considered recovery is subject to debate. Some patients recover to the point that they can resume work and other activities, but continue to experience periodic flaring of symptoms. Some patients recover completely with time, and some grow progressively worse. Chronic fatigue immunodysfunction often follows a cyclical course, alternating between periods of illness and relative well-being. The Centers for Disease Control continues to monitor and study patients."

One thing that seems to be clear is that CFID patients with coexisting conditions, such as FM, do have greater disability.[91] Although complete recovery may not be possible for some, there is hope for improvement through recognition of symptoms, understanding aggravating and alleviating factors, and application of a solid, consistent treatment program.

The relationship of cause and treatment is a continuing debate. We don't yet know all of the answers, but with your help, knowledgeable physicians can help you identify achievable treatment objectives.

Living in the present with optimism for the future is what supplies the fortitude for achieving goals. By educating, identifying, planning, and participating in a positive treatment plan, the prognosis for improving activities of daily living is possible.

Summary Exercise: CFID

Can you briefly describe the key points listed below?

- Definition of CFID
- History and demographics of CFID
- Symptoms
- Personal testimony (a narrative of your own experience)
- Etiology
- Diagnostic criteria
- Prognosis

What do you do if you experience a new, undiagnosed symptom?

What did you learn from this section that will affect your life?

Your Inventory of Symptoms

Which of the following symptoms do you have? (Check all that apply.)

Diagnostic Criteria

Both of the following symptoms must be present for a diagnosis of CFID.

- ☐ Chronic fatigue of new onset not alleviated by rest
- ☐ Symptoms that have persisted for at least six or more months and do not predate the fatigue

Four or more of the following symptoms must be present for a diagnosis of CFID:

- ☐ Cognitive impairment, substantially reduced short-term memory, or loss of concentration (brain fog—difficulty processing information or finding words)
- ☐ Throat soreness—unexplained inflammation without secretions
- ☐ Lymph node tenderness
- ☐ Muscle pain (myalgia)—persistent and reproducible on repeated examination
- ☐ Joint pain, multiple, without swelling or redness (arthralgias)
- ☐ Headaches of a new type, pattern, or severity
- ☐ Non-restorative sleep
- ☐ Post-exertional malaise (ill feeling) lasting more than twenty-four hours

Other Symptoms that May Accompany CFID

- ☐ Alcohol intolerance
- ☐ Allergies or sensitivities to foods, alcohol, odors, chemicals, medications, or noise
- ☐ Chills and night sweats
- ☐ Chest pain
- ☐ Chronic cough
- ☐ Gynecological problems, including PMS and endometriosis
- ☐ Irritable bowel, abdominal pain, nausea, diarrhea, or bloating
- ☐ Irregular heartbeat
- ☐ Jaw pain
- ☐ Difficulty maintaining upright position (orthostatic instability, dizziness, balance problems, or fainting)
- ☐ Low-grade fever or low body temperature
- ☐ Muscle twitches
- ☐ Paresthesias—abnormal sensations (burning, numbness, or tingling)
- ☐ Psychological problems (depression, irritability, mood swings, anxiety, or panic attacks)
- ☐ Ringing in the ears (tinnitus)
- ☐ Seizures
- ☐ Sensitivity to heat and/or cold
- ☐ Shortness of breath
- ☐ SICCA-like symptoms (mucosal dryness, such as dry mouth and eyes)
- ☐ Visual blurring, eye pain or dry eyes
- ☐ Weight loss or gain

Chronic Myofascial Pain—Nerve to Muscle

Chronic myofascial pain is a disease that affects the chemicals that cross between nerve endings and muscles. It is literally, a disease at the neuro-muscular junction—nerve to muscle.

Definition

Chronic myofascial pain, or CMP, is a chronic disorder in which myofascial trigger points (TrPs) cause sensory, motor, and autonomic symptoms. This condition may develop in muscles that are overstressed, overused, or injured. Different from isolated incidental occurrences of trigger points that can happen to normal individuals, CMP develops when TrPs are apparent in several quadrants of the body and have become chronic. The trigger points may be active, latent, or secondary.[92]

Chronic myofascial pain (CMP) is a term used by Devin J. Starlanyl, author of *Fibromyalgia and Chronic Myofascial Pain: A Survival Manual.* In the original publication of this book, the term "myofascial pain syndrome" was used; however, this commonly used term has led to confusion. Many people in the health care community, particularly those who treat temporomandibular dysfunction (TMJ/TMD), use the acronym MPS, implying that myofascial pain syndrome is not widespread throughout the body.[93] A person can have trigger points in the face that affect the temporomandibular joint, but to imply that trigger points occur only in the facial area could not be further from the truth. It is extremely important to understand that the term MPS is not synonymous with TMJ/TMD, which will be discussed further in the next chapter.

---

peripheral nervous system: the part of the nervous system that is outside the central nervous system and consists of two branches: the autonomic, or involuntary nervous system, and the voluntary nervous system.

autonomic nervous system: controls organ function or involuntary actions either by sympathetic or parasympathetic response impulses. The caretaker of the body.

voluntary nervous system: the branch of the peripheral nervous system that includes both motor and sensory nerves, controls muscles, and carries information to the brain via nerve cells in the form of electrical charges and chemical messages.

Chronic Myofascial Pain and Sensitization of the Central Nervous System

When information relayed to the brain via the spinal cord is disrupted by chemical mis-messaging, as suggested in studies of FM, CFID, migraine, or any other condition related to central sensitization, TrPs can get in on the action, too.[94, 95] Chemical changes in neurons do occur in response to chronic pain. This wind-up phenomenon will be called CMP, stage II, and is the subject of a new textbook for physicians,[96] but what is important for you to know is that the longer the TrPs go untreated, the more difficult they will be to treat, and there is an increased chance they will be perpetuated by a broken biofeedback loop. The constant bombardment on the CNS from sustained TrPs can extend the area of dysfunction. The body constantly strives to maintain balance, and relies on an accurate exchange of information between the periphery and the brain. Do all that you can to keep this loop intact by treating CMP before it becomes a central sensitization problem.

Myofascial Trigger Point

A myofascial trigger point (TrP) is a self-sustaining, irritable area in the muscle that can be felt as a nodule in a taut band. This irritated spot causes the muscle to gradually shorten, interfering with the motion function of the muscle and causing weakness and pain. Trigger points differ from tender

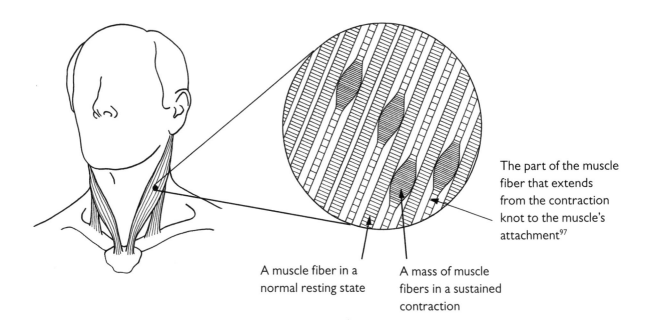

The part of the muscle fiber that extends from the contraction knot to the muscle's attachment[97]

A muscle fiber in a normal resting state

A mass of muscle fibers in a sustained contraction

Trigger point—a hypersensitive bundle or knot of muscle fiber within a taut band of muscle

points in that generally they refer pain to other parts of the body and can usually be felt with the hand (palpated) unless the muscle is too rigid from intense muscle involvement, or the trigger point is in a deep muscle or under bone. The tender points of FM or myalgias associated with CFID do not restrict motion or cause localized muscle weakness. If they do, the patient should also be evaluated for the presence of CMP. Trigger points in CMP are well defined and often radiating—the pain radiates out to other parts of the body.

In CMP, you can have pain in your hand that is activated by a trigger point in the hand, the forearm, or further up the arm. Specific trigger points can be mapped according to pain and symptom referral patterns. They have no relevance to the size of the muscle, and in some cases, small muscles can cause more problems than larger ones.

In response to a stressor, excessive amounts of the neurotransmitter acetylcholine is released from our nerves to our muscles at the motor end plate, the neuromuscular junction. Trigger points develop in the form of hypersensitive "contraction" nodules located in a taut band of muscle.

Active Trigger Point

An active TrP is a myofascial trigger point that causes pain at rest. It is always tender, causes shortening of the muscle, weakens the muscle, and causes patient complaints of referred pain on direct compression. An active trigger point can elicit a visible local twitch response when adequately stimulated by compression or needle insertion. It can produce referred motor and autonomic phenomena, generally occurring in the TrP referral zone. An active TrP can also cause the referral zone to become tender.[98]

COMMON ABBREVIATIONS

MPS: myofascial pain syndrome

CMP: chronic myofascial pain

MTP: myofascial trigger point

TrP: trigger point

Secondary Trigger Point

A secondary TrP is one that develops in a second compensating muscle. A compensating muscle is one that is trying to make up for the malfunction of the muscle affected by primary trigger points.[99] In other words, when a primary trigger point causes muscle dysfunction, the opposing muscles become stressed. These opposing muscles become overloaded because they are attempting to carry the entire load of the muscle work needed to perform a task. When staring at a computer screen your head starts to drift forward after a while, particularly if you spend hours there. You may have primary TrPs in muscles on the front of your neck, which may or may not be making their presence known. As your head starts drifting forward, putting less stress on the primary TrPs because of the slackening, the muscles on the backside of your neck are being stretched and stressed in an effort to keep your face from falling onto your keyboard. The sustained overstretching of these muscles causes secondary trigger points to develop in the muscles on the back of your neck. (This is an important reason to pay attention to posture as an aggravating factor, to be discussed in chapter 4.)

Secondary (compensatory) myofascial trigger points develop in muscles that are trying to take up the workload for the muscle affected by a primary TrP. Secondary TrPs can be on the same or opposite side of the body. Pain may shift as secondary TrPs are "uncovered." You are unraveling the "crime scene," eventually revealing the criminal—the primary TrP(s)—making them available for treatment.

Satellite Trigger Point

A satellite trigger point is a type of secondary TrP that develops in a muscle of the primary trigger point's referred pain area.[100] The following example illustrates some possible referral patterns for TrPs that develop in the neck, which may clarify what is meant by a satellite TrP. (For specific TrP referral zones for specific TrP[s]—a specific place in a specific muscle—please refer to one of the books suggested in the resource section.) When a TrP develops in a referral area, it is called a satellite TrP. Think of it this way: A satellite in space receives a scrambled signal from somewhere on Earth. If the problem is with both the base station and the satellite (TrPs in both locations), both need to be fixed. Repairing the satellite TrP alone is not going to remedy the problem; you must treat both. If you treat only the satellite TrP, your referred symptoms will return and you will think the treatment was unsuccessful. Understanding referral zones, TrP definitions, and the importance of

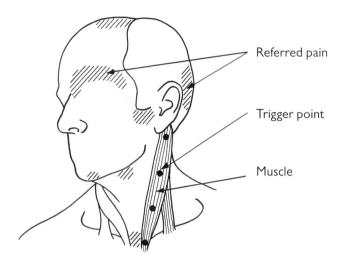

Referral zones (referred pain) and satellite TrP location. A secondary trigger point found in a referral zone is called a satellite TrP.

locating each one of these points is imperative to proper treatment and relief of symptoms.

Devin Starlanyl believes that the primary trigger point (the one that really launches the whole event) may not start screaming until you start treating the one that is painful, which may very well be an active satellite TrP. This can be very difficult and frustrating for the patient and the practitioner unless they both understand what is happening. When I have treated an "acting out" trigger point, other ones "pop up," or so it seems. This is because I actually treated a screaming satellite TrP. In reality, the primary trigger point wasn't treated at all. Remember, the satellite TrP is in the primary TrP referral zone, which can be (but isn't necessarily) well away from the primary TrP site. Because of this, "People may give up, thinking that their condition is worsening," says Starlanyl. "Sometimes, due to the nature of a specific injury, the primary TrP can be suggested by history and exam, but it may be under layers of other TrPs, calcified, or fibrotic, tissue. It takes time, patience, and knowledge, and cannot be rushed."[101]

referred pain: pain that manifests in a different part of the body from the origin of the problem.

referral zone: an area of pain directed by a primary trigger point (TrP).

Latent Trigger Point

Latent TrP(s) can lie in wait and ambush you when you least expect them. This type of trigger point is painful only when there is pressure on it. A latent TrP can restrict muscle movement and cause stiffness and weakness that persist for years after apparent recovery. Unless restricted motion or weakness causes you to start rubbing around to find the source, a latent TrP may go unnoticed. When you stumble upon a sore, hypersensitive nodule in a muscle that does not refer pain anywhere, you have found a latent trigger point. Now you have discovered the source of your restricted motion and weakness. Dormant latent TrPs can be reactivated by overstretching, overuse, or injury. Treat TrPs when you discover them, because some seemingly minor event, such as chilling, can cause a latent TrP to transition to an active trigger point.[102] Once the TrP transitions from latent to active it will be painful all the time and can cause referred pain. Treatment is discussed in chapter 4.

Once you know about the different types of trigger points (TrPs), it is easier to understand their cause and effect. If you don't know how to treat TrPs or how to track them down, you might think your condition is declining, with no hope for recovery. But chronic myofascial pain is not a progressive illness. A progressive disease is one that continues to worsen and doesn't respond to treatment. Chronic TrPs may never be totally dormant, but they are always treatable. You can get rid of them, even if only temporarily. They return when you neglect self-care measures. It might take a while to see improvement, but treatment does alleviate symptoms.

History

The real pioneer in the study of chronic myofascial pain as we know it today is Dr. Janet Travell, later joined by Dr. David Simons. Travell discovered as early as 1940 that by applying pressure to a trigger point, she could establish and predict referred pain patterns. After successfully treating President John F. Kennedy for residual effects from bouts with myofascial pain and longstanding back problems, she was the first woman and first non-military doctor to be appointed to the post of White House physician. Dr. Travell is considered to be an expert authority, and her work and dedication continue to be internationally referenced.[103]

---

myofascial medicine: the study of muscle and soft tissue.

Although Dr. David Simons started his medical career as a military clinician and research scientist, since 1965 he has been practicing physical and rehabilitative medicine. Dr. Simons, a world leader in myofascial medicine, continues to lecture and advocate for research in this "new field" of medicine. Drs. Travell and Simons co-authored *Myofascial Pain and Dysfunction: The Trigger Point Manual*, Vol. 1, published in 1983, and Vol. 2 in 1992. The revised edition of Vol. 1 was published in 1999.[104]

Thanks to their dedication to scientific study and education, we now know that specific trigger points cause specific pain patterns and symptoms.

Demographics

Chronic myofascial pain is often misdiagnosed or not diagnosed at all. It is not considered gender prevalent, but there may be a genetic predisposition to the development of the taut bands found in CMP.[105] Many of the perpetuating factors of TrPs are genetic, such as short upper arms, short lower legs, curvature of the spine, or some metabolic dysfunctions. People with skeletal structural defects or lack of symmetrical bone structure seem to be at higher risk for developing chronic myofascial pain. Structural causes include both inherited problems and acquired defects from injury, surgery, post-polio syndrome, or poor posture.

Dr. John Whiteside, M.B.B.S., (Bachelor of Medicine, Bachelor of Surgery, U.S. equivalent, M.D.), Fellow of the Australian College of Nutritional and Environmental Medicine has lectured with Dr. Simons and is working on an advanced training course for medical practitioners. Dr. Whiteside believes that approximately 70 percent of all pain is primarily myofascial in origin. The remaining 30 percent has other causes but is normally associated with a secondary myofascial pain syndrome.[106]

Do not follow where the path may lead. Go instead where there is no path, and leave a trail.

AUTHOR UNKNOWN

Diagnostic Criteria

Pain is a warning sign from your body that something isn't right. You and your physician should make sure there is nothing life threatening causing your pain, which means running tests to rule out conditions that could cause the same or similar symptoms. There are three variables at work here:

1. Your physician may not be trained to recognize TrPs and referral patterns (most are not).

2. TrPs may be hidden and difficult to pinpoint.
3. You may be a poor historian.

Diagnosis can sometimes be very complicated and is often delayed because myofascial disorders are generally poorly understood in the medical community. As previously mentioned, there are no two identical people. The perpetuating factors that cause TrPs can, and do, vary greatly among us. Some of us work at computers, others have been in a car accident, some may be professional athletes, and the list goes on. The important thing to remember is that trigger points can be activated by acute overload on the muscle involved, or by chronic overuse of the affected muscle. This can be directly or indirectly due to overwork, over-stretching, fatigue, trauma, muscle injury, or not protecting muscles from the external environment.

The diagnosis of CMP involves multiple factors. One characteristic of TrP disease is a history of pain resulting from a muscular insult, direct or indirect, that has outlasted the causative event. Hyperirritable trigger points (TrPs), usually felt in a taut band, restrict motion and cause pain at the end of the range of motion. Chronic myofascial pain can be long lasting with development of secondary TrPs, and may (but doesn't necessarily) involve multiple quadrants. A person might have CMP that involves only the head and neck area, yet has lasted for six years. People with head and neck TrPs may or may not experience other eventual muscle involvement, but should these patients be excluded from the category of CMP? Dr. Simons and Devin Starlanyl think not. Generally, chronic symptoms are those that persist for six months or more; however, the word "chronic" may have a different application when it comes to TrPs. Chronic in this case means that the symptoms have outlasted their usefulness as a warning sign. We can expect there will be a more thorough definition and explanation of chronic myofascial pain in the third volume of *Myofascial Pain and Dysfunction: The Trigger Point Manual*, which is presently being written by Dr. David Simons with contributions by Devin J. Starlanyl, and will combine Volumes 1 and 2.[107] It will be a valuable medical textbook for physicians and other health care providers.

Myofascial trigger points (TrPs) can vary and can occur in any part of any layer of any muscle. They can be felt unless they are in a rigid taut band, buried in a deep muscle, or trapped behind bone. They constrict movement, cause weakness, and/or refer pain that is typical to the location of each specific trigger point. When a latent trigger point cannot be found because it is too deep or behind bone, you will notice tightness, limited movement, or weakness. When an active TrP cannot be felt because of its obscure location, it can be backtracked from the pain referral zone. The trigger point location depends upon a good historical account of your symptoms and a complete, comprehensive, hands-on exam. Locating trigger points that lie deep beneath layers of muscle or under bone depends on the restriction of motion, weakness, or pain referral pattern of the muscle involved. A trigger point can refer pain to more than one place. These are the reasons it is important for the person examining you to look for several indicators.

central TrP: a trigger point in the mid-fiber region, the belly of the muscle.

attachment TrP: can be a trigger point in the taut muscle band near where the muscle tapers and the fascia, or muscle covering, narrows to form the tendon. Attachment trigger points can also be in the actual tendon or ligament, but their mechanism is different from what we are discussing.

The person evaluating you for CMP will look at your history (identifying possible causative or perpetuating factors), the presence of palpable TrP(s), particular pain referral patterns, and any weakness or restriction of motion. Finding the right health care provider (HCP) is extremely important. We will talk more about how to do that later in the book.

Your physician is going to need a clear and concise history in order to have a good understanding of your TrP issues and determine the correct diagnosis. Once again, an isolated event can cause severe disabling pain and dysfunction, but when successfully treated, it will not lead to a chronic myofascial pain state (CMP) if there are no perpetuating factors, or the perpetuating factors are brought under control.

Perpetuating factors include, but are not limited to, posture-risk furniture, ill-fitting shoes, paradoxical breathing patterns, poor diet, immobility, and environmental factors such as pollution and poor lighting. Changing perpetuating factors when possible, along with improving management of those that cannot be changed, increases the likelihood of pain management.

paradoxical breathing pattern: abnormal chest wall and belly movement that restricts full inhalation into the lungs.

Muscles come in many shapes and sizes according to what motion they are responsible for performing. Sometimes trigger points can linger in hidden areas, such as smaller, less well-defined muscles that are located deep in the muscle structure of the body. Often they are in muscles that can't be readily accessed, and can only be diagnosed by trained professionals using careful palpation skills. Therefore, the skill of the practitioner at palpation will determine the success of the exam, which is paramount in diagnosis and treatment.

The following symptoms, along with an in-depth history and a hands-on physical exam, are all part of a CMP diagnosis.

Symptoms as Part of Diagnostic Criteria[108]

- A taut muscle band that you can feel
- Exquisite spot tenderness of a nodule in a taut band
- Patient's recognition of current pain complaint by pressure on the tender nodule
- Painful limit to full stretch of range of motion

Other Symptoms that May or May Not Be Present

Symptoms depend on many variables, among which are the specific TrPs involved; the presence of nerve, blood vessel, or lymph entrapment; and the presence of coexisting conditions. The following list is not all-inclusive, but meant as a guide for understanding the way untreated trigger points can affect the body.

Skeletal muscles are those that give our body its shape. The symptoms listed in this section may indicate trigger points in any of them.

- Back pain
- Breast pain and/or hypersensitivity
- Bladder difficulties—pain, frequency, inability to empty, and/or urinary incontinence
- Cardiac arrhythmia—rapid heartbeat or fluttery/jumpy feelings
- Chest pain associated with chest wall movement or touching
- Disequilibrium—lack of coordination, problems with balance, or dizziness
- Dropping things unexpectedly, weak grasp
- Dry mucous membranes (eyes, nose, mouth, vaginal, gastrointestinal)
- Ear—pain, itching, ringing (tinnitus)

- Eye—pain, excessive tearing, reddening, eyelid twitches
- Facial related—pain, sleep drooling, teeth grinding, choking on saliva
- Gastrointestinal (GI) disturbance—pain, bloating, burping, constipation, nausea, cramping, diarrhea, food intolerance
- Growing pains in children
- Gynecological symptoms—pain; menstrual cramping; delayed, irregular, or missed periods; bleeding irregularity
- Headaches—frequent or severe
- Joint dysfunction—ankle, hand, elbow, frozen shoulder, knee, hip, wrist, sacroiliac (SI)
- Muscle cramps, such as upper and lower legs; at nighttime in the calf
- Muscle tightness, such as hamstring
- Pain with repetitive movement, stretching, or contracting muscles
- Paresthesias, unexplained—numbness, burning, or tingling
- Pelvic—groin, buttock, hip, rectal, or genital pain
- Radiating pain
- Sexual dysfunction—painful intercourse (women and men), impotence (men)
- Shortness of breath and pain with deep breathing
- Sinus problems, stuffy or runny nose, chronic or dry cough
- Soreness or pain, unusual (such as on the top of your head, when wearing a heavy head covering; or from writing by hand)
- Stiff neck
- Swelling from entrapment of blood vessels by trigger points
- Throat problems—pain or soreness when swallowing or chewing
- Visual disturbances

gynecological: pertaining to female anatomy

impotence: inability to achieve or maintain erection

urinary incontinence: inability to control urine

Some Other Indirectly Related Symptoms

- Depression from chronic untreated pain
- Fatigue as a result of chronic muscle tension and sleep disruption

Some of these symptoms may signify something wrong within your organ system. They could indicate a life-threatening event and the symptoms may be explained by something other than TrPs. As with all the symptoms discussed in this book, if these are new ones for you or you do not have a history of CMP, pay close attention to them *after* other problems have been ruled out.

CAUTION

If you have a history of heart problems or suspect your symptoms may be due to something other than known trigger points, seek immediate treatment.

Many non-pain symptoms are caused by active TrPs. Myofascial trigger points in the sternocleidomastoid muscles at the front of the neck cause changes in balance, vision, and hearing, and can produce nausea and dizziness. Trigger points in the pectoral muscles on the front of the chest can cause heart palpitations. Trigger points in the abdominals and in the long back muscles can cause bowel and gynecological problems.

Trigger points can cause phenomenon such as local vasoconstriction, ringing in the ears, knee buckling, ankle jerking, jaw pain, headaches, numbness, tingling, burning, hypersensitivity, excessive tearing, excessive salivation, persistent nasal congestion, secretions, and swelling.[109] Myofascial symptoms are common, but not commonly diagnosed.

ETIOLOGY OF TrPs

Muscles can develop TrPs because of accident, surgery, poor posture, repetitive motion stress, or even chronic tension,[110] and among other problems can cause changes in balance, gait, vision, and hearing, and can even affect the body to the point of nausea and dizziness. Untreated TrPs can also cause bowel and gonad-related problems,[111] heart arrhythmia (uneven heart beat), and difficulty breathing.[112]

There are several theories regarding the cause of myofascial pain and trigger points. Trigger points have been evaluated both clinically and scientifically, and it is now definitively known that TrPs cause myofascial pain.[113] Scientific evaluation has been achieved by biopsy, dissection, **electrophysiology,** ultrasound imaging, and **histological** and microscopic exam. Furthermore, newer studies indicate an intensified pain state in TrP patients associated with abnormal brain activity, suggesting a

---

electrophysiology: The study of electric currents in cells and tissues.

histology: The study of the anatomy dealing with the minute structure, composition, and function of tissues.

central sensitization as seen in FM and CFID patients.[114]

Because of the ability to use objective data to retrieve information, the diagnosis of chronic myofascial pain does not totally rely upon subjective (from you, the patient) criteria. Dr. David Simons asserts that "myofascial trigger points are identified electrophysiologically by characteristic spontaneous electrical activity (SEA), and histologically by contraction knot." He believes that "this is a result of excessive release of the neurotransmitter acetylcholine from the nerve terminal of the motor end plate."[115] Because of the relationships revealed among dysfunctional nerve activity, ultrasound imaging of local twitch response, and contraction knots biopsied in the trigger point of muscle fiber, trigger points can be defined as a neuromuscular disease.

Dr. C. Z. Hong penned an article in 2002 stating that a trigger point has both a sensory and a motor component. These can be demonstrated by locating tenderness, locating a referred pain pattern, and demonstrating a local twitch response by mechanical stimulation. He also believes sensitivities can be widely distributed in the muscle but seem to be mostly concentrated in the end plate,[116] the end of the neuron that releases the neurotransmitter acetylcholine to the muscle. An active location is a site from which spontaneous electrical activity (SEA) can be recorded, in much the same way that heart electrical activity is recorded on an EKG. The spontaneous electrical activity from the trigger point is essentially the same electrical activity recorded from an abnormal end plate that would be reported by a neurophysiologist.

Trigger points are always found in taut bands of muscle and are histologically related to contraction knots caused by excessive end plate release of acetylcholine, the substance that acts as a neurotransmitter at nerve endings. Hong concludes that trigger points appear to be the result of "a serious disturbance of the nerve endings and the contractile mechanisms at multiple dysfunctional end plates."

There is also the energy crisis theory. This theory suggests that when the tissue is deprived of normal metabolic activity, oxygen deprivation occurs and increases the metabolic demand already in short supply. The energy crisis concept, investigated by Dr. Simons, does not refute the theory of end plate dysfunction, but is part of it.[117]

Acetylcholine and other chemicals are transmitted within the human body via the nervous system. These neurotransmitters determine the elasticity of tissue by sending and receiving information along the neurological pathway, the two-way road from the peripheral nerves to the central nervous system. This would be much like ingoing and outgoing messages along an information highway. We suspect that trigger points found in CMP are due to the localized area craving oxygen, because the muscle of the residing TrP gets an ongoing message that there is an energy crisis, and forces the body to respond.

Another hypothesis suggests there may be a dysfunction in one of the ion channels, specifically the ryanodine-receptor-calcium channel. (These channels in various forms are found in excitable animal tissue—in both muscles and neurons—and they mediate calcium within the cell. Calcium reception is a necessary step for muscle contraction.) In very simple terms, when the channel controls don't function properly (as in channelopathy—a dysfunction of the channel), all kinds of problems can occur, as if a floodgate is opened. This hypothesis may explain excessive release of acetylcholine and calcium, and the excessive motor end plate noise noted in previous studies on TrPs.[118] Hypotheses and studies on cellular TrP formation are important to us. Each piece of information is a puzzle piece and the more pieces to the puzzle we have, the clearer the picture becomes.

The aforementioned exams have been performed during research. To help in clarifying your own situation, you should request a thorough physical exam by a health care provider who is qualified to diagnose CMP. To date, the only way to receive a diagnosis of CMP is through a clinical exam that includes palpating the abnormal muscle knots and bands, perceiving the twitches that occur (sometimes just to touch), and identifying distinctive consistent pain and symptom referral patterns.

Personal Testimony

The muscle twitches mentioned at the end of the etiology box above remind me of the need to explain the different types of twitching you may experience. My myofascial release therapist, a physical therapist who specializes in soft tissue treatment, had a student with her one day, and I, being a teacher myself, always welcome students. While my therapist was working, the student stood behind me to observe. I heard her say to my therapist, "You need to come here," to which the therapist responded, "What is it you see?" The student repeated, "I think you need to come here." My therapist looked at me and smiled; we were both impressed by the student's acute observation skills. My whole back was dancing to a tune, and of course I knew this because I could feel it, but the student? Well, it obviously was her first experience. My therapist explained to her that my myofascia was acting out in response to the therapy. Although it is not a pleasant experience, I was glad for the diversion and to be a part of this student's learning opportunity.

The visible muscle twitching that the student observed on my back is called fasciculation. Fasciculation occurs when there is a spontaneous discharge of impulses within a bundle of skeletal muscle, kind of like a strobe light. Why? No one seems to know the causative mechanism. This involuntary muscle twitching, has been reported in CFID patients and my own rheumatologist has told me that other FM patients have complained of this. It may be the result of those coexisting conditions, in me. Please don't become confused; the muscle twitching I just described is not the "twitch response" seen in TrP release. A TrP "twitch response" is a localized twitch of the TrP as it is directly treated, either by direct pressure, dry needle, or injection therapy.

Trigger points associated with CMP are well understood, because unlike the pain of FM and CFID, they usually can be seen or felt, and we know there is a disruption at the neuromuscular junction. This, however, does not explain why the trigger point develops. As discussed above, it could be from some type of nerve chemical disruption between the nerve ending and the muscle it affects, in the ion channels that direct the flow of charged particles, or both. It could be linked to a disruption within the sympathetic nervous system itself, or maybe not, but we're sure to get a better understanding of why this disruption occurs as scientists continue to explore. One thing is for certain—we are getting closer every day to finding the cause of TrPs. When that happens, treatment directed at the cause instead of the effect (the TrP) will be developed, and that prospect is music to my ears.

Entrapment

Trigger points in the myofascia cause taut ropy bands that can physically entrap nerves, blood vessels, or lymph vessels. The entrapment by taut muscle bands can occur between muscle and bone, or muscle and another muscle. When this happens, any structures located within or around the taut band can be affected.

Nerves provide power to your body, just as electricity provides power to your house. Myofascial trigger points are in taut bands of muscle. When these taut bands of muscle "entrap" a nerve, the nerve cannot perform its function. You could equate it to a lightbulb flickering due to intermittent power disruption during an electrical storm. Usually the entrapment does not cause a total power outage, just a modified one. The result is nerve pain (neuralgia), numbness, tingling, and other unusual sensations.

neuralgia: pain in a nerve or along the course of a nerve or nerves; usually sharp, spasm-like pain that can recur at different intervals.

Among its other functions, blood transports oxygen from the lungs to various parts of the body. Oxygen is nourishment for our body parts and is required for cellular metabolism. When blood vessels are entrapped, the resulting decreased blood flow deprives cells of oxygen and nutrients. When blood vessels cannot carry blood freely, the fluid backs up into the tissue and causes swelling, poor circulation to the area, and compromised healing.

When lymph vessels are entrapped, the free flow of lymph is obstructed. Lymph is the liquid collected from tissues and returned to the blood via the lymph system. Among other duties, this system is responsible for recirculating fluid from tissues to blood and helping rid the body of waste, such as bacteria and toxins. When the lymph system is dammed up, fluid extracted from the surrounding tissue, with its load of bacteria and toxins, is unable to escape.

Treating the TrPs involved in CMP frees nerves, blood vessels, and lymph vessels, and resolves symptoms.

Other Disorders

Chronic myofascial pain is a great imitator. Often the pain seems indicative of some inflammatory process; however, research shows us that this is not the case. Other inflammatory disorders that cause muscle pain do exist and can render the same type of pain as that found with CMP. This is why it is important to be diagnosed expeditiously by an experienced practitioner familiar with this disorder and the criteria for proper diagnosis. It is equally important to understand that other conditions may coexist with, or aggravate, CMP.

meralgia paresthetica: a condition of pain, numbness, and tingling in the anterior (front) and lateral (outside) aspect of the thigh; most often caused by TrPs.

Prognosis

Treatment of individual isolated events of trigger points has been quite successful. However, when treatment is delayed because of failure to identify TrPs or address perpetuating factors, or there is a possible underlying genetic tendency (still under investigation), full-blown CMP can develop. When this happens, both latent and active TrPs become more resistant to treatment. The TrPs may last a lifetime even if perpetuating factors such as the effects of kyphosis, lordosis, or scoliosis are brought under control and appropriate care is provided.

Your goal should be to bring trigger points under control with proper myofascial treatment, supervised exercise, medication, and avoidance of perpetuating factors. If you have aggravating or perpetuating factors that cannot be changed, such as a structural abnormality of one leg shorter than the other, abnormal spinal curvature, short upper arms, post-polio effects, or any other health disorder, certain modifications can be made. This would include remedies such as shoe lifts, assistive devices, and controlling metabolic disturbances. If you have to deal with rebounding TrPs because perpetuating factors are out of your control, taking action is the key to success for at least temporary relief.

In review, trigger points are always present in CMP and there are multiple factors involved in making a diagnosis. These factors are as follows: TrPs in taut bands of muscle fiber that can be felt and that hurt when touched; painful limits with full range of motion; restricted movement causing weakness or referred pain that has persisted beyond the initial event, despite bringing perpetuating factors under control; and the presence of primary, secondary, and/or latent TrPs. Myofascial trigger points can be perpetuated by surrounding factors, including anatomical abnormalities, other health problems, poor posture, additional trauma, surgeries, or inadequate coping strategies. The goals of TrP treatment are to restore normal resting length of the muscle, restore endurance, and restore strength of the muscle involved. They *will not*, however, resolve without proper treatment. Start your action plan today!

Summary Exercise: CMP

Can you briefly describe these key points?

- Definition of CMP
- History and demographics
- Symptoms
- Personal testimony
- Objective findings
- Subjective findings
- Etiology
- Genetics
- Prognosis

What do you do if you experience a new, undiagnosed symptom?

What did you learn from this chapter that affects your life?

Your Inventory of Symptoms

Which of the following symptoms do you have? (Check all that apply.)

Diagnostic Criteria

The following two criteria must be present for a diagnosis of CMP.

☐ A history of pain as a result of muscular insult that has outlasted the causative event

☐ Persisting trigger points

Symptoms that Contribute to Diagnostic Criteria

☐ A taut muscle band that you can feel

☐ Exquisite spot tenderness of a nodule in a taut band

☐ Patient's recognition of current pain complaint by pressure on the tender nodule

☐ Painful limit to full stretch of range of motion

Other Symptoms that May or May Not Be Present

☐ Back pain

☐ Breast pain and/or hypersensitivity

☐ Bladder difficulties—pain, frequency, inability to empty, and/or urinary incontinence

☐ Chest pain associated with chest wall movement or touching

☐ Disequilibrium—lack of coordination, problems with balance, or dizziness

☐ Dropping things unexpectedly, weak grasp

☐ Dry mucous membranes (eyes, nose, mouth, vaginal, gastrointestinal)

☐ Ear—pain, itching, ringing (tinnitus)

☐ Eye—pain, excessive tearing, reddening, eyelid twitches

☐ Facial related, pain, sleep drooling, teeth grinding, choking on saliva

☐ GI disturbance—pain, bloating, burping, constipation, nausea, cramping, diarrhea, or food intolerance

☐ Growing pains as a child

☐ Gynecological symptoms—pain; menstrual cramping; delayed, irregular, or missed periods; bleeding irregularity

☐ Headaches, frequent or severe

☐ Heart (cardiac) arrhythmia—rapid heartbeat or fluttery/jumpy feelings

☐ Joint dysfunction—ankle, hand, elbow, frozen shoulder, knee, hip, wrist, and/or sacroiliac

☐ Muscle cramps—upper and lower legs; nighttime in the calf

☐ Muscle tightness, such as hamstring

☐ Pain with repetitive movement, stretching, or contracting muscles

☐ Paresthesias, unexplained—numbness, burning, or tingling

☐ Pelvic—groin, buttock, hip, rectal, and/or genital pain

☐ Radiating pain

☐ Sexual dysfunction—painful intercourse (women and men), impotence (men)

☐ Shortness of breath and pain with deep breathing

☐ Sinus problems—stuffy or runny nose, chronic or dry cough

☐ Soreness or pain, unusual (such as the top of your head, when wearing heavy head covering; or from writing by hand)

☐ Stiff neck

☐ Swelling from entrapment of blood or lymph vessels by TrPs

☐ Throat problems—pain or soreness when swallowing or chewing

☐ Visual disturbances

Indirectly Related Symptoms

☐ Depression from chronic untreated pain

☐ Fatigue as a result of chronic muscle tension and sleep disruption

Chapter Summary

FM/CMP–FM/CFID—Is It a Double Cross?

It appears that FM can coexist with CFID and/or CMP, and CFID can coexist with FM; however, CFID and CMP are seldom discussed together. This does not mean they don't occur together; only that studies have not been done regarding this specific connection. However, FM is a perpetual central sensitization state that sets the stage for the development of chronic TrPs, causing chronic myofascial pain in the periphery, which in turn perpetually bombards the CNS, thus increasing the sensitivity of the brain and other CNS tissue. It is a vicious cycle. If FM and CFID are both centrally mediated, which is becoming more evident, then one could easily conclude that CMP can, and most likely does, coexist with CFID, and could explain the unexplained myalgia associated with it. This would be just like the peripheral input from migraine, irritable bowel syndrome, or any other of the many possible coexisting conditions. The presence of CMP in these patients must be considered.

Chronic pain disorders are not limited to FM, CFID, or CMP. Some other syndromes under this umbrella are Gulf War syndrome, multiple chemical sensitivity syndrome, and post-polio syndrome. Although awareness of all these illnesses is essential to research and education, only the relationship of FM, CFID, and CMP are the focus of this book. The question is: How strong are the interconnections among these three?

There are commonalities to be sure, but also substantial differences. Glial cell activation is a possible source of FM pain and can be seen in pathological pain states in general.[119] Fibromyalgia evidence indicates a dysfunction in the central nervous system and possibly the autonomic nervous system. Chronic myofascial pain research is strong enough to upgrade its distinction from a syndrome to a myofascial disease of the peripheral nerve end plate at the neuromuscular junction. Chronic fatigue immunodysfunction symptoms are often discussed with FM. They may share some overlapping qualities, but these two conditions are, and have been, exclusively set apart. Central nervous system involvement is being studied in both FM and CFID; however, the primary symptom of FM is diffuse pain, and the primary symptom of CFID is fatigue.

glial cell: one of two types of cells found in the CNS, the other being neurons. Also called glia, these cells provide support and nutrition, maintain homeostasis, form myelin (to protect the nerves found in the CNS), and participate in signal transmission. Glia are believed to also secrete certain neurotransmitters.

All three disorders have specific diagnostic criteria as previously discussed. The diagnostic criteria for each of them are very separate and distinct, so it would be unreasonable to lump them together as the same illness. Their differences are clear.

It is easy to see it is not all in a name. All three disorders need better terms that reflect their causes, rather than their symptoms. Does the term we are "labeled" with matter? I think it does. That is why I refer to chronic fatigue syndrome as "chronic fatigue immunodysfunction." Once the causes of FM and CFID have been identified, maybe we will see better defining terms. Dr. Simons will offer a definition of the chronic myofascial pain from TrPs in the next edition of *The Trigger Point Manual*. For now, we can make a difference by advocating for a name change.

Chronic fatigue immunodysfunction does not appear to be a peripheral nerve disorder. Rather, as in FM, there seems to be a disruption in both the central and autonomic nervous systems. Since these two conditions both exhibit this disruption, they are often discussed simultaneously. It has been suggested that neuroendocrine abnormalities may be an important indication in the pathogenesis of both FM and CFID. In the introduction to a Turkish study of healthy, FM, and CFID patients, cortisol levels were found to be low in both the FM and CFID groups. But in the subgroup of FM and CFID participants who did not present symptoms of depression, cortisol levels were lower in the CFID group. It was found that depression coexisting with FM and CFID may lower cortisol and LH (a gonadal hormone). Alternatively, low cortisol could lead to the depressive symptoms seen in these patients.[120] Here again, which came first the cart or the horse? There may be similarities and overlap in the etiologies of FM and CFID, yet they remain distinctly separate.[121]

Can chronic fatigue aggravate FM? Absolutely! Can FM aggravate CFID? Clearly! Can FM and CMP cause chronic fatigue? Yes, both FM and CMP can cause chronic fatigue; however, fatigue and chronic fatigue immunodysfunction are two different things. Even electrocardiograms are showing there is a difference between FM and CFID.[122] Is the fatigue associated with FM and CMP the same as the chronic fatigue of CFID? No! Does FM and/or CMP cause CFID? Absolutely not! Chronic fatigue seen in FM patients is *not*—I repeat, *not*—the same as chronic fatigue immunodysfunction, also known as chronic fatigue syndrome.

The primary symptom of CFID is chronic fatigue, but does everyone with FM also have a chronic sore throat and swollen lymph nodes, or some type of infectious or exposure process as a trigger? No. Untreated trigger points *can* cause a sore throat, but this does not mean, even remotely, that the sore throat associated with CFID is caused by trigger points, unless the CFID patient also has CMP, in which case the presence of TrPs should be ruled out. Non-restorative sleep affects 33–80 percent of CFID patients versus more than 95 percent of FM patients, yet chronic fatigue immunodysfunction patients have greater fatigue. There is also a higher acute onset in CFID compared to FM.[123] And although trigger points can be located all over the body of a CMP patient, trigger point pain is not the same as the body-wide pain of FM.

Science has proven that these disorders are real. New studies of FM show scientific evidence of a disruption in the pain pathway using objective data such as a functional MRI.[124] CFID has been identified through brain mapping and sleep studies. Elevated substance P has been found in spinal fluid of FM patients, but is not present in CFID patients.[125, 126]

The TrPs of chronic myofascial pain have been scientifically defined and proven by biopsy and the presence of electrophysical abnormalities. It is thought by some that the clustering of symptoms in some patients and the coexistence of disorders, such as multiple chemical sensitivity, FM, CFID, and Gulf War illnesses, may have more than a casual resemblance. They may be closely related in their disruption of the chemical messaging system between the brain and body, affected by the HPA axis and autonomic nervous system.[127] FM, CFID, and CMP are diagnosed by distinctive criteria, and although there may be overlapping symptoms, there are also symptoms that are unique to each of these disorders. Therefore, logic would imply that although they may exist together, making a diagnosis more difficult, they are not one and the same.

Researchers need to understand the importance of screening all study participants for all three disorders, so that results are not skewed.

Uncomfortable as they may be, symptoms are actually a good thing—they are your body's alarm system. Ignoring them would equate to not responding to a fire alarm. Think about it.

Fibromyalgia and chronic fatigue syndrome are known to exist in children. You may have been one of them. Children are underdiagnosed even more than adults are. This is partly because they are such poor historians, but also because adults tend to dismiss children's symptoms. If you think about how these symptoms affect your activities of daily living, think what they can do to a child. They disrupt their play, their interactions with friends, and their ability to concentrate in school, and a disruption to all these things can lead to behavioral problems. It is heartbreaking for children to go untreated—in pain, fatigued, and broken—just because we don't know enough.

Fibromyalgia, chronic fatigue immunodysfunction (chronic fatigue syndrome), and chronic myofascial pain all disrupt our normal activities of life, emotional stability, and spiritual well-being. It is most important to find a physician who is familiar with these disorders. Much relies upon your ability to give an accurate, comprehensive history that is clearly communicated so that the physician understands your needs. This includes an account of your present and past symptoms, previous medical care, a complete physical exam, and reliance upon objective and subjective findings (see chapter 2).

There are common goals in collecting objective and subjective data. Other examinations or referrals may be made by your physician to rule out, or rule in, coexisting conditions or conditions that can mimic FM, CFID, or CMP. The outcome relies upon subjective data given by the patient and objective criteria, such as laboratory findings, radiographic testing, MRI, CT scan, and neurological examination and testing. Subjective criteria will depend upon your input, because it relies upon information received from you, the subject. It is important that you understand the differences among the criteria so that you can take an interactive part in your own health care. Subjective findings will be discussed extensively in the chapter relating to your physician and health care worker.

Feel free to copy any of the worksheets you complete and share them with your physician. The worksheets include information to be used as a guide. We are all unique and have individual needs, so be sure to add any other known conditions particular to you.

The differences between FM, CFID, and CMP are more than a matter of semantics. How are they different? What are the similarities? The good news is the scientific community is recognizing them all. With that recognition comes advocacy, funding, and research. We need to find a way to get the information provided by the research out to the clinicians in the medical community.

Until the origin of all three of these disorders is known, we can contribute to the benefit of all by speaking out and participating in the march against chronic pain. It is not normal to experience constant widespread pain and tenderness. The general population experiences any one of these symptoms intermittently. The added symptoms of flu, fatigue, and memory difficulties also manifest in the general population from time to time. But who among us would want to have all these symptoms together, all the time? Nobody. That is why chronic pain patients must persevere. Don't give in, join in. You can play an important role, and the information you need to accomplish this can be found in chapter 3.

Glossary of Terms Introduced in Chapter 1 that Describe Pain

algology: The science and study of pain; *algo* is a prefix of Greek origin, based on the word *algos,* meaning "pain." An algologist is one who studies algology.

allodynia: Pain from stimuli that are not normally painful. The pain may occur somewhere other than in the area stimulated. Allodynia means "other pain."

analgesia: The absence of a pain response to a type of stimulation that normally would be painful, particularly when there is no loss of consciousness.

angina: Pain resulting from a strangulation of the blood supply to the heart muscle. Usually used to describe pain associated with cardiac disease.

arthralgia: Joint pain; pain where two bones meet.

central pain: Pain associated with a lesion (disruption) of the central nervous system.

deafferentation pain: Pain caused by elimination or interruption in sensory (afferent) nerve fibers, such as a result of lesions of peripheral nerves or a disruption in the central nervous system.

dermatome: The segment of skin or subcutaneous tissue supplied with sensory (afferent) nerve fibers.

distal: Away from the point of origin.

dysesthesia: An unpleasant, abnormal sensation, whether spontaneous or evoked. Compare this term with pain and with paresthesia. Special cases of dysesthesia include hyperalgesia and allodynia. A dysesthesia is always unpleasant, whereas a paresthesia is not.

hyperalgesia: An increased response to a stimulus that is normally painful.

hyperesthesia: Abnormal, increased sensitivity to stimulation.

hypoesthesia: Abnormally diminished sensitivity to stimulation.

myalgia: Muscle pain. Muscles are bundles of specialized cells that contract and produce movement when activated by the nervous system.

neuralgia: Pain in a nerve or along the course of a nerve or nerves. Usually sharp, spasmlike pain that can recur at different intervals.

neuritis: Inflammation that attacks the peripheral nerves linking the brain and spinal cord to muscles, skin, organs, and all other parts of the body.

neuropathic pain: Pain caused by a functional or pathological change in the peripheral nervous system. Also used to denote pain as a result of a nonspecific lesion, as opposed to an inflammatory lesion.

neuropathy: A disturbance of function or pathologic change in a nerve. Ascending neuropathy progresses from the feet upward; descending neuropathy starts proximally and descends downward from the affected area toward the distal extremity; entrapment neuropathy is any group of neuropathies that puts mechanical pressure on the peripheral nerve; progressive hypertrophic interstitial neuropathy is slow, progressive, familial disease that causes thickening of peripheral nerve trunks and posterior roots leading to atrophy of distal parts of the legs (also called Dejerine's disease).

nociceptor: A receptor preferentially sensitive to a noxious stimulus or to a stimulus that would become noxious if prolonged.

pain: A feeling of distress, suffering, or agony caused by stimulation to specific nerve endings. Usually a protective mechanism that alerts the sufferer to early tissue damage somewhere in the body.

pain threshold: The level that must be reached for a stimulus to be recognized as painful.

paresthesia: An abnormal sensation of burning or prickling.

radiculalgia: Pain resulting from irritation of spinal nerve roots.

radiculopathy: A disturbance in a nerve root or nerve roots.

radiculitis: Inflammation of a spinal nerve root, especially the part between the spinal cord and the spinal canal.

referred pain: Pain in a different part of the body from where the problem originates.

sciatica: Neuralgia along the sciatic nerve track located in the buttocks, but pain may refer down the nerve track and affect distal portions of the body.

somatic: Pertaining to, or characteristic of, the body.

trigger point: A self-sustaining, irritable area in the muscle that can be felt as a nodule in a taut band.

2

Communicating Your Health Care Needs

Relating your health care needs to your health care providers can have a positive or negative impact on your outcome. The goal is to find the right people to ensure positive results.

By the end of this chapter you should be able to:

- Use common terms to describe your symptoms.
- Identify what may aggravate your symptoms.
- Identify conditions that perpetuate the symptoms of your FM, CFID, and/or CMP.
- Define the physician-patient relationship.
- Identify the primary component of a productive health care relationship.

Unfortunately, it is all too human to deny or disbelieve what is not understood. This is why it is so important to relate information accurately to your health care workers. We fear what we do not understand, and what we feel comfortable with, we accept. It is up to you to establish a working relationship with your health care provider so that everyone involved will be comfortable with your assessment and your treatment plan.

For every doubting Thomas there is someone who actively responds to our needs by educating and advocating for FM, CFID, and CMP. Research indicates these disabling disorders are all identifiable conditions and should not be dumped into a "wastebasket diagnosis."

On occasion, many of us feel we are somehow to blame for our symptoms; we develop feelings of distrust, sadness, or anger. If your health care professional makes you feel guilt or shame for your diagnosis, seek help elsewhere.

You have every right to be treated with compassion and confidence. Tips on how to find appropriate health care providers will be discussed later in the chapter.

Being able to relate your health needs with confidence is necessary in creating the kind of physician-patient relationship you'll need to determine your diagnosis and make proper referrals to other health care team members. You must feel comfortable that your physician behaves ethically and keeps your medical information confidential. Trusting your doctor is the first step toward the development of productive communication.

With the uncertainty of the health care market and constraints placed on our medical providers, it is imperative that we all become proactive in our own health care. By learning to collect our own data and acquiring effective communication skills, we can take a major role in the outcome of our physical and mental well-being.

Misdiagnosis and delayed diagnosis are common with disorders such as FM, CFID, and CMP, so it is important that we communicate our symptoms effectively in order to begin an appropriate therapeutic treatment plan as soon as possible. Early diagnosis is the most common factor for optimal recovery.

Relating Your Symptoms and Health History

Learning how to relate your symptoms and give a detailed description of your health history is the first step in developing rapport with your health care provider (HCP).

Having worked through the previous exercises, you should now be able to identify your symptoms and what they indicate for you with a certain amount of reliability. This section is dedicated to helping you understand how to relate your symptoms and health history to your health care team. It is important that you be able to determine if your exam is accurate and thorough, that proper documentation of your complaints is made, and that appropriate referrals are conducted.

Symptoms

Your health care professional needs to know how you feel. It is important to avoid vague or misleading words, such as "seems like" and "might be," unless you can further elaborate in terms of severity and character. Describe your complaints in such a way that the person you are communicating with will understand what it feels like to be in your body. Present your account as if you are painting a picture with words. Relate as accurately as possible the time frame and conditions of the onset of your problems.

Identify what actions make you feel better or worse. Ask yourself, "What have I done that improves or aggravates my symptoms?" Describe what everyday life is like for you. Ask yourself, "How are my symptoms affecting my daily living?" Use descriptive adjectives and language that will give a clear image of how you feel.

DESCRIBING YOUR SYMPTOMS

Some words that may be helpful in describing symptoms are:

aching	discolored	irritable	progressive	sudden
acute	dizzy	irritated	pulling	superficial
agitated	dry	itchy	pulsating	swollen
agitating	dull	jarring	racing	symmetrical
anxious	electric	jittery	radiating	taut
blanched	exhausted	jumpy	random	tender
blistering	external	lax	raw	tense
blotchy	extreme	lethargic	recurring	throbbing
blurring	feathery	light	red	tick
bruised	feverish	light-headed	referred	tingling
burning	flaccid	limited	restless	tired
burping	fluctuating	localized	rigid	tormenting
ceaseless	flu-like	mottled	ringing	trapped
chilling	flushed	nagging	runny	twisting
churning	fluttering	nauseating	sad	twitching
chronic	forgetful	needles	scalding	unbalanced
clenching	frequent	nervous	scattered	unbearable
cold	gnarling	numb	searing	unequal
comes and goes	gnawing	often	seldom	unrelenting
confused	gradual	one-sided	sensitive	unstable
constant	grinding	on fire	sharp	vibrating
contracting	gripping	painful	shooting	vise-like
cramping	hard	palpitating	slurred	vomiting
crawling	heavy	patchy	sore	warm
creeping	hot	penetrating	spasm	wasting
crippling	immobilizing	persistent	spotted	waxing, waning
deep	incessant	piercing	static	weak
depressed	inflamed	pins	stiff	weeping
dejected	in knots	poking	stinging	whirling
diffuse	intense	positional	strong	widespread
digging	intermittent	pounding	stuffy	woozy
disabling	internal	prickly	stumbling	wormy

Let me share an experience of working in the emergency department. It relates the stories of two different people with two very different scenarios, both in excruciating pain.

Patient 1 presented with a hand wound, much like a deep paper cut. He was pale, crying, and hyperventilating, and had to be immediately placed in a wheel chair; he was nearly unconscious. He described his pain as the most "awful" pain he had ever experienced.

Patient 2 presented an hour later with an ax wound to his foot that caused blood to ooze from his boot and leave bloody footprints on the floor. He adamantly refused a wheel chair. He stated that although the pain was pretty "awful," he had experienced worse.

Two different people, two very different scenarios; yet, they both described their injuries with the same term.

Because the problems in this story involved injuries that were quite visible to the examiner (objective data), the interventions and treatments were easily determined. When dealing with "invisible" disorders such as FM, CFID, and CMP, the examiner must rely on you to describe your symptoms, giving them "subjective data" to determine the severity, necessary treatment, tests, and/or referral.

Table 2.1. Relating Symptoms

ONSET

When did each symptom or problem begin? Does it happen at a certain time of the day? What was going on when you started having problems; were you at work, active, or inactive? At that time were you experiencing a major life event, such as marriage, divorce, death, moving your home or office, or a new job?

DURATION

How long does the symptom last? Does the symptom last minutes, hours, days, or weeks? Is it constant or does it come and go? What are the chronological events of your symptoms?

SEVERITY

How intense is the pain? Is the intensity constant or does it come in waves of severity? (See pain scale in table 2.2.)

CHARACTER

How does the pain feel? Is it sharp or dull? Is it hot or cold? Describe it.

LOCATION

What part of your body is affected by the symptom or symptoms?

OTHER

Are you able to work, play, sleep, and eat? Do the symptoms affect your ability to interact with others?

Rating Pain

Rating pain is purely subjective. Even the same patient may rate pain differently at different times; however, the pain scale is the best tool we have to determine some idea of how another person is feeling. It is difficult for us to use the 1–10 pain scale, because our symptoms vary frequently and we can hurt at different scores at different places at different times. Many variable factors play a part in the dynamics of chronic pain compared to acute pain, for which the 1–10 scale was originally devised. Physical pain is charted by most medical professionals on a scale of 1–10, with "1" being the least amount of pain you can remember, and "10" being the worst pain you have ever felt. This rating is purely subjective, because the rating is totally determined and related by you, the subject.

Table 2.2. Pain Scale

Barely noticeable			Tolerable				Intolerable		Unable to function
0	1	2	3	4	5	6	7	8	9	10
No pain									Worst pain imaginable

1–2 Barely noticeable—doesn't interfere with normal routine

3–6 Tolerable—interferes with daily activities minimally to moderately

7–9 Intolerable—interferes with daily activities moderately to significantly

10   Unable to function in daily activities

Determining Your Benchmark

To establish a baseline for rating your pain, you need to have a benchmark. For instance, a severity score of 10 for me is pain that is equal to that of shingles, refractory migraine, or shoulder reconstruction. These are situations where I cannot or could not function. If you were able to drive yourself to the doctor's office, your pain is probably not a 10.

By observing your body language and other nonverbal clues, health care providers (HCPs) are able to assess and document your pain tolerance and reaction to painful stimulus. With this particular method of charting, the examiner is able to document objective data. For example, are you guarding a painful area? Do you walk with a limp because of a painful extremity? Are you unable to make certain movements without grimacing or crying out? Do you frown when the examiner touches a painful area on your body? These are all reactions the examiner can observe, so do not try to be stoic. Let your HCP see how you normally tolerate your symptoms, and don't dismiss them to your HCP if you are normally unable to dismiss them at home. Don't minimize or maximize your discomfort. If you maximize your reaction to pain, others may see you as a malingerer and your pain complaints will be dismissed, regardless of how you really feel. Honesty is your best policy.

malingerer: a person who engages in willful, deliberate, and false exaggeration of symptoms to attain a consciously desired end.

The Anatomical Diagram

Investigators Staud, Price, Robinson, and Vierck (Department of Medicine, McKnight Brain Institute, University of Florida-Gainesville) found that anatomical pain diagrams are most useful for evaluating clinical pain. They found the diagram more useful than counting FM tender points for assessment of intensity and pain effects on emotions.[1] This does not surprise me, and its use should also be considered for FM, CFID, and CMP patients.

The anatomical diagram is helpful for communicating what is not visible to the eye. Becoming familiar with the chart at the end of the chapter may help you describe your symptoms. Include a statement, such as, "These are my trigger points," "This is where I hurt," or "This denotes my pain." Please use this along with the other assessment tools provided. These guides will help your doctor understand how your pain affects your activity, and will provide a time-saving way for your doctor to document in your chart. The right doctor will appreciate this input from you.

In my professional experience, I have found that patients frequently downplay the severity of their pain, for fear they will not be believed. It is important that you communicate how you feel on both your best and worst days, regardless of how you might be feeling the day you see your physician or nurse.

Remember that the key to effective communication is trust, and trust is built on truth.

Man seems to be a rickety poor sort of a thing, any way you take him; a kind of British Museum of infirmities and inferiorities. He is always undergoing repairs. A machine that was as unreliable as he is would have no market.

MARK TWAIN

Your relationship with your HCP usually begins with a medical history interview. Your physician or nurse practitioner will be the one to complete your history and give you a physical exam.

There are several components to your medical history, and you can expect to be asked certain questions in an orderly fashion. Other professionals on your treatment team will probably ask you some of the same questions in a more informal way, especially if they do not have access to your physician's medical records, so prepare yourself for some redundancy. Always appreciate that the person you are speaking with may not have previous knowledge of your condition.

Relating your medical history can become overwhelming to people with a chronic condition. It seems we are always repeating ourselves. This is why keeping our own records and making copies to share with others is not only helpful for them, but can also save us time and energy, which is often a very valuable commodity.

The following is a brief outline for data collection of your medical history.

- Chief complaint and/or present problem. This is a short statement of why you are seeking a medical evaluation. Your HCP will ask, "Why are we seeing you today?" (Example response—"I'm in pain.")
- Presenting problem. This is a more detailed account of why you are seeing the doctor. The physician will ask you to give a more in-depth description of your symptoms. (Example response—"My pain is everywhere; it is widespread and I cannot seem to keep my thoughts straight or keep up with my normal activities because of it. The pain has been going on for days and I feel swollen, although you cannot see it. I feel worn out.")
- Past medical history. This will include your general health, childhood illnesses, last menstrual period, onset of puberty, adult illnesses, immunizations, hospitalizations, surgeries, medications, allergies to medications, environment or chemical exposure, sexually transmitted diseases, and any blood transfusions you may have received and your reactions.

- Family history. This portion of the history will include questions regarding your family's known illnesses, such as FM, CFID, CMP, diabetes, arthritis, heart disease, high blood pressure, cancer, tuberculosis, stroke, gout, kidney disease, thyroid disease, asthma, blood disease, stroke, or any other familial disorder.
- Psychosocial history. In this area of the history, expect to be asked about personal status, such as, where you were born, where you live, cultural background, education, diet, gender preference, sexual activity, position in the family, marital status, habits, hobbies, home conditions, occupation, environmental issues, military record, religious preference, and mental health issues.

Procedures for documenting medical history may vary somewhat among physicians, but the content is the same. Do not expect a complete interview with every doctor's visit. Doctors may ask you to update their records every year or two just to make sure your record is complete. Remember that physicians and nurses are very adept at collecting information, and they begin this process, formally or informally, from the moment they enter the room.

Medication History

An up-to-date medication log or journal is an easy way to keep track of information you will need to share with people on your health care team. It is important to relate your medication allergies or adverse reactions, as well as medication, vitamins, and herbal remedies you are currently taking.

How should you organize the medication log? Allergies and sensitivities to medications should top your list. Next, list current medications, amount, and frequency. This should include regularly scheduled medications, as well as those taken on an as-needed basis, such as antihistamines during allergy season, pain medication during a flare, or for an acute problem. Also include the purpose of taking the medication, such as for sleep, pain, or depression. The approximate date you started taking the medication is important. If the medication is helpful, what percentage of the time or intensity does it alleviate the symptom? Last, but certainly not least, you should include any significant medications you are no longer taking, including the date and reason you stopped. This will assist you and your doctor in prioritizing your medication regimen. With this information, it is less likely time will be wasted trying medications already determined to be ineffective. At the end of this section you'll find a useful medication log form that you are free to copy.

Be sure to let your doctor know if you are experiencing any problems with a certain medication. Include sensitivities such as stomach upset, or if it keeps you awake. It is unlikely you will continue a medication to which you are sensitive. Due to the nature of FM and CFID, chemical sensitivities can be caused by either the inert (inactive) or the active ingredients. You may actually tolerate the same medication from a different manufacturer, depending, of course, upon the reaction you experience. Your physician, with your input, should help you determine that.

The goal is to learn how to achieve a good health care relationship, so you get the care you deserve.

Identifying Aggravating and Alleviating Factors

By documenting everything that makes a difference in your well-being, you are identifying your aggravating and alleviating factors. This includes any treatment, medication, activity, or even a new doctor.

By identifying aggravating factors you increase the likelihood of finding something you can do to help.

---

aggravating: anything that causes a symptom to worsen.

alleviating: anything that lessens or abates the symptom.

Although there are certain predisposing conditions that cannot be changed, identifying them brings knowledge, and that is your tool.

General Aggravating and Predisposing Factors
- Activity level—too little or overexertion
- Allergies, uncontrolled
- Anxiety or depression
- Barometric pressure changes or fluctuations
- Chemical exposure
- Coexisting conditions—by nature or poor self-care
- Coping mechanisms—lack of healthy ones, or inappropriate ones
- Diet deficiency—improper diet or consumption of specific, known food triggers
- Exercise—too much, too little, or the wrong kind
- Infection

- Medications
- Metabolic and endocrine dysfunction (thyroid problems, hypoglycemia, diabetes, anemia, mononucleosis)
- Neglect of spiritual or emotional needs
- Poor posture
- PMS
- Rapid body position changes
- Seasonal affective disorder (SAD)
- Situational crisis
- Skeletal structural deformities and lack of corrective measures
- Sleep disorders, including sleep apnea, sleep deprivation, disrupted sleep, and non-restorative sleep
- Stress management—lack of, or inappropriate coping
- Symptom neglect
- Tight clothing, including ill-fitting shoes
- Trauma
- Treatment plan non-participation, or lack of a plan
- Trigger points—neglect
- Unhealthy environmental exposure (excessive sun, smoke, allergens, noise)
- Unprotected exposure to cold

Some aggravating factors can be changed and others cannot, but modifications can be made. Examples of factors that cannot be changed but may be addressed with personal awareness or environmental modifications include allergies, barometric pressure changes, metabolic and endocrine dysfunction, PMS, bruxism, and skeletal structure malformation (unless due to TrPs).

Bruxism is a fancy term for grinding teeth. This condition can aggravate facial trigger points, interfere with restorative sleep, cause teeth erosion, and, among other things, contribute to migraines. If you catch yourself grinding your teeth during the day, concentrate on sending relaxation messages to your jaw. Heighten your awareness of and then release that tightening of those special little muscles that allow us to have expression, nourishment, and speech (especially before sleep). Assistive devices, such as a nighttime mouth guard, can inhibit some of the pain associated with the disorder and can help keep proper alignment, which may abate the development or recurrence of TrPs, and help if you also have TMJ/TMD, discussed later.

Learning to identify predisposing factors as an element of your aggravating factors is a useful tool.

Inappropriate management of aggravating factors can trigger multiple symptoms, so that one particular aggravating factor to the pain associated with FM, CFID, or CMP often becomes difficult to identify. It is important that you learn to identify specific triggering events, create a plan, and determine the proper tools for fixing the problem. A productive carpenter would not start a project without putting it on the drawing board. A well-thought out plan will help you determine what tools are needed to complete each task that arises.

Coexisting conditions are often unchangeable, but they are manageable. For example, a structural skeletal problem is often an aggravating factor to pain, but proper posture, physical therapy, physical aids, therapeutic devices, and meditation can help bring the maximum benefit from a treatment plan. So don't be discouraged.

It may not always be easy to define what your aggravating factors are, but you can certainly get a lot further through work and perseverance than by ignoring your symptoms or having a health care worker dismiss them.

You may have to do a juggling act. For instance, when I treat resistant TrPs while also dealing with unexpected FM symptoms, it can cause a serious flare of body-wide pain to the depths of my inner core, with many of the other symptoms that accompany it. This, in turn, results in a flare of CFID, lowering my resistance to infection and increasing general malaise. Sometimes the best thing to do is treat the condition that needs the most attention. As my mom said, "The wheel that squeaks the loudest is the one that gets the grease." Let your body teach you. When something is out of whack, look for possible causes and then follow through. Prioritize and follow your gut instinct when it comes to your health. Only you know how you feel. No one else can do that for you.

I'm not going to vacuum 'til Sears makes one you can ride on.

Roseanne Barr

Coexisting Conditions

The purpose of reviewing possible coexisting conditions is to help you understand their significance. Why is it so important? Coexisting health problems can exacerbate each other. It is important to identify what makes what worse, and this includes multiple disorders in the same person. An accurate and complete account of your condition to your physician and other health care team members will provide the information needed to make your treatment plan as comprehensive as possible.

Other diseases can coexist with, aggravate, or mimic symptoms of FM. These conditions include osteoarthritis (OA), cervical and lower back degenerative diseases, rheumatoid arthritis (RA), systemic lupus erythematosus (lupus), ankylosing spondylitis, hypothyroidism, thoracic outlet syndrome (TOS), polymyalgia rheumatica, Lyme disease, chronic fatigue syndrome (CFID), prolapsed mitral valve, HIV infection, myofascial pain syndrome, Sjogren's syndrome,[2] Raynaud's, and livedo reticularis (mottled skin).[3]

Some symptoms related to mental difficulties may also coexist. It is important to note, however, that these related symptoms or disorders, unless otherwise diagnosed, are a result of chronic pain, and not the other way around. These include anxiety, depression, irritability, and other mental disruptions.

---

coexisting: a disorder that exists in addition to another.

mimicking: a disorder that acts like another, but is not the same. It is a disorder with similar symptoms, but different etiology, or cause.

Devin Starlanyl, an author and an expert in both FM and CMP, agrees that other conditions or symptoms can accompany or perpetuate FM and/or CMP.[4] Likewise, some of the symptoms of FM or CMP may be attributable to another condition all together.

Because FM causes body-wide pain, it is easy to see why similar conditions could be confused with it. Even though the following can also cause diffuse body-wide pain, they do not have the specific anatomical tender point patterns seen only in FM. They are:

chronic myofascial pain, Gulf War syndrome, HIV infection, lupus (systemic lupus erythematosus), Lyme disease, multiple sclerosis, neurally mediated hypotension (NMH), post-polio syndrome, yeast infections/candida[5] . . . and hypometabolism.[6]

Some disorders may have symptoms that overlap or perpetuate those of FM. Remember, the distinctive symptom of FM is body-wide, diffuse pain with tender point patterns. Even though some of these are painful conditions or can engender an overall feeling of illness, none of the following meet the FM diagnostic criteria. They are as follows:

arthritis (AS, OA, and RA), complex regional pain syndrome (CRPS), depression as a result of chronic pain, interstitial cystitis, irritable bowel syndrome (IBS), lupus (systemic lupus erythematosus), migraine headache, polymyalgia rheumatica, posttraumatic stress disorder (PTSD), Raynaud's phenomenon or symptoms, reactive hypoglycemia, and restless leg syndrome (RLS).[7]

As you stack one block upon another, you decrease stability and increase the possibility the whole pile will topple over. The same holds true with additional conditions in the same patient. These disorders can wreak havoc, and the more you have, the more difficult it is to deal with FM, CFID, and/or CMP. That is why it is important to pay close attention. To understand how these might affect you, see the note in each of the conditions following in this chapter.

The trigger points of CMP cause specific, localized pain and dysfunction, and because of this can be confused with some of the conditions listed below. By their nature, other conditions (tension, fatigue, musculoskeletal misalignment, or muscle stress) can also aggravate or perpetuate CMP. (Please find how they may relate to the following conditions in the descriptions of the coexisting disorders following this introduction.)

Even though some of these are painful conditions, none of the following meet the TrP diagnostic criteria of lumpy bumpy knotted up muscle fibers that refer pain in specific patterns as seen in CMP. They can, however, be misdiagnosed in the presence of TrPs. Conditions that can be confused with CMP are as follows: arthritis (including AS, OA, and RA), carpal tunnel syndrome, complex regional pain syndrome (CRPS), hypermobility syndrome, interstitial cystitis, irritable bowel syndrome (IBS), post-polio syndrome, restless leg syndrome, temporomandibular dysfunction, and vulvodynia (chronic vulvar pain).[8]

You may also find with CMP that other conditions can coexist. The pain of untreated or under-treated trigger points is sometimes incorrectly attributed to these disorders: bursitis, intervertebral disc problems, dyslexia, foot problems (fallen arches foot drop, hammertoe), gastric upset, headaches, inner ear dysfunction, joint difficulties, sciatica,[9] neuralgia, plantar fasciitis (pain caused by inflammation in the sole of the foot), thoracic outlet syndrome, and FM.[10]

Your doctor may test you for some of the disorders in the following paragraphs, because some of their symptoms may overlap with your condition and mask the appropriate diagnosis.

A study was done on sets of twins with chronic fatigue of greater than six months and sets of twins without complaints of chronic fatigue. "The chronically fatigued twins were found to have higher rates of fibromyalgia and irritable bowel syndrome. The strongest associations were observed among chronic fatigue, fibromyalgia, irritable bowel syndrome, chronic pelvic pain, multiple chemical sensitivities, and temporomandibular disorder."[11] "Coexisting conditions must be identified and treated before CFID can be diagnosed; it is a condition [determined by] exclusion."[12]

Commonly found conditions in patients with CFID are: infection (such as mycoplasma, chlamydia, and human herpes virus 6),[13] allergies, cardiac arrhythmias, depression, FM, Hashimoto's thyroiditis, interstitial cystitis, irritable bladder, irritable bowel syndrome, migraine, CMP, neurally mediated hypotension (related to blood pressure) and postural orthostatic tachycardia syndrome (POTS, a heart-related disorder), prolapsed mitral valve, multiple chemical sensitivity, Raynaud's, SICCA-like symptoms, and TMJ/TMD.[14]

There is also a noted correlation in certain British patients of Gulf War syndrome with multiple chemical sensitivity and CFID.[15]

According to the CDC, "there are a large number of clinically defined, frequently treatable illnesses that can result in fatigue." Diagnosis of any of these conditions would exclude a definition of CFID, unless the condition has been treated sufficiently and no longer explains the fatigue and other symptoms. These include: hypothyroidism, sleep apnea and narcolepsy, major depressive disorders, chronic mononucleosis, bipolar affective disorders, schizophrenia, eating disorders, cancer, autoimmune diseases, hormonal disorders, sub-acute infections, obesity, alcohol or substance abuse, and reactions to prescribed medications.[16]

The importance of identifying your own coexisting conditions is to help you zero in on ones that may be aggravating your FM, CFID, or CMP. Your treatment plan for any of these three may also need to include treatment for other aggravating disorders.

The material here is not intended to replace sound medical assessment and advice. Questions regarding these conditions or diseases should be discussed with your doctor, who will make the diagnosis based on medical findings.

Allergies

Scientists are researching neuroendocrine-immunological responses (the way the immune system works). It is suspected that allergies, which are abnormal reactions by the immune system to ordinarily harmless substances, may be an important triggering event for FM and CFID.[17]

Allergies can range in severity from mildly bothersome to life threatening. The normal immune system ignores harmless substances, for example, food; and fights threatening ones, such as bacteria. A person develops an allergic reaction when the immune system cannot differentiate the good guys from the bad guys and releases histamine, a chemical antigen that attacks the harmless substance as if it were a threat to the body's normal function. This inappropriate histamine release produces many of the symptoms associated with allergies.

An allergen is any substance that triggers an allergic reaction when it is inhaled or swallowed, or comes into contact with the skin. The most common allergens are pollen, mold spores, dust mites, animal dander, foods, insect bites, drugs, and environmental factors. However, people can have adverse reactions to such things as fragrance, hygienic products, and medications.

Allergy symptoms are in response to an abnormal neurotransmitter, specifically, histamine. You may recall that FM is predominately believed to be due to a disruption of our biochemical responses. Because of this, we may have allergies but not react normally to the skin tests used to diagnose specific allergens. Dr. Starlanyl believes this may be due to an allergic reaction that lacks, or for some reason does not utilize, the immune mechanism (IgE).[18]

What lies behind us and what lies before us are tiny matters compared to what lies within us.

WILLIAM MARROW

Anxiety

Anxiety causes a feeling of uneasiness, apprehension, or dread, often associated with restlessness and changes in physical responses. Most people experience anxiety at various times and find healthy ways to deal with it. It is when they can no longer deal appropriately with feelings of anxiousness, or the symptoms become chronic, that it's time to seek professional help and guidance.

Physical responses to anxiety include sweating, a rise in blood pressure, palpitations, increased heart rate, accelerated breathing, and feelings of generalized stress. Someone with an anxiety disorder may also experience an increase in muscle tension, causing pain and stiffness, and/or a decrease in intestinal blood flow, which can result in nausea or diarrhea.

Anxiety disorders include phobias, panic attacks, generalized anxiety disorder, obsessive-compulsive disorder, agoraphobia, and posttraumatic stress disorder. Anxiety can be caused by several different biochemical abnormalities, and treatment includes medication, psychotherapy, cognitive-behavioral therapy, systematic desensitization, biofeedback training, and hypnosis.

Those of us with FM, CFID, or MPS may experience anxiety as the result of trying to deal with our symptoms. When we are fatigued and in pain, it is easy to become "out of sorts." Some of this could even be a side effect of some of our medications. (I took medication to treat my insomnia, and, like many people with FM and CFID, I had an unusual reaction. It caused extreme agitation, anxiety, accelerated heart rate, and lack of sleep. When I stopped taking the medication, the extreme anxiety-like symptoms went away.)

It is important to identify the source of your anxiety so you can incorporate lifestyle changes and activate healthy coping mechanisms to minimize the "side effects" of chronic pain.

Arthritis

Two protective structures support joint health: the cartilage and the synovium. Cartilage is a rubbery material that protects bones and facilitates easy, painless joint movement. Synovium is a thin membrane that provides fluid that acts as a lubricant to joints. When cartilage or synovium wear out, arthritis occurs. Arthritis is an inflammatory condition involving the joints. It is not to be ignored; any type is painful and can be a serious aggravating factor when it coexists with FM, CFID, and/or CMP.

Included in the arthritis family are:

Ankylosing Spondylitis

Ankylosing spondylitis (AS) is a form of chronic inflammation of the spine and the sacroiliac joints, and it is predominantly associated with back pain and stiffness. The cause is unknown, and symptoms predominately begin to appear in a person's twenties. Over time the spine becomes stiffer, and eventually the vertebrae (bones in your spine) may grow or fuse together. It is progressive, especially if left unattended, and can lead to poor posture and deformities.

Symptoms include stiffness and pain in the lower back, buttocks, and hips upon waking in the morning or after a period of inactivity; back pain relieved by movement and exercise; difficulty bending the spine; pain in the hips and difficulty walking; pain in the heels and soles of the feet;

bent-over posture; and straightening of the normal curvature of the spine.

Other symptoms of AS are fever, loss of appetite and weight, fatigue, eye swelling, redness and pain, sensitivity to light, difficulty taking a deep breath, and disruption in the flow of the electrical impulses that cause your heart muscle to contract. Treatment consists of physical rehabilitation and medication used to treat arthritis.

The stiffness and pain upon waking in the morning or after a period of inactivity is similar to FM symptoms, and the joint pain (arthralgias) may be confused with that symptom in CFID. Trigger points of CMP can cause malfunction and pain, and you may remember from the first chapter that they also cause lumps and bumps in soft tissue. However, none of these are disorders of the joints.

Osteoarthritis

Osteoarthritis (OA), also called degenerative joint disease, is distinguished by degeneration of cartilage, loss of bone tissue at the margins, and changes in the protective synovial membrane. Like degenerative disc disease, OA occurs as part of the normal aging process, but degeneration may occur prematurely in some individuals. OA is most often caused by undue stress on the joints over years. A common type affects the distal joints of the fingers, predominately in women. Symptoms are joint deformity and pain, and can vary from mild to severe, depending upon the progression of the disease.

If the joint degeneration is diffuse, the body-wide pain can sometimes be attributed to FM or vice versa; however, arthritis of all forms is an inflammatory condition, whereas FM is not. The joint pain seen in CFID is not associated with swelling and redness, and should not be confused with osteoarthritis.

Rheumatoid Arthritis

Rheumatoid arthritis (RA) is a chronic inflammatory disease that causes pain, swelling, stiffness, and loss of function in the joints, and generally occurs in a symmetrical pattern. It primarily involves the peripheral joints, which are the finger joints, wrists, toes, and knees. Rheumatoid arthritis affects not only joints, but also their surrounding muscles, tendons, ligaments, and blood vessels, and can affect other parts of the body as well. Another feature of RA is that symptoms vary in intensity and duration from person to person. The disease may come on slowly or appear suddenly. Some people have a worsening period, or flare, followed by periods of symptom remission. Still others have severe disease that is active most of the time, lasts for many years, and progresses to serious joint damage and disability.

---

symmetrical: even, balanced.

The cause of RA, like FM and CFID, is unknown, but it is categorized among the autoimmune disorders, and symptoms may also occur in other parts of the body besides the joints.

Some symptoms of RA overlap with FM, CFID, and CMP. These include fatigue, pain, malaise, weakness, and neuropathy—similar to FM and CFID; vague joint symptoms, weight changes—similar to CFID; and joint dysfunction and muscle weakness—similar to CMP. However, RA is also an inflammatory condition associated with heat in the affected joint and localized joint swelling, whereas FM, CFID, and CMP are not. In determining appropriate treatment, it is important not to confuse RA with these three.

Bursitis

Bursitis is inflammation of the bursa, a small, fluid-filled sac situated in a place where friction would otherwise occur. Bursae, plural for bursa, facilitate the gliding or cushioning wherever your bones, tendons, and ligaments move against each other, particularly near joints. By reducing friction, bursae help our joints operate smoothly through the full range of natural movement.

Although bursitis is initially an acute condition, it can develop into a chronic problem causing continued pain, inflammation, swelling, and restricted movement of the specific joint involved, such as the shoulder, elbow, knee, or hip.

Bursitis is usually diagnosed because of the pain it causes. However, everywhere there is a bursa, there is also a tendon connecting the muscle to the bone, facilitating movement. From repetitive movement or over use, trigger points can develop that appear to be bursitis. The treatment for bursitis is to reduce inflammation, but if the pain is coming from an untreated TrP, that treatment will be of no use to you. Before you give in, become frustrated, or get your stomach eaten up by a medication that isn't helping, check out those trigger points.

Bruxism—Teeth Grinding

Teeth grinding may be a factor in quality of sleep,[19] which is disrupted in FM and CFID.

Bruxism can be a major contributor to facial TrPs. If you grind your teeth and have unexplained facial pain, be sure to check out those trigger points.[20]

Candidiasis

Fungi cause candidiasis, also known as yeast infection. Candida are normal flora of the mouth, skin, intestinal tract, and vagina, but can cause a variety of infections in any of these areas or in the respiratory tract. This yeast can cause a systemic infection, and although rare, it can infect the heart lining.

Intestinal yeast has been linked to small bowel bacterial overgrowth (SIBO) causing excessive gas, bloating, abdominal pain, and altered bowel habits.[21]

In the mouth, yeast in oral mucosa is linked to thrush.

Yeast infections can occur with FM and overgrowth may increase the symptoms of bloating, brain fog, abdominal complaints, and muscle aches associated with FM and CMP. It can also exacerbate the usual symptoms of FM and CMP.[22] It has been identified as a possible trigger to CFID, and some association has been made with chronic candidiasis syndrome.[23] Yeast infections should always be treated, but you can also exercise preventive lifestyle choices.

To help prevent vaginal yeast, avoid vaginal douching, keep the area dry, and use a blow dryer after showering. Wear 100 percent cotton underwear dried on high heat, and avoid nylon panty hose. If you are a carbo junkie, change your diet. There are other reasons for this that will be discussed later, but understand that excessive sugar and carbohydrate intake have been linked to a higher risk of developing yeast overgrowth.

Insulin resistance and some medications may perpetuate yeast or leaky gut.[24] Antibiotic use should be avoided when possible, as antibiotics are indiscriminate and kill off our "protective" flora along with offending microorganisms. Of course, there are times when their use is needed. Just be aware that when you must take antibiotics, candidiasis may occur and need to be treated. Talk to your doctors if you are prone to yeast infection with antibiotic use, so that you can get appropriate treatment.

There are specific tests to check for candidiasis-initiated responses by the body, called IgG, IgA, and IgM antibodies.

Carpal Tunnel Syndrome

Carpal tunnel syndrome is caused by the compression of the median nerve as it passes through a bony canal that is covered by a broad ligament in the wrist. It is associated with weakness that sometimes extends to the elbow. Repetitive motion injury and inflammatory forms of arthritis are the most common causes.

Trigger points can also press on nerves and cause paresthesias, such as numbness, tingling, or electric shock-like feelings. TrPs also cause weakness of the muscle supplied by the entrapped nerve. Because of this, many people who are thought to have carpal tunnel syndrome actually have untreated trigger points. As the saying goes, "Don't be late, investigate." If you have CMP and trigger point treatment doesn't resolve your problems, you may need further evaluation by a surgeon.

Complex Regional Pain Syndrome (also called Reflex Sympathetic Dystrophy Syndrome)

Complex regional pain syndrome (CRPS) is a chronic condition characterized by severe burning pain, pathological changes in bone and skin, excessive sweating, tissue swelling, and extreme sensitivity to touch in an upper or lower limb following injury. It is also known as algodystrophy, causalgia syndrome, posttraumatic dystrophy, reflex neurovascular dystrophy, and Steinbrocker syndrome.

One theory is that CRPS may be caused by an overactive sympathetic nervous system that causes irregular blood supply to areas of the body.[25] Although the exact cause is unclear, a number of factors may contribute to the symptoms, particularly changes in autonomic nervous system function.

The pain is typically more intense and severe than would be expected from a seemingly minor injury. In the early stages there may also be redness, tenderness, and swelling. Range of motion of joints may be limited. In some patients, as the condition progresses and pain worsens, range of motion is further restricted and weakness occurs. The skin may appear cool and clammy, and may become glossy. The pain is often worse at night.[26]

Because the symptoms of CRPS can affect the entire body, it may be confused with FM and/or CFID. The range of motion restriction may be confused with CMP. The reverse is also true, in that people with FM/CMP complex are often incorrectly diagnosed as having CRPS.[27]

If CRPS persists beyond the first stages it becomes difficult to diagnose. During later stages, some of the early symptoms may not be present. This is a prime example of why the history of your symptoms is so important. Those that may seem of no importance to you can make a big difference to the diagnostician.

Costochondritis

Inflammation of the cartilage between the ribs and breastbone is called costochondritis. Costochondritis causes chest pain, particularly with deep inspiration or when pressure is applied. This chest wall pain and inflammation may result from a virus, but often the cause is unknown.

Because costochondritis causes pain between the ribs, it may be confused with the tender points of FM. It can also be confused with untreated trigger points present in the area or in the resulting referral zone. Chest pains have also been associated with CFID.

Costochondritis is an inflammatory condition and the treatment differs entirely from either FM or CMP.

Degenerative Disc Disease

A disc is a flat, circular capsule made of a soft, gelatinous substance covered by a tough, fibrous material that serves as a shock absorber. The discs act like cushions between the spinal vertebrae (bones) that make up the spine, providing protection and flexibility. Spinal discs also protect the nerve roots that extend out from the spinal cord, which is protected by the spinal vertebrae. As discs begin to age there is a gradual loss of flexibility, and the discs start to harden and lose their resiliency and protective qualities. This process is known as degeneration.

vertebrae: bones that line up to make the spine. They provide structure and protect the spinal cord, which passes through them.

neuritis: degeneration of nerves that link the brain and spinal cord with muscles, skin, organs, and all other parts of the body.

neuropathic pain: pain caused by a functional or pathological change in the peripheral nervous system.

neuropathy: any functional disturbance or pathological change in the peripheral nervous system; also used to denote nonspecific lesions, in contrast to inflammatory lesions.

radiculalgia: pain as a result of a distribution of spinal nerve roots.

radiculopathy: a disturbance in a nerve root, especially the part between the spinal cord and the spinal canal.

The rate of spinal disc degeneration varies among individuals. With added stress it is possible for the inner material to swell and bulge through a weakened spot in the tough outer covering, causing its shape to become distorted. Disc degeneration can also cause an actual tear or rupture of the fibrous capsule.

The pressure resulting from a bad disc causes pain (neuropathic), inflammation, and swelling of all the structures around it. The disc material can injure the spinal cord if the defect is central. If the defect is to the outside of the spinal column, the protrusion (herniation) affects the nerves that project from the spinal cord out through the vertebrae. When this happens it can produce extreme, debilitating pain and the damage can be irreversible. However, not all herniated discs press on nerves, and it is entirely possible for a person to have deformed discs without any pain or discomfort.

Causes for premature degeneration are overexertion, stress on the spine from unconditioned physical activity, and structural malformation. Spinal misalignment puts sustained pressure on the intervertebral discs from the vertebrae. Such prolonged pressure can be caused by lordosis, kyphosis, scoliosis, and TrPs in the intervertebral and supporting muscles. Myofascial trigger points make the intervertebral muscles tight and can cause the vertebrae (back bones) to shift, contributing to disc degeneration.

Symptoms that indicate a disc has degenerated or herniated include sharp pain in the back that sometimes extends down one or both legs immediately upon, or shortly after, exertion or injury; inability to bend or straighten your back, accompanied by severe pain; gradual development of neck or lower-back pain; intense pain on arising, or when sneezing or coughing; and numbness or tingling in an arm or leg, with possibly a progressive loss of strength in the extremity.

intervertebral: between two vertebrae.

kyphosis: exaggerated front to back curve of the thoracic spine (hunchback).

lordosis: exaggerated forward spinal curvature of the low back (swayback).

scoliosis: lateral curvature of the spinal column (S shape, side to side).

Treatment may include medication, physical therapy, acupuncture, manipulative therapy, trigger point therapy, spinal injections, or even surgery.

Degenerative disc disease can be very painful. It is diagnosed by specific tests, such as an MRI. It can coexist with, and be a great aggravator of, FM, CFID, and CMP.

Trigger points can mimic every symptom of degenerative disc disease. If your physician has ruled out degenerative disc disease, or you do not respond to the usual treatments for the disease, please consider the presence of untreated TrPs. Trigger points occurring in muscles—intervertebrals; quadratus lumborum; piriformis; or gluteus maximus, medius, and minimus—could be the culprit.

Depression

The scientific term for depression is dysthymia, but it is most often referred to as the blues, dejection, discouragement, gloom, moodiness, and sadness.

When you suffer from a chronic pain disorder, it is not unusual to expect secondary depression, anger, fear, withdrawal, or anxiety (depression and chronic pain will be covered more extensively in chapter 4). When these psychological disturbances are secondary to disorders such as FM, CFID, or CMP, it's easy to fall prey to the role of victim. Be careful not to let a secondary reaction become a primary problem. It is important that you address mental health, as well as your physical health.

Depression is a disorder in which someone experiences a mental state of sadness, despair, discouragement, change in appetite or weight, difficulty sleeping or oversleeping, physical slowing or agitation, energy loss, inappropriate guilt, difficulty thinking or concentrating, and feelings of worthlessness or hopelessness. At their most severe, symptoms include recurring thoughts of death or suicide. Severity, duration, and the presence of particular symptoms determine the type of depression. It is usually preceded by some stressful life event, such as chronic illness. In men, depression is often experienced as anger and irritability.

The feelings of despair and hopelessness associated with depression can occur as the result of any chronic illness. This is because you are in a grieving process for the loss of your previous functioning. It can be a result of, rather than the cause of FM, CFID, or CMP.

When depression persists and impairs daily life and relationships, it may be an indication of a more serious problem that requires professional help from a licensed psychologist. The psychologist may see the need to refer you to a psychiatrist if medication is indicated.

Foot Problems

Both the foot and ankle are comprised of a complex array of bones, tendons, joints, muscles, soft tissues, ligaments, nerves, blood and lymph vessels, and skin. Any of these tissues may be damaged or affected by disease, resulting in foot and/or ankle problems. The causes of most incidents of foot pain are poorly fitting shoes; however, other conditions can also cause foot pain, such as pronation, weather changes, gait disturbance, one leg shorter than the other, high-impact exercising, TrPs, and injury. Other conditions that cause foot pain include corns, calluses, blisters, muscle cramps, acute knee and ankle injuries, plantar fasciitis, plantar warts, bunions, hammertoes, arthritic conditions, osteoporosis, diabetes, diseases that affect the nervous and circulatory systems, pregnancy, obesity, diseases that affect muscle and motor control, and some medications.

gait: step, walk, or stride.

plantar: bottom aspect of the foot.

pronation: inward roll of foot on walking.

Plantar Fasciitis

Plantar fasciitis is inflammation of the thick, fibrous band of tissue that extends from the heel of the foot to the toes, supporting the muscles of the bottom of the foot and helping the foot to function properly. This disorder is usually due to injury of the plantar (sole) fascia (connective tissue). When the plantar fascia becomes overstretched, tiny tears can riddle its surface, and the associated inflammation causes swelling and pain. The pain can be severe, especially in the morning. Does this sound familiar? This is not to be confused with morning foot pain and/or swelling associated with FM and neurotransmitter dysfunction, paresthesias often associated with CFID, or specific foot-related TrPs of CMP.

Excessive pounding on the bottom of the feet; improper shoe support; foot structure abnormality, such as pronation; and some forms of arthritis can cause it. This condition is often treated with medications for inflammation and pain.

Tarsal Tunnel Syndrome

Tarsal tunnel syndrome is a complex of symptoms resulting from compression of the posterior tibial or plantar nerves in the tarsal (foot bone) tunnel. The tunnel provides passage for the nerves, tendons, and vessels that supply the foot. When the bony tunnel is constricted for some reason, symptoms of tarsal tunnel syndrome occur. Symptoms are pain, numbness, and tingling on the bottom of the foot. Tarsal tunnel symptoms can be caused by untreated TrPs.

Other Causes of Foot Pain

I have read about FM patients complaining of burning feet and neuropathic-like symptoms. I do have this problem, but I also have CMP. In fact, TrPs in the calf can cause similar symptoms. So before you assume that you have to "learn to live" with these symptoms, be sure you check out possible trigger points.

Don't be late, investigate!

Many perpetuating factors of foot problems can be changed; but some, such as blood sugar problems and neurotransmitter imbalances, cannot. You have no control over hammertoes, or having one leg shorter than the other, but you can lessen the stress put on skeletal deformities by using orthotics. A shoe lift when you have one leg shorter than another will bring your entire body into proper alignment, not only correcting the immediate deformity but a myriad of other problems as well, such as spinal, knee, and hip problems. This could be a major improvement to bringing perpetuating problems under control if you have CMP.

TrPs also occur in the feet, or in places that refer to them. They can aggravate any existing foot condition or be the result of it. Look for trigger points that could be causing some of your foot pain or dysfunction.

If you have a primary foot problem, you are at risk for developing TrPs secondary to your adaptive mechanisms, one of them being altered gait. They can coexist.

Gulf War Syndrome

Gulf War syndrome (GWS) affects a subset of patients who participated in the Persian Gulf War. The symptoms are suggestive of CFID, except that these are Gulf War veterans. Because such symptoms have occurred in other veterans groups, some experts suspect that posttraumatic stress syndrome may be responsible for the symptoms in some cases. Some researchers identified an unusual bacteria-like organism known as Mycoplasma fermentans in nearly half the veterans who suffered from Gulf War syndrome. Other possible causes among these veterans include multiple immunizations, oil well fire contaminants, and sleep apnea.[28, 29]

Some of the symptoms of GWS overlap with FM and CFID. This does not mean you must have been in the Persian Gulf to have FM or CFID; it means you must have been in the Persian Gulf to have GWS. In addition, many of the symptoms of GWS may be due to coexisting trigger points.[30] The nature of the work of the military is suggestive of perpetuating factors for CMP.

Severe Headaches

Headache means, simply, "pain in the head." Headaches are a symptom, not a disease, and may be caused by various factors.

Vascular type headaches are sometimes described as classic migraine, common migraine, cluster headache, or hemiplegic migraine.

Classic Migraine

A classic migraine is a recurrent, throbbing headache accompanied by anorexia (loss of appetite), nausea, vomiting, fatigue, and sensitivity to light, noise, and smells. Attacks are commonly one-sided and their onset may be indicated by an aura. Classic migraines can last for hours and can occur one to several times a month.

aura: a sharply defined, transient visual, sensory, motor, speech, or cognitive symptom that occurs before a migraine attack.

Common Migraine

A common migraine is one without an aura that presents as a throbbing pain or constant ache when lying still. It is usually one-sided, often shifting sides from one attack to the next. A common migraine can occasionally affect both sides of the head. Location is at the temple, in the forehead area, and sometimes has a suboccipital component. Common migraines can vary widely in frequency. An attack may last for several hours to several days.

occipital: bone in the back lower part of the skull.

Cluster Headache

A cluster headache is an intensely painful vascular headache that occurs suddenly and lasts from thirty to sixty minutes. It is predominantly one-sided, and usually associated with flushing, sweating, runny nose, and increased tears. It is named for its repeated occurrence in groups, or clusters. It is a constant penetrating, and occasionally throbbing, headache. Pain is located in and around the eye, over the temple and forehead areas, and sometimes in the occipital region.

Hemiplegic Migraine

A hemiplegic migraine is a vascular headache symptomized by motor phenomena that persist during and after the headache. This headache occurs in patients with a history of classic or common migraine. The headache, when accompanied by hemiplegia (one-sided weakness, or paralysis), is usually more severe. Motor or sensory problems, pre- and post-attack, persist through the headache phase and may continue for several days afterward.

Migraine headaches as a coexisting condition intensify the central sensitization process of FM. This patient subset group not only has the added pain of migraines, but greater FM pain, compared to patients who do not have migraines.[31]

Headaches of new onset are part of the diagnostic criteria for CFID. Therefore, if you have, or suspect you have, CFID, report your symptoms. Any new headache should be examined by a physician. There can be life-threatening causes of headache, if it is new.

Tension and neck pain trigger migraines, or migraine-like symptoms. If tension is a perpetuating factor for your CMP, treating TrPs may be of benefit for migraine eradication. The same is true if you have cervicogenic headaches originating in bone or soft tissues of the neck and referring pain to the head. Tension and cervicogenic headaches can be primary or secondary, but the important thing to focus on here is that both of these headache types can either be caused by TrPs, or activate TrPs. Try to avoid stress and treat TrPs appropriately at their first sign. Believe it; they don't go away on their own. I recommend *Trigger Point Therapy for Headaches & Migraines,* by Valerie DeLaune, which is listed in the resource section of this book.

A number of factors including, stress, allergies, particular foods, alcohol, hormonal fluctuations, and weather changes can perpetuate certain headaches. The important thing is to identify the cause of your headaches so the appropriate treatment can be initiated. For stress-related headaches, check out the treatment section of this book and learn to make active lifestyle changes to reduce the stress in your life. If you know your headaches are aggravated by allergies or hormonal fluctuations, there may be medication available. Unfortunately, barometric pressure changes that precipitate weather-related headaches are not something you can change. But if you know extreme weather is about to occur, you can work a little harder at relieving some of your other perpetuating events. For instance, it you also have sinusitis and live in an arid climate, you might try a humidifier; if extreme humidity is a causative factor for you, a dehumidifier might help.

HIV Infection and AIDS

AIDS is an acronym for acquired immune deficiency syndrome. It is caused by HIV infection that slowly destroys the body's immune system. The immune system is responsible for helping the body fight off germs and cancer, and plays a very important role as the body's main defense mechanism.

HIV virus destroys an important kind of blood cell called the T cell, which is a critical part of the immune system. As the virus attacks the T cells, they die off and the body loses its ability to fight off other invading diseases. When people with HIV get these infections or when their T-cell levels get too low, they generally develop AIDS. Usually it takes many years with HIV for the body to develop AIDS.

The symptoms of HIV are flu-like and include, but are not limited to, fever and fatigue lasting for a week or two. Symptoms occur several weeks after exposure to the virus through contact with body fluids of an infected person. The transmission can occur from having sex without a condom; sharing needles and/or syringes to inject drugs; pregnancy, delivery, or breast-feeding; tattooing, electrolysis, or piercing with a contaminated needle; transfusing contaminated blood products; or organ transplantation.

The flu-like symptoms of AIDS or HIV overlap with those of both FM and CFID. This disorder must be ruled out if you are at high risk for exposure. Be sure to let your doctor know if you fall into this category.

Both FM and CMP may occur in HIV patients.[32]

Hypermobility Syndrome

Joint hypermobility syndrome is abnormally increased mobility of joints that allows them to stretch beyond the limits of their physiological movement. It can be caused by an abnormality in the chemical structure of the body's connective tissue, Ehlers-Danlos syndrome (EDS). In hypermobility syndrome the joints, muscles, tendons, skin, and ligaments are lax and fragile. The fragile skin and unstable joints found in EDS are the result of faulty collagen.

Some people with FM also have joint hypermobility. It bears mentioning here, because stretching is often indicated to help mobilize stiffness. You don't want to overstretch your muscles if you also have joint hypermobility. While rehabbing after reconstruction of a hyper-mobile shoulder, which required a lot of stretching, I nearly undid the surgeon's entire repair job. As he told me, "Celeste, our goal is not for you to be able to unhook your bra from behind; it is to keep your shoulder in place, so don't be too aggressive."

Joint hypermobility and skin disorders have been more frequently observed in children with CFID than in otherwise healthy children.[33]

When I was pregnant I was rather proud of the fact that I never developed stretch marks. However, everything in life is a trade off. I have had to have my shoulder reconstructed, and have chronic hip problems because of hypermobility. When joints have little stability it is easy for TrPs to develop, entrapping nerves and causing other difficulties. So believe me when I caution that if you have hypermobility syndrome, often referred to as being double-jointed, you are also a prime target for the development of TrPs. Stay alert, don't desert!

Hypoglycemia

Hypoglycemia is characterized by an abnormally low level of sugar (glucose) in the blood. The condition may result from an excessive rate of removal of glucose from the blood, or from decreased secretion of glucose into the blood. An overdose of injected insulin or overproduction of insulin from the Islets of Langerhans in the pancreas can result in increased utilization of glucose. In this case, glucose is removed from the blood at an accelerated rate. Any instance of decreased circulating blood sugar is considered hypoglycemia. Initial symptoms of hypoglycemia are mental confusion, increased pulse rate, increased blood pressure, sweating, anxiety, dizziness, headache, and weakness. In severe cases of insulin overdose, shock may result, causing hallucinations, coma, and death.

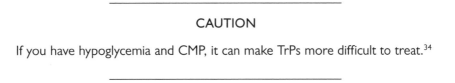

CAUTION

If you have hypoglycemia and CMP, it can make TrPs more difficult to treat.[34]

Reactive Hypoglycemia—Insulin Intolerance

Reactive hypoglycemia (RHG) is a form of hypoglycemia that occurs from two to three hours after eating a high carbohydrate meal. The rapid release of carbs, followed by rapid glucose absorption in the digestive tract causes a large amount of insulin production. Reactive hypoglycemia causes the body to overcompensate and results in hypoglycemia (diminished circulating blood sugar available for cellular energy). This prompts symptoms of hypoglycemia. Conventional blood testing is not sufficient for checking reactive hypoglycemia.[35]

Reactive hypoglycemia may accompany FM and CMP in a certain subset of patients, and may lead to insulin resistance.[36]

Some of the symptoms resulting from FM and CFID—such as, fatigue, headache, and mental confusion—overlap with hypoglycemia, but it is neither the cause nor the result of either condition.

Primary treatment for both hypoglycemia and reactive hypoglycemia remains diet, although your doctor may also prescribe medication.

Hypothyroidism

The thyroid gland is a butterfly-shaped organ located in the front of the neck, just over the windpipe. It produces iodine-containing hormones, such as thyroxin. Thyroxin regulates the rate at which body cells use energy and produce heat. When these hormones are low, a person is said to have hypothyroidism.

Several disorders can cause hypothyroidism, and there are several types, but the symptoms are generally the same. These symptoms are physical and mental sluggishness, fatigue, dry skin, weight gain, hair loss, cold sensitivity, muscle cramps, constipation, irritability, and in more serious cases, enlargement of the tongue and/or thickening of the skin. Mental "sluggishness" and cold sensitivity are also seen in FM and CFID; however, these are just coincidentally similar symptoms. Because you have brainfog and are sensitive to cold, it doesn't mean you are hypothyroid (low on thyroid hormone). Nor does being hypothyroid mean you also have FM or CFID, but you can have hypothyroidism concurrent with FM or CFID. Weight gain may be present in any of the three disorders, but it can be explained by inactivity due to pain and fatigue, or certain medications used to treat FM, CFID, or CMP.

Hypometabolism–Thyroid Resistance

Hypometabolism is not the same as hypothyroidism. In this case the thyroid is working appropriately, but the body isn't utilizing the thyroid hormones. Like reactive hypoglycemia, thyroid hormone levels are normal but they are resisted in the peripheral tissue; this is thyroid resistance. As suggested in chapter 1, some FM and CFID patients have hypometabolism.

The role of thyroid resistance in the fibromyalgia patient is being investigated, and thyroid autoimmunity has been associated with FM severity.[37] It may also contribute to the development of TrPs.[38]

Hashimoto's Thyroiditis—Autoimmune Thyroiditis

Hashimoto's thyroiditis is a condition known to coexist—although not exclusively—in a certain subgroup of CFID patients. It is a type of auto-immune thyroid disease, meaning the body's immune system attacks and destroys the thyroid gland. Its characteristics are inflammation of the thyroid gland, fatigue, depression, cold sensitivity, weight gain, muscle weakness, thickening of the skin, constipation, dry or brittle hair, muscle cramps, increased menstrual flow, and goiter. Some patients may not have any symptoms.

goiter: enlargement of the thyroid. Even when goiter is present, the thyroid may produce below normal, normal, or above normal amounts of hormones.

Infection (Viral and Bacterial)

Infection is an invasion and reproduction of unwanted microorganisms in body tissues. These hurtful microorganisms cause injury to cells and threaten the normal balance of cellular metabolism. The invading infection may be caused by a virus or by bacteria.

Infection can be a triggering event in some cases of CFID. The question of a possible immunological disruption in the disorder is present in a certain subgroup of CFID patients. This requires them to be acutely aware of their difficulty in warding off invading organisms. If you fall into this class of patients, please take care to report signs of infection—redness, heat, or swelling of the insulted area—and cold or flu symptoms (different from your usual problems). Don't rely on your body to take care of it naturally.

Inner Ear Dysfunction

Inner ear dysfunction is any disturbance in the labyrinth, which includes the vestibule, cochlea, and semicircular canals. The bony portion of the labyrinth, the osseous labyrinth, is composed of a series of canals tunneled out of the temporal bone. The vestibule (a name that denotes space) is an oval cavity in the middle of the labyrinth; the cochlea is concerned with hearing; and the semicircular canals regulate the sense of balance. Vertigo or dizziness caused by inner ear dysfunction may be confused with other disorders known to cause the same symptoms. There can be several causes of inner ear dysfunction, and many of them are easily treated.

---

equilibrium: sense of balance.

labyrinth: the inner ear, including the vestibule, cochlea, and semicircular canals.

vertigo: dizziness, spinning sensation.

Trigger points have also been noted to cause loss of coordination, dizziness, loss of balance, ear pain, and ringing in the ears.[39] If conventional treatments do not work and you have not previously been diagnosed with CMP, look into it.

Interstitial Cystitis and Irritable Bladder

Interstitial cystitis (IC) is an inflammation of the bladder without infection. Its cause is unknown but it may be associated with an autoimmune or allergic response. It is not the same as cystitis due to a urinary tract infection. You may also hear interstitial cystitis referred to as sterile urine cystitis. Chronic inflammation of the bladder can create ulcers in the lining and cause scarring, which leads to stiffening of the bladder wall. These occurrences to the bladder structure cause chronic pelvic pain and urinary disturbances. Interstitial cystitis has been found in certain FM patients, and it is speculated that IC, which has traditionally been considered a bladder disorder, may also be centrally mediated.[40] This might help explain why certain disorders seem to be more prevalent in FM and CFID patients than in the general population.

Irritable bladder can manifest in frequency, phobia (a persistent fear that you will need to urinate, causing you to get up several times in the middle of the night, or fear that you are contracting an infection), and chronic infection, and may have associated symptoms that may or may not be associated with interstitial cystitis.[41]

Yeast overgrowth or trigger points may cause irritable bladder and female urethral syndrome symptoms.[42] Yeast overgrowth can also occur in the bowel. If you are a carbo junkie, changing your diet and adding a probiotic, such as acidophilus, may help. Overwhelming yeast overgrowth needs medical intervention. In the case of trigger points, a gynecological urologist, a doctor that specializes in female urological problems, will be more astute at noting internal vaginal or rectal tissue abnormalities (possibly including trigger points), and can prescribe pelvic floor physical therapy. The highly specialized physical therapist will treat pelvic floor trigger points and will educate you on what you can do to help. If you have irritable bladder and routine tests do not explain your symptoms, please check out both of these.

Irritable Bowel Syndrome

Irritable bowel syndrome (IBS), or spastic colon, refers to a noninflammatory intestinal disorder that is characterized by recurrent cramping abdominal pain, bloating, mucous in the stool, and diarrhea and/or constipation (some people experience both).

The predictability of an attack is not always evident. I have spent many a night, all night, with abdominal cramping, followed finally by water-loss diarrhea. It depletes the body's normal fluids and leaves me exhausted and weak. I carry a coffee can in the car at all times because of the unpredictability. I don't know why I can be begging to have a bowel movement before leaving the house, only to have it trigger by the sound of the car running. Of course this happens only after we are well away from the house. It is embarrassing and uncontrollable.

The cause of IBS, like the causes of FM and CFID, is unknown, and there is no cure. Doctors call it a functional disorder because there is no sign of disease when the colon is examined. While IBS can cause a great deal of discomfort and distress, it does not cause permanent damage to the intestines and does not lead to other diseases, such as cancer. But that doesn't make dealing with it any easier.

Irritable bowel symptoms are often seen in FM, CFID, and CMP patients. Some aggravators are low fiber or poor diet, lack of routine bowel habits, trigger points, medication and food sensitivities, yeast overgrowth, menstruation, and stress. Irritable bowel may also be a disorder that is centrally mediated.

Paying attention to what perpetuates the attack might give you some feeling of control.

Leaky Gut Syndrome

The purposes of the bowel are to break down food into nutrients and eliminate waste or unwanted products. Leaky gut syndrome (LGS) causes body-wide symptoms because of holes in the intestinal barrier. Due to this breakdown, the bowel does not function normally and does not filter out some harmful substances, such as bacteria, toxic waste products, food additives, infectious agents, and inflammatory substances. These irritants initiate an immune response, causing inflammation. With this disruption to normal bowel function, the immune system leaves the gut open to infections and yeast overgrowth, causing not only gastrointestinal symptoms like bloating, gas, diarrhea, and abdominal pain, but other feelings of ill health as well. Leaky gut syndrome is seen in irritable and inflammatory bowel disorders and has been linked to other diseases. Opportunistic pathogens (harmful substances) of specific types take advantage of other factors, such as poor diet, stress, and antibiotic use, which may weaken the immune system response.[43]

Some of the neuromuscular symptoms of leaky gut are similar to those seen in FM and CMP.[44] It can coexist with any condition; however, it does not cause FM or CMP and is not caused by them. Because of the many possible triggering events of CFID and the nature of LGS, it cannot be absolutely ruled out as a causative factor in some CFID patients. If you have LGS, it can be a most unwelcome addition to your list of aggravating conditions.

Treatment, includes restoring the gut's friendly acidophilus bacteria, restricting foods with chemical preservatives, avoiding alcohol, ingesting fiber and magnesium to speed intestinal motility, avoiding NSAIDS (nonsteroidal anti-inflammatory medications) that upset the intestinal lining, limiting caffeine and yeast products, and avoiding sugar and saturated fats. A new antibiotic is now available by prescription that treats bacterial infections in the intestinal tract only.

Lupus—Systemic Lupus Erythematosus and Discoid Lupus

Systemic lupus erythematosus (SLE), commonly known as lupus, is an inflammatory autoimmune disease in which the body's immune system mistakenly attacks its own tissues. It causes a deterioration of the connective tissues in various parts of the body, including the skin, muscle, heart, lungs, kidneys, joints, and nervous system. Lupus can range from mild to severe. Symptoms include fever, abdominal pain, muscle pain, and joint pain. Lupus of this type is a serious disorder.

Some symptoms of SLE may overlap with FM, CFID, CMP, or other conditions known to be present in some patients. However, it is very important that you understand that SLE is not the same. It is a serious disease that can be life threatening. There is a specific test to detect it, so if you experience any of the symptoms and have not been screened for it, please contact your physician.

Another form of lupus is discoid lupus, or lupus myositis. It affects the skin and is not a generalized connective tissue disorder. Often a person with discoid type has a butterfly rash over the nose and face, which is photosensitive. The rash is not, however, always confined to the face.

Patients with lupus can develop secondary FM.[45]

Livedo Reticularis

Idiopathic, or primary, livedo reticularis refers to blue mottling of skin, usually on the legs. The condition may be caused by swollen blood vessels, may get worse when the temperature is cold, and has been noted in some FM patients.[46]

Lyme Disease

Lyme disease (LD) is caused by the spirochete bacterium, Borrelia burgdorferi. The infection is passed to humans by the bite of an infected tick carrying the microorganism. Symptoms include a "bull's eye" rash at the site of the bite, malaise, fever, headache, muscle aches, and swollen lymph nodes. Untreated Lyme disease can result in symptoms occurring months or years after the initial exposure and causing damage to the heart, joints, and nerves of infected individuals. Symptoms can imitate other diseases and can be misdiagnosed.

Because Lyme disease is also known as a great imitator, it is important for your doctor to run the appropriate test before making a diagnosis of FM, CFID, or CMP.

Meralgia Paresthetica

Meralgia paresthetica is a condition characterized by pain, paresthesia, and numbness on the lateral aspect of the thigh. These symptoms usually occur on only one side. Damage to the nerve is caused from overstretching or compression of the lateral femoral cutaneous nerve, which is a sensory nerve arising from the lumbar (low back) vertebrae L2 and L3 nerve roots.

Hyperextension of the hip (as seen in hypermobility syndromes), lumbar lordosis (exaggerated curvature of the low back), and spinal structural deformity may cause nerve damage. Ischemia of the nerve also results because of its entrapped position in the inguinal ligament. This lack of proper circulation is aggravated by things like wearing tight pants or maintaining a prolonged crouching position. Although symptoms usually resolve spontaneously, the condition may last indefinitely.

---

lateral: to the side, sidewise, the opposite of medial.

ischemia: deficiency of blood due to constriction or obstruction.

paresthesias: abnormal sensations.

Okay, but what else can cause these symptoms? That's right! A trigger point—one of many located in the muscle that attaches from the hip bone, then wraps around to the inside of the knee bone—can also cause this type of response.

Meralgia paresthetica was the name they gave my symptoms. For me the symptoms are burning, sensitivity to light touch, numbness, and itching (did I say itching?). They told me it would go away. It never has. I did discover that some of my symptoms were caused or aggravated by the development of chronic TrPs in the area. Once I determined this, I knew exactly how to get some relief for the pain and dysfunction. I still have recurrences but with my theracane or therapeutic balls as my best friends and constant companions, they are not disabling.

Multiple Chemical Sensitivity

Multiple chemical sensitivity is an illness characterized by adverse reactions to common environmental materials.

These chemicals include pesticides, perfumes, inks and dyes, painting products, laundry agents, home building products, soaps and deodorants, drugs, home and clothing fabrics, tobacco smoke, office machine toners, processed food products, and many others. Illnesses that can be affected by environmental exposures include asthma and allergies, fibromyalgia, chronic fatigue immunodysfunction, migraines, epilepsy, electrical sensitivity, and candidiasis. Symptoms of chemical sensitivity are headaches, joint and muscle pain, gastrointestinal problems, flu symptoms, rashes, hair loss, memory and concentration impairment, depression, sleep and seizure disorders, hyperactivity in children, and mucous membrane irritations. The overlapping of symptoms is obvious, but exposure to chemicals is the key element in diagnosis. This disorder sometimes coexists with FM and CFID.

Multiple chemical sensitivity, like FM, CFID, and GWS, is considered a syndrome because of the frequent clustering of symptoms. More studies are indicated regarding the physical and psychological attributes of symptoms. It might make it easier to accept our symptoms if we knew we could do something about at least some of them. We need to feel that we are in control, and being able to identify and avoid certain chemicals known to aggravate our pain and fatigue can provide that feeling.

Multiple Sclerosis

Multiple sclerosis (MS) is a progressive disease of unknown cause that affects the central nervous system (brain and spinal cord). It destroys the protective covering, called the myelin sheath. The loss of this protection causes a slowing of electrical impulse transmission, thereby impairing nerve conduction. The destructive process causes formation of scars or plaque that can be seen on radiographic studies, such as an MRI, of the central nervous system.

---

myelin: the whitish protective coating over nerve components in the central nervous system. It is believed to influence the rate of impulse transmission in the brain and spinal cord, CNS, where they are predominantly found.

gray matter: unmyelinated nerve components found in abundance in the autonomic nervous system, outside the CNS.

The prognosis of MS is variable and unpredictable. The amount of disability and discomfort varies with the severity and frequency of attacks, and with the portion of the central nervous system affected by each attack.

Symptoms of MS are those you would expect with nerve signal disruption: tingling sensations of the extremities (paresthesias), numbness of the extremities, dizziness, uncontrollable tremors, slurred speech, blurred or double vision, loss of vision, walking/gait abnormalities, hearing loss, muscle weakness, poor coordination, unusual fatigue, muscle cramps and spasms, bladder and bowel dysfunction, sexual dysfunction, paralysis, confusion, and forgetfulness. Pain is not a primary or initial complaint with MS.

Because some symptoms of MS overlap with FM, CFID, and CMP, you can expect your doctor to do certain tests. The breakdown of the protective myelin sheath on the nerves of a person with MS is picked up on an MRI, and you might expect to be referred to a neurologist. Multiple sclerosis does not cause FM, CFID, or CMP, or vice versa, but they can coexist.

Neuralgia

Neuralgia is pain along the tract of a nerve or several nerves. The pain is usually sharp and spasm-like and may recur at any time. Neuralgia is caused by inflammation of, or injury to, a single nerve or nerve group. Sciatica is considered to be a type of neuralgia because it is pain along the tract of the sciatic nerve. Neuralgia is also associated with CFID, CMP, arthritis of the spine, degenerative disc disease, diabetes mellitus, and gout.

If a trigger point is pressing on a nerve, this, too, can cause pain and other associated symptoms distal to the area the nerve supplies. What's the rule? Don't be late, investigate!

Neuralgia-Inducing Cavitational Necrosis

Neuralgia-inducing cavitational necrosis is caused by cavities in the jawbone leading to destruction. It occurs after tooth extraction and is often missed on X-rays until significant damage is done. It is the result of a lack of blood supply to the area usually as a result of trauma or from an untreated trigger point inside the mouth.[47] There can also be other causes, such as tissue being left behind with extraction or surgical removal, a weakened immune system, a poorly functioning thyroid, poor nutrition, or smoking. Chronic osteoporosis can also impede healing. Use cautionary measures to prevent necrosis after having a tooth extracted. The treatment, if necrosis occurs, is surgical removal of the bone and tissue involved.

Neurally Mediated Hypotension

Neurally mediated hypotension (NMH) has been noted in a certain subset of FM[48] and CFID patients.[49] It manifests in low blood pressure that doesn't go up with standing or exercise, and is seemingly caused by a miscommunication between the heart and the brain. In these patients the normal equalization process of increased heart rate with low blood pressure to pump more blood, hence oxygen, is out of whack. People with NMH have a surge of increased heart rate, but don't maintain it normally. It can occur after standing or sitting for prolonged periods, when blood pools in the legs due to gravity; being in a warm environment, which causes the blood vessels to dilate; after exercise or an emotionally charged event, when your heart rate goes up until the stressful event subsides; and after eating, when blood has been shunted to the gut to digest food. Symptoms are related to the sudden drop in blood pressure and include dizziness, weakness, sweating, disorientation, or even fainting. The fatigue associated with NMH can last for days after moderate activity. Treatment is aimed at controlling aggravating factors and increasing plasma volume.

Postural Orthostatic Tachycardia Syndrome

Postural orthostatic tachycardia syndrome (POTS) occurs when the patient affected has a heart rate increase of thirty or more beats per minute within thirty minutes or less, when moving from a prone position to a standing position. It is a diagnosis of exclusion, meaning any other causes of this tachycardia (rapid heartbeat) must be ruled out first. It is usually accompanied by frequent spells of NMH.

Osteoporosis

Osteoporosis occurs when the body fails to form enough new bone, or when too much old bone is reabsorbed by the body, or both.

Osteoporosis is not considered a common coexisting condition; however, it is frequently associated with FM, particularly in perimenopausal women.[50] Therefore, it should not be ignored. Early detection, exercise, calcium and vitamin D3 supplementation, and bone mineral enhancing medication may be indicated.

Peripheral Neuropathy

Peripheral neuropathy (PN) is a fancy word that means an abnormal nerve signal outside the central nervous system. It can often be related to diabetes, prolonged peripheral artery disease (from oxygen deprivation secondary to decreased blood supply to peripheral nerves), MS, autoimmune disorders (that affect nerve tissue), nerve trauma, toxic exposure, nutritional deficiencies, and alcoholism. Peripheral neuropathy symptoms have also been associated with FM, CFID, and CMP.

Peripheral neuropathy-like symptoms—numbness, tingling, pins and needles, sensitivity to touch, or muscle weakness—can be the result of untreated trigger points. CMP patients with entrapped nerves are sometimes misdiagnosed with peripheral neuropathy. Trigger points, which are treatable, need to be considered as a cause before a definitive diagnosis of neuropathy is made.

Of course, PN that is secondary to diabetes or something similar would not benefit from trigger point therapy unless the patient also has trigger points. TrPs often develop due to the stress of physical work, trauma, and disease processes. I don't mean to imply that treating trigger points would make a primary disease go away, but it may be something worth exploring.

To date, nothing seems to help PN other than addressing the underlying disease process, adopting a nutritionally sound diet, avoiding exposure to toxins, following a physician-supervised exercise program, eating a balanced diet, correcting vitamin deficiencies, and limiting or avoiding alcohol consumption.

Piriformis Syndrome

The piriformis is a very small, deep muscle that extends from the side of the sacrum (lowest backbone, tailbone) to the top of the thighbone at the hip joint, passing over the sciatic nerve. When a short or tight piriformis is stretched, it can compress and irritate the sciatic nerve, causing the pain of sciatica. Referred pain from the piriformis is felt in the sacrum, buttocks, and hip. A tight piriformis muscle can also put pressure on the pudendal nerve and cause pain in the groin, genitals, or rectum. In severe cases, piriformis syndrome could be responsible for buttock atrophy. The pain can cause altered gait and guarding, which can cause development of secondary musculoskeletal difficulties.

Treatment of piriformis syndrome calls for releasing the entrapped sciatic nerve. I have found myofascial release and specific TrP treatments to be beneficial.

Polymyalgia Rheumatica

Polymyalgia rheumatica (PMR) is an inflammatory disorder of unknown cause that is characterized by muscle pain and stiffness on both sides of the body, most commonly in the shoulder, neck, and hip regions. Stiffness is particularly noticeable in the morning. This disorder may develop quickly or gradually. Without treatment, polymyalgia rheumatica may go away in one to several years, but with treatment, the symptoms disappear quickly. However, there is a risk of giant cell arteritis in people with polymyalgia rheumatica, and that can have serious repercussions if not treated.

Because muscle pain and stiffness are associated with PMR, it could be confused with FM, CFID, or CMP. However, it is a different condition all together. Polymyalgia rheumatica is inflammatory in nature and responds to anti-inflammatory medications.

Giant Cell Arteritis

Giant cell arteritis, also known as cranial arteritis and/or temporal arteritis (inflammation of the temporal artery), is a disorder that results in swelling of arteries in the head (most often the temporal arteries), neck, and arms. This swelling causes the arteries to narrow, reducing blood flow. With proper treatment the disease is not threatening. Untreated, however, giant cell arteritis can lead to serious complications, including permanent vision loss and stroke. Early symptoms of giant cell arteritis may resemble the flu. As the condition progresses, people are likely to experience headaches, pain in the temples, and blurred or double vision. Pain may also affect the jaw and tongue. These symptoms should not be confused with FM, CFID, or CMP, and should be investigated by a physician, especially when there is a history of PMR.

Post-Polio Syndrome

Post-polio syndrome/sequelae (PPS) can affect polio survivors, sometimes striking many years after recovery from polio. It is characterized by a further weakening of the previously involved muscles and is usually a slow, progressive condition. It often occurs after a physical or emotional trauma, illness, or accident.

The primary symptoms of PPS are fatigue and exhaustion. Other symptoms include muscle atrophy, muscle stiffening or weakness, painful joints and muscles, sensitivity to cold and heat, sleep disorders, difficult breathing and/or swallowing, and/or muscle twitching.

Symptoms of post-polio sequelae may vary and are not predictable.

Symptoms such as fatigue, stiffening, weakness, pain, cold sensitivity, and sleep disorders could be attributed to both PPS and FM, if you are known to have both.

Similarities with CFID have also been noted and reviewed.[51] Symptoms such as muscle twitching and difficulty breathing or swallowing can be attributed to both PPS and untreated TrPs. Remember, body structure and posture can perpetuate CMP, and many polio survivors have abnormalities of both.

Posttraumatic Stress Disorder

Posttraumatic stress disorder (PTSD) is a syndrome that causes "general numbing of emotions." It can re-injure the individual mentally by causing a reliving of some past traumatic event. Posttraumatic stress disorder can affect how well a person copes with pain and/or responds to treatment, particularly if the person also has FM or CFID.

One hypothesis is that there may be similar etiology—elevated nitric oxide/peroxynitrite—among posttraumatic stress disorder, fibromyalgia, chronic fatigue syndrome, and multiple-chemical sensitivity.[52]

Prolapsed Mitral Valve

Ten percent of the population is affected by mitral valve prolapse (MVP), and one study suggests as many as 75 percent of FM patients have it.[53] Study participants are being recruited for studying the connection between MVP and chronic fatigue syndrome at the National Institutes of Health.

The mitral valve controls the flow of blood into the left ventricle (one of four chambers) of the heart. Normally when the left ventricle contracts to push blood out to the body, the mitral valve closes to keep blood from regurgitating back into the left atrium (the left chamber just above the ventricle) and the blood flows out through the aortic valve. The job of the heart's valves is to maintain the flow of blood in one direction, ensuring proper circulation. In mitral valve prolapse, the shape of the valve is abnormal and doesn't allow the valve, or gate, between the atrium and ventricle to close all the way during the contraction of the heart. This backflow of blood into the atrium from the ineffective valve is called "mitral regurgitation." The regurgitation of blood may cause a sound, or murmur, that can sometimes be heard with a stethoscope.

atrium, left: the upper left chamber of the four heart chambers. The left atrium collects the blood returning from the lungs, after the blood collects oxygen.

left ventricle: the lower left chamber of the four heart chambers, which is the largest and has the thickest muscle tissue. Its purpose is to receive blood from the left atrium, which sits on top of the left ventricle, and squeeze (pump) the oxygenated blood out through the aorta to all parts of the body via the arteries.

palpitation: a feeling of rapid, irregular, or fluttering heartbeat.

People who experience symptoms may have brief episodes of palpitation or chest pain that is not typical of heart attack or coronary artery disease. A few people may experience fatigue, shortness of breath, light-headedness, or loss of consciousness. An extremely rare occurrence is sudden death.

Certain precautions should be taken when mitral valve prolapse is present, and these should be discussed with your doctor. Otherwise, it is usually considered a benign (nonthreatening) disorder.

If you have hypermobility as a coexisting condition, it is important for you to know that your mitral valve could also be lax (prolapsed).

Raynaud's Phenomenon or Disease

Raynaud's phenomenon is a disorder of small blood vessels that respond excessively to stimuli. This causes poor blood flow, usually in the fingers, but may also affect the toes and nose. It exists in a particular subset of patients with FM.[54]

When this condition occurs by itself, it is called Raynaud's disease, or primary Raynaud's phenomenon. When it occurs along with other diseases, such as scleroderma, rheumatoid arthritis, systemic lupus erythematosus, polymyositis, dermatomyositis, Sjogren's syndrome, or mixed connective tissue disease, it is called secondary Raynaud's phenomenon.

Symptoms occur when tissue is deprived of the blood's oxygen from the vasospasm; the skin first turns white from insufficient blood, then blue from insufficient oxygen. As I can personally attest, certain areas are more prone to an attack, such as fingers, toes, and nose. During the attack there may be numbness of the affected part. When the arteries relax and blood flows back in, the skin then turns red and there may be associated pain, burning, or stinging.

CAUTION

- Treating cold intolerance and neurally mediated hypotension is important, since so many people with FM and CFS/ CFID have these problems. It is important to understand that treatment for both is focused on prevention. For cold intolerance, dress in warm clothing and stay warm. Vasodilator type medications may be indicated in more severe cases.
- In the case of Raynaud's, re-warm slowly.
- For neurally mediated hypotension, the goal is to improve circulation with low-impact aerobic exercise. To avoid dizziness, change body position gradually.

The cause is unknown, but some abnormality of the sympathetic nervous system seems to be present. The attacks are precipitated by cold or, occasionally, by emotional upset.

Myofascial TrP nerve entrapment can worsen symptoms.[55] If you have CMP and Raynaud's, be sure to check those trigger points; you may be able to lesson the severity of an attack.

Raynaud's can cause excruciating pain, especially during re-warming. It predisposes you to frostbite, so take care to use preventive measures. Avoid alcohol consumption, especially in cold weather; caffeine; and smoking. There are certain medications to avoid if you have Raynaud's, so be sure to consult with your physician or pharmacist.

Restless Leg Syndrome

Restless leg syndrome (RLS) describes a condition in which uncomfortable sensations are experienced in the lower legs during periods of rest, especially before sleeping. The symptoms are accompanied by an overwhelming urge to move the legs. Movement seems to provide temporary relief of a "creepy," "crawly," or "weird" feeling. Although these sensations are usually not painful, they are annoying and unrelenting. The symptoms often lead to serious sleep deprivation, fatigue, and depression.

The cause is unknown. It has been associated with pregnancy, diabetes, multiple sclerosis, rheumatoid arthritis, iron-deficiency anemia, caffeine intake, poor leg circulation, certain vitamin and mineral deficiencies, and FM, and can be perpetuated by untreated TrPs. Restless leg syndrome can also be a potential side effect of some prescription medications.

The syndrome is separate from, but often associated with, involuntary leg movements during sleep, called periodic limb movements.

Periodic Limb Movement Disorder

Periodic limb movement (PLMD) can coexist with FM. It is characterized by involuntary jerks of the legs and/or arms during sleep. Most experts believe PLMD results from a recurrent central nervous system processing disruption that causes a disturbance in the normal brain wave patterns and results in lack of restorative sleep. Hmm, sound familiar?

Sciatica

Sciatica is inflammation of the sciatic nerve, marked by pain and tenderness, which usually starts in the buttocks and extends down the rear of the thigh along the course of the nerve, and on through to the lower thigh and calf. The pain along the sciatic nerve tract can even extend from the lower back to the sole of the foot. Movements that compress the sciatic nerve, such as standing, lifting, sitting, bending, or straining, may aggravate the pain.

Usually, no specific direct trauma can be blamed for sciatica. A herniated or bulging disk in the low back is the primary cause.

Piriformis syndrome and untreated TrPs can be misdiagnosed as sciatica, which can delay appropriate treatment.

SICCA-like symptoms and DEMS (Dry Eye, Dry Mouth Syndrome)

Do you get all "gunked up" when you have sinus congestion? Wouldn't you just love to be able to blow your nose and get something out? Are your eyes red most of the time and do your eyelids feel like sandpaper as they blink over your dry eyes? Does your mouth feel like someone stuffed it with cotton? This collection of symptoms—dry eyes, nose, and mouth are SICCA-like symptoms. A group of patients presenting with SICCA symptoms were expected to test positive for Sjorgens, but did not. Instead a subgroup with DEMS was noted and these subjects tended more toward FM and CFID.[56] From what I have been able to unravel, when dry eye, dry mouth, and dry nose symptoms are accompanied by lymphocytic infiltration of the exocrine gland it is called SICCA complex (see Sjogren's following). Some references interchange SICCA with dry eye, dry mouth (DEMS), and dry nose symptoms and some use the term SICCA interchangeable with Sjogren's, so I am reporting the information here as I see it, and will call dry eyes, nose, and mouth SICCA-like symptoms.

Specific TrPs can also cause dehydration in one or more areas if they entrap lymph, blood vessels, and, perhaps, ducts. The resulting dryness could be mistaken for SICCA-like symptoms.[57]

So what can help? Increased water intake (unless contraindicated by another medical condition), lubricating eye drops, and saline nasal spray will help. There are also some new products available by prescription to help increase your tears. If you have extremely dry nasal secretions, you may find nasal "douches" helpful, as I did. Limit known dehydrating items from your diet, and when possible, limit medications known to "dry you out." If TrPs are involved, treat them.

Sjogren's Syndrome

Sjogren's syndrome is an autoimmune disorder that primarily causes chronic dry eyes and dry mouth.

It generally occurs in two ways: primary and secondary. Primary Sjogren's syndrome occurs by itself and is not associated with other diseases. Secondary Sjogren's syndrome occurs with rheumatic diseases, such as rheumatoid arthritis, systemic lupus erythematous, polymyositis, and some forms of scleroderma.

Sjogren's syndrome can also cause problems in other parts of the body, including the joints, lungs, muscles, kidneys, nerves, thyroid gland, liver, pancreas, stomach, and brain.

Sjogren's syndrome affects everyone differently; however, the most common early symptom is severe dry mouth and eyes. Other symptoms include swollen salivary glands; dental cavities; dry nose, throat, and lungs; vaginal dryness; fatigue; muscle weakness; confusion and memory problems; dry skin; and paresthesias. Some patients develop cancer of the lymph tissue.

The symptoms of Sjogren's can be confused with FM and CFID. It is not the same, nor is it treated in the same way.

Temporomandibular Dysfunction

Temporomandibular dysfunction (TMD/TMJ), once known as temporomandibular joint syndrome, or TMJ, occurs when the muscles used in chewing and the joints of the jaw fail to work in coordination with each other. Sometimes symptoms occur for no obvious reason. Temporomandibular dysfunction is often associated with complaints of chronic muscular headaches and craniofacial pain. Pain can also extend to the ears, neck, and shoulders. Some people experience clicking and grinding noises during movement of the jaw, limited or asymmetrical (uneven) jaw movement, and pain and tenderness of the jaw muscles.

craniofacial: pertaining to the head and neck.

Among the causes of TMD are teeth clenching or grinding (bruxism); structural abnormality, such as a poor bite; accidents that damage the bones of the face or jaw; untreated trigger points; occasionally diseases, such as arthritis; or no obvious reason.

If you have TrPs causing TMD, treat them prior to getting dental work. They can cause dysfunction of the temporomandibular joint, which can affect the outcome of a visit to the dentist.[58] When TrPs are present they can restrict jaw motion and disrupt your normal bite. This could result in dental disaster if your dentist is forming fillings or crowns to a misaligned temporomandibular joint.

Tendonitis

Tendonitis is inflammation or irritation of the tendon, a band of fibrous tissue that connects muscle to bone. The natural tendency to favor the painful area can lead to stiffness and loss of flexibility and mobility. Tendonitis can become a chronic problem due to scarring of the tissues from continued overuse. If you are told you have tendonitis, rest the involved area and give it a chance to heal before it becomes a chronic problem. Chronic inflammation of the tendon can cause permanent damage.

Almost any tendon in the body can be affected, but those located around the knee, foot, ankle, elbow, and shoulder are the most frequently identified.

Tendonitis, like bursitis, is usually diagnosed because of the pain it causes. Everywhere there is a muscle, there is a tendon connecting that muscle to the bone. Because of this fact, trigger points can develop in the area from repetitive movement or over-use. Treatment for tendonitis is to reduce inflammation. If the pain is coming from an untreated TrP, the treatment is trigger point therapy (see chapter 4). You can have both tendonitis and TrPs, or tendonitis may be diagnosed when it is actually CMP. Don't be late, investigate!

Thoracic Outlet Syndrome

Thoracic outlet syndrome (TOS) is an abnormal condition characterized by numbness and tingling of the fingers, arm fatigue, and loss of grip strength. Some type of compression of the brachial plexus nerve trunks or blood vessels causes the symptoms of TOS. Pain may be in the shoulder, arm, or hand, or in all three locations. Hand pain is often most severe in the fourth and fifth fingers. Other causes include carpal tunnel syndrome, drooping shoulder girdle, abnormal first rib, or herniated cervical (neck) disc.

---

brachial plexus nerve trunks: bundled nerves that separate and pass into the arms from the neck.

tendon: the extension of fibrous tissue covering muscle that connects muscle to bone.

Thoracic outlet syndrome may be incorrectly diagnosed or coexist with CMP. Several muscles can be affected by TrPs that cause the same symptoms in a taut band of muscle fiber. Muscles that can be affected are brachioradialis, serratus anterior and posterior, pectoralis major, subscapularis, the scalenes, flexor digitorum, and dorsal interosseous.

Vulvodynia

Vulvodynia is pain in the external female genitalia. It can be caused by untreated pelvic floor trigger points.[59] Oragel may help numb the pain of vulvodynia. As discussed under irritable bladder, there are pelvic floor treatments available. If you find TrPs in the pelvic floor (between the vagina and rectum, or the vulva, sitting on a therapeutic ball can be used to treat them. I would suggest that you use a soft chair to avoid applying too much pressure to the area.

Summary of Interactions with Coexisting Conditions

As previously discussed, FM and CMP have very specific patterns that make them easier to diagnose than CFID, which can only be diagnosed after many of the listed conditions have been eliminated. That does not mean, however, that some of these conditions cannot coexist in the same patient.

By treating the primary condition and identifying aggravating and alleviating factors, you can minimize your symptoms. For instance, migraine and cluster headaches can have a significant myofascial pain component. Fibromyalgia patients battle recurring headaches. Periodic limb movement can coexist with FM. Carpal tunnel symptoms, thoracic outlet syndrome, irritable bladder, neuralgia, piriformis syndrome, and sciatica can intensify the trigger points of CMP or be caused by them. Untreated trigger points, if you have CMP, can increase the pain cascade of any other pain disorder.

Many of us also have symptoms that can be confused with symptoms of other disorders; for example, problems with coordination. This does not mean we have multiple sclerosis, Parkinson's disease, inner ear dysfunction, or any of the other disorders that can cause balance problems. Over and over again I hear testimony from others that many of us have problems staying upright. Have you ever heard the term, "like a bull in a china shop"? That is exactly what I feel like, with bruises to prove it. I tend to bump into things or walk with an altered gait, so sometimes people stare as if I'd just staggered out of a bar! You've probably already experienced this if you are reading this book. As to why we seem to have more coordination problems than the average bear, or suffer from some symptoms that go along with other disorders, I am not sure. Possibly it is because of the susceptibility to cold, a disruption in the central nervous system, or lack of oxygen from poor breathing patterns. On the other hand, it could be from untreated trigger points that directly affect, or have referral patterns to, the muscles responsible, or from coexisting conditions. Or it may just be the nature of the beast.

One of the most common tender points in FM is in the frontal rib area. This is not to be confused with costochondritis, which is an inflammation between the ribs that can be caused by virus or injury; or with the myofascial trigger points of CMP that can also cause pain in the rib or chest area. As you can see, it's easy to mistake a symptom for something else.

Some diseases may be more prevalent in FM, CFID, or CMP individually; however, this certainly does not mean that these conditions cannot coexist in all three. Coexisting conditions are different from one person to another because we are all unique individuals, so you may find you have a coexisting condition other than those identified here. Unless cloning of human life occurs, it is safe to say that this will always be true.

As discussed, some of these diseases or conditions can often coexist with and aggravate FM, CFID, and/or CMP; others may merely have similar symptoms. This is why it is so important to find a doctor familiar with our conditions. With proper consultation and treatment, you may find the help you need to alleviate some of your aggravating factors. Depending upon your myriad conditions, the treatment regimen may vary, and rightly so. The treatment for one may not be seen by your doctor, or you, to outweigh the risks of exacerbating one of your other conditions, so don't compare notes with support group members too feverishly.

Talk to your doctor about the role any other conditions may play in your comprehensive treatment plan.

Communicating with Your Physician and Other Health Care Providers

Finding the right people for your health care team is not an easy task, but with a little help, it can be a rewarding journey. It is important for your team members to know what your health care needs are, and it is equally important for them to know how to help you with your unique treatment and specific requirements.

The overall goal for you and your health care team is to create a regimen aimed at improving your mental, physical, emotional, and spiritual well-being. For the plan to be successful it must also be measurable. In other words, if the plan is working you should see improvement in your ability to perform daily activities, you should feel good about yourself, and your spirits should remain positive.

If you find a good doctor, stick with him 'till you die.

AUTHOR UNKNOWN

Recognizing Resistance

Historically the role of the doctor in the physician-patient relationship has been paternalistic, with the patient dependent solely on the physician's authority. The patient blindly trusted there would be benefit from the physician's recommendations. If the patient possessed enough knowledge to suggest health care preferences, those were generally overridden or ignored by the physician.

There are still some doctors who believe these disorders are psychological in nature. Dr. Muhammad Yunus, a well-known researcher in the field of FM and CFID, refers to this belief as disturbed physician syndrome (DPS). He says, "It is the physicians who are psychologically disturbed because they ignore the data, and whatever data there is, they manipulate it to say what they want it to say."[60]

The mindset Dr. Yunus refers to does exist in some health care providers. Learning to recognize this attitude in members of your health care team could have a tremendous effect on your life.

The last thing you need to have to deal with is dismissal of your complaints, which only compounds your problems. If more HCPs were educated in soft tissue disorders and the psychological effects of chronic pain, this "all in your head" attitude would not exist. If you feel up to the task, and you feel comfortable with your HCP, you may want to work with that person. Such seeming resistance could be an honest lack of knowledge.

In a study done at Simon Fraser University on "Chronic Pain and the Doctor-Client Relationship,"[61] patients (clients) suggested doctors don't take the time needed to reevaluate their knowledge. One doctor admitted he felt anxious when patients displayed too much knowledge. Patients felt as though the doctors were always hurried, but doctors felt that patients were impatient because they wanted immediate pain control before their interview. Wow, no kidding.

To serve as focus points for further analysis, the Simon Fraser study abstract lists ten topics identified by physicians and patients.

- Doctors do not get enough information from patients.
- Doctors need better listening skills.
- Doctors and patients do not know enough about chronic pain.
- Doctors and patients do not have enough time for dialogue.
- Medicine is not an exact science.
- Patients do not have enough energy to go to the doctor, communicate efficiently, and so on.
- Clients' symptoms are discounted.
- Chronic pain is an invisible disability.
- Doctors and clients need to have a dynamic, working, active "partnership."

These findings are similar to the findings in a British study reported in *Social Science & Medicine,*[62] which suggests medical care is evaluated less on the doctor's ability to treat CFID and more on the doctor's ability to communicate and use interpersonal and informational skills. They also found that lack of interpersonal communication skills was an obstacle to the development of a therapeutic doctor-patient relationship.

Dr. Bernie Siegel, a surgeon and author renowned for his work in body-mind communication, wrote in his book, *Peace, Love and Healing,* "When doctors look at their patients they are trained to see only the disease. That is why so many of us need to be reminded that there is a human being in the room with us."[63]

Health care provider: "You look good today."

Patient: "Thanks, I must be doing a good job of hiding my pain."

Today a paternalistic, authoritative relationship between the physician or other HCP and the patient/client should not be tolerated. It should be an equal partnership with interactive roles that will lead to optimal health and well-being for both the patient and the HCP. Whether they like it or not, physicians are pushed into time constraints by insurance companies, limiting effective communication with the patient. This forces them to rely heavily on the patient's understanding of her or his own disorder. The role of physician and patient has changed, and until the health care system improves, both must accept it and move forward.

If your disorder is CMP, FM, or both, you will find informative and educational physician and health care provider handout sheets in Dr. Devin Starlanyl's, *The Fibromyalgia Advocate.* (See resource section.)

Following is an excerpt from a letter I wrote to my brother when he doubted the reality of my fibromyalgia because of medical literature that suggested it was not a real medical condition.

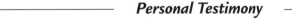

Personal Testimony

Dearest Brother,

Mom told me that somehow you came upon information that dispels the existence of FM. Yes, it is classified as a syndrome, not a disease. Just like rheumatoid arthritis and many others. That is because in order to be classified as a disease, researchers must know what causes it, and they don't. A syndrome is an exact set of symptoms that remain constant throughout the community of people affected.

I do believe it is possible that you have FM, even though it is less common in men. It could be possible that you also suffer chronic myofascial pain. This has been upgraded from a syndrome to a disease at the neuromuscular junction. Unlike FM, which scientific evidence (funded by the National Institutes of Health studies, and others) points to as a disruption in the central nervous system, CMP (chronic myofascial pain) causes knotting in the muscle tissue itself.

Doctors who make claims that these conditions don't exist have obviously not put their hands on a patient or they couldn't make such uneducated assumptions. Any health care provider who doesn't believe FM, CFID, and CMP exist is not continuing their education and should not advertise it. Unfortunately, doctors in the United States are under-trained in conditions that have been statistically proven to cause more time off work and more disability than any other medical condition.

You can go to www.PubMed.com and type in fibromyalgia, chronic fatigue syndrome, or chronic myofascial pain and see all the research going on in this field, and what the studies are showing. If they didn't exist, all these people, from doctors to scientists to our government, would have figured that out by now. Anybody can make claims from not believing to having a miracle cure, but nobody can dispute scientific fact.

Love, Sis

Disillusionment is a good thing. Because of it I can see what is real, in and around me.

WILLIAM ELLIOTT

Overcoming Resistance

It is important to let your health care providers know you'd like to take a proactive role in your health care and be a primary member of the health care team. By agreeing to be a part of the changes taking place in health care administration, you recognize that your physician and HCPs operate with many insurance and health care restraints that were not present in the days of authoritative health care delivery models. All of your HCPs should appreciate the benefits of a proactive patient. Along with that role, however, comes a certain amount of accountability. You should be able to rely upon your health care providers and they should be able to rely upon you. Building confidence brings about a trusting, productive relationship that benefits both patient and HCP.

Health History and Agenda

By keeping a notebook you can provide your HCP with a written, brief, current health history and an agenda for your meeting. This will help you utilize your time together more efficiently. (See the Useful Tools section at the end of this chapter.)

In addition to the history you give your HCP as previously discussed in this chapter, you should document such things as marital status, work status, home life adaptations, symptoms, and how you feel you are coping. Also include a chronological chart of past doctors, listing specialty, test results, treatments, and outcomes.

Example

Marital status: Married, 40-year-old female. Two children at home; son aged 20 and daughter aged 18.

Work status—present: Unemployed due to on-the-job injury to shoulder while lifting 40-pound crate.

Past work history: Factory worker for 20 years, cut hours back to part time after 15 years due to pain and inability to continue in this line of work on a full-time basis.

Life style adaptations: Require assistance for tasks that used to be routine, such as opening jars, shopping, and vacuuming. Riding in a car causes extreme pain to my neck and low back, and trips are limited to one-hour intervals with frequent rest stops. I am no longer able to bowl, play racquetball, or play golf due to past injuries and pain. Hobbies are now sedentary in nature, such as playing backgammon and watching movies. I use a brace for the deformity of my left shoulder, a TEN's unit, and topical ointment for the pain in my shoulder, low back, and hips.

Symptoms: This is where you should list your symptoms. You may want to use your previously completed symptom inventory or incorporate it here. This information will help the HCP get a better understanding of how much your symptoms interfere with your daily activities.

Coping: Include here what you do to cope with your pain and/or fatigue. Do you read self-help books, participate in spiritual activities, learn new hobbies that are less stressful, go to talk therapy, belong to a support group, or use diversion tactics in order to get through a day, week, or month?

The chronology chart should include specific criteria as follows:

- Date of service
- Health care provider's name
- HCP's specialty, such as family physician, specialist, therapist, or nurse practitioner
- Primary reason for seeing the HCP
- Outcome of the visit, such as tests ordered, therapy initiated, new medications, and so on
- Test results
- Referrals and outcomes of referrals

Sample Chronology Chart

1970–1985, Dr. Joe Blow (general practitioner)
General health care
Neck pain
Migraine
Menstrual difficulties
MRI neck = bulging disc C4-5
MRI head = negative
Pelvic sonogram = pelvic inflammatory disease

1986–Present, Dr. Ralph Head (neurologist)
Migraine
Neck Pain
Brain mapping = negative except for migraine
EMG arms = radiculopathy C4-5

1986–Present, Dr. Mighty Friendly (general practitioner)
General health care

9/2001—Dr. Friendly
Neck pain
Low back pain
Supportive care, medication, and PT = helpful

9/2002—Dr. Friendly
Left shoulder injury
MRI left shoulder = torn rotator cuff
Referral orthopedic

11/2002—Dr. Funny Bone (orthopedic)

Left shoulder injury

EMG left arm = nerve problem

12/2002—Dr. Funny Bone

Left shoulder surgery—in rehab

Although this chronology is only necessary for your initial visit, it is a good idea to keep it up to date and review it with your physician on an annual or semiannual basis, depending upon any changes and your health care needs.

Agenda for Progress (The Planning Board)

Your agenda should include all the things you want to discuss with your health care provider. Write down questions as you think of them. Recopy them in order of priority, state as such, and provide your physician with a reference copy. Try to simplify your questions so that they require only a short answer. Open-ended dialogue requires more time, and time will be in short supply. The agenda will keep your visit on track and you will not leave wishing you had remembered to ask something else. After you get accustomed to using this format, you may not need to be so specific; key words that prompt your discussion may be sufficient. Also expect that if your list can't be reasonably accommodated, you will need to address the remainder of your concerns at another scheduled visit. This is why it is important to prioritize your needs. The agenda is also a useful tool for your physician, who will not have to try to recall all of your information when charting in your medical record after having seen twenty to thirty patient that day. Embrace with caring and concern the understanding that you are not the only patient your HCP sees, and that a refresher course on your health care concerns will likely be needed.

Utilize resources, such as your physician's nurse. If you are able to establish a good rapport, the nurse can be a valuable asset to you.

Keep one copy of your health history, worksheets, chronological chart, and agenda for yourself and two for your health care provider. Your HCP may choose to use what you provide as a worksheet and place it in your record. If your physician and other HCPs are willing to work *for* you, they should be willing to work *with* you. Their reception of this information will indicate if they want to be part of your health care team. If they are intimidated, don't take it personally. Give them time. Once they learn how much your contribution saves in documentation and that you are not substituting your knowledge for their sound medical advice, they will appreciate it. If, after a reasonable courting period, you are still not sure the HCP appreciates your proactive role, it may be time to move on and find one who does.

Tips for Finding the Right Doctor

- Refer to local agencies for referral; for example, the Arthritis Foundation.
- Network within a support group.
- Check credentials with the physician's specialty board.
- Set up a compatibility interview.
- If possible, have someone accompany you to get a second opinion of the physician-client exchange.
- If you feel you need a doctor to be readily available, ask questions such as, "How long does it usually take to get an appointment?"
- Think about the location of the doctor's office. Is it convenient for you?
- Decide if the doctor's office hours are compatible with your needs.
- The right doctor is one who listens.
- The right doctor explains things so that you understand them.
- The right doctor treats you with respect.

The Interview

Patients generally decide for themselves which of their physician instructions are compatible with their existing belief system. Also important to patients is that the recommended treatment plan can be easily incorporated into their everyday lives. If there is a conflict, the physician may feel the patient is non-compliant or doesn't trust the evaluation. In turn, the patient may feel that the plan is so complex that it's overwhelming. If there is some reason you are not able to participate in the outlined treatment plan, such as conflicting spiritual beliefs or lifestyle issues, you should let your HCP know so that alterations in the plan can be made to accommodate you. Remember, in order for the plan to be successful, it should be developed by you and your physician together. It should also have the capacity to be reevaluated and changed to meet your needs. If your HCP cannot see that your input is necessary, that person may have a problem giving up the authority role, which would impair the communication system.

TIPS FOR FACILITATING EFFECTIVE COMMUNICATION

- Assume a position of comfort.

- Establish eye contact.

- Listen without interrupting.

- Show attention with nonverbal cues, such as nodding.

- Allow expression of feelings.

Patient and Physician Rights

Each state and most health care delivery organizations have a Patient's Bill of Rights. The patient's rights may vary from state to state, or organization to organization, but as a health care consumer you have some entitlement. You have the right to:

- Respectful care
- Be informed about your illness, treatment options, and risks
- Refuse a treatment, as permitted by law
- Privacy and confidentiality

Doctors sometimes encounter a patient whose needs or demands are too great, or are outside the realm of the physician's expertise. Whichever it is, it can detract from a therapeutic relationship. When no agreeable compromise can be reached, the physician-patient relationship may need to be severed. In this case the physician cannot abandon the patient but must provide the patient with resources to obtain ongoing medical care.

By learning how to effectively communicate your health care needs you increase the likelihood of finding compassionate, caring health care team members who make you feel comfortable with their knowledge and mutual consideration. The healing power of body, mind, and spirit is greatly enhanced by a good, solid relationship between health care provider and patient.

Summary Exercise: Clear Expressions

List at least five common terms used to describe your symptoms.

_____

_____

_____

_____

_____

Check the applicable aggravating or predisposing factors and list any others you have identified.

Some General Aggravating and Predisposing Factors

(Identify by checking those that apply to you.)

- ☐ Activity level—too little or overexertion
- ☐ Allergies, uncontrolled
- ☐ Anxiety or depression
- ☐ Barometric pressure changes or fluctuations
- ☐ Chemical exposure
- ☐ Coexisting conditions—by nature or poor management
- ☐ Coping mechanisms—lack of healthy ones, or inappropriate ones
- ☐ Diet deficiency—improper diet or diet consisting of specific known food triggers
- ☐ Exercise—too much, too little, or the wrong kind
- ☐ Infection
- ☐ Medications
- ☐ Metabolic and endocrine dysfunction (for example, thyroid problems, hypoglycemia, diabetes, anemia, mononucleosis)
- ☐ Neglect of spiritual or emotional needs
- ☐ Poor posture
- ☐ PMS
- ☐ Rapid body position changes
- ☐ Seasonal affective disorder
- ☐ Situational crisis
- ☐ Skeletal structural deformities and lack of corrective measures
- ☐ Sleep disorders, including sleep apnea, deprivation, and disrupted sleep order
- ☐ Stress management—lack of or inappropriate coping

☐ Symptom neglect

☐ Tight clothing, including ill-fitting shoes

☐ Trauma

☐ Treatment plan for the disorder—lack of any or lack of participation

☐ Trigger points—neglect

☐ Unhealthy environmental exposure (excessive sun, smoke, allergens, noise)

☐ Unprotected exposure to cold

☐ Other_____

_____

Use the following to describe each of your symptoms. For documenting severity use the 1–10 scale, ten being the most severe. If there are fluctuations in the severity of your symptoms, it would be good to note that and give a range.

ONSET	DURATION	SEVERITY	CHARACTER

Describe corrective actions you take to help your symptoms.

SYMPTOM	ACTION

Check the conditions for which you have been diagnosed.

☐ AIDS/HIV infection

☐ Allergy

☐ Ankylosing spondylitis (AS)

☐ Anxiety

☐ Bursitis

☐ Bruxism

☐ Candidiasis

☐ Carpal tunnel syndrome

☐ Complex regional pain syndrome (CRPS)

☐ Costochondritis

☐ Degenerative disc disease

☐ Depression

☐ Foot problems

☐ Gulf War syndrome

☐ Headaches, severe

☐ Hypermobility syndrome

☐ Hypoglycemia

☐ Reactive hypoglycemia

☐ Hypothyroidism

☐ Hypometabolism

☐ Infection (viral and bacterial)

☐ Inner ear dysfunction

☐ Interstitial cystitis or irritable bladder

☐ Irritable bowel syndrome (IBS)

☐ Leaky gut syndrome

☐ Lupus—systemic lupus erythematosus (SLE)

☐ Lyme disease (LD)

☐ Meralgia paresthetica

☐ Multiple chemical sensitivity

☐ Multiple sclerosis (MS)

☐ Neurally mediated hypotension (NMH)

☐ Neuralgia

☐ Neuralgia-inducing cavitational necrosis

☐ Osteoarthritis (OA)

☐ Osteoporosis

☐ Peripheral neuropathy

☐ Periodic limb movement (PLMD)

☐ Piriformis syndrome

☐ Plantar fasciitis

☐ Polymyalgia rheumatica (PMR)

☐ Post-polio syndrome (PPS)

☐ Posttraumatic stress disorder (PTSD)

☐ Prolapsed mitral valve

☐ Raynaud's phenomenon or disease

☐ Restless leg syndrome (RLS)

☐ Rheumatoid arthritis (RA)

☐ Sciatica

☐ Seasonal affective disorder (SAD)

☐ SICCA-like symptoms

☐ Sjogren's syndrome

☐ Temporomandibular dysfunction (TMD/TMJ)

☐ Tendonitis

☐ Thoracic outlet syndrome (TOS)

☐ Vulvodynia

Describe your relationship with your doctor. Does your doctor work with you to address your health care needs?

_____

_____

_____

_____

_____

_____

_____ promotes effective communication with your doctor and is the basis of a working relationship between physician and patient. (Trust)

You should avoid words that are vague and misleading when describing your symptoms. What are some words you would use to describe your symptoms?

_____

_____

_____

_____

_____

_____

Useful Tools
for
Communicating with
Health Care Providers

The following forms will help you document your condition accurately and communicate clearly with health care providers, so that you can receive the most appropriate and effective care for your particular health care needs. Feel free to photocopy these forms before filling them out so that you will have blank forms available for updating your records or for communicating with new health care practitioners.

- Medication Log
- Symptom Inventory Survey
- Anatomical Diagram of Pain
- Health History Log

Medication Log

For _____

Date completed/updated_____

Medication Allergies

(Reactions include rash or hives, shortness of breath, swelling, or loss of consciousness.)*

MEDICATION	REACTION

*As opposed to an outright allergy, which produces immediate acute symptoms, a sensitivity to a medication produces milder, less immediate symptoms that are not life-threatening—for example, upset stomach, headache, or inability to sleep—but are unwanted side effects that would prevent you from taking the medication. Sensitivities to medications can be noted on the second part of this form.

Medications

Name	Start date	Dose	Schedule	Taken for	Response	% helps	Stop date and why

Reviewed with Dr._____ on_____

Symptom Inventory Sheet

Date _____ Name_____ SS#_____

Symptom History (Circle one for each category)

IN GENERAL, OVERALL PAIN IS

| severe | moderately severe | moderate | moderately tolerable | tolerable |

AS A GENERAL RULE, ACTIVITY LEVEL IS

| very poor | poor | moderately poor | moderately good | good |

ENERGY IS GENERALLY

| very poor | poor | moderately poor | moderately good | good |

SLEEP QUALITY IS USUALLY

| very poor | poor | moderately poor | moderately good | good |

SLEEP AMOUNT IS USUALLY

| 2–4 hours | 4–6 hours | 6–8 hours | 9 or more hours |

FEEL RESTED

| never | usually | sometimes | always |

CONCENTRATION/MEMORY IS GENERALLY

| very poor | poor | moderately poor | moderately good | good |

LIST KNOWN AGGRAVATING FACTORS

_____

_____

_____

_____

_____

_____

Specific Pain History

Rate your pain using the 1–10 pain scale below.

NONE									WORST EVER	
0	1	2	3	4	5	6	7	8	9	10

	TODAY	PAST WEEK	PAST MONTH	PAST SIX MONTHS
At its least	_____	_____	_____	_____
At its most	_____	_____	_____	_____

Circle the number that best describes how your pain has interfered with each of the following categories:

ACTIVITIES OF DAILY LIVING

0	1	2	3	4	5	6	7	8	9	10
None										Completely

RELATIONSHIPS WITH OTHERS

0	1	2	3	4	5	6	7	8	9	10
None										Completely

ENJOYMENT OF LIFE

0	1	2	3	4	5	6	7	8	9	10
None										Completely

Rate the efficacy of treatments or medications using the scale provided below.

NO RELIEF									COMPLETE RELIEF	
0%	10%	20%	30%	40%	50%	60%	70%	80%	90%	100%

List types of treatment and rate percentage of relief provided by each type. *(For example, list medications, exercise, physical therapy, and pain management techniques.)*

TYPE OF TREATMENT	% RELIEF
_____	_____
_____	_____
_____	_____
_____	_____
_____	_____

Anatomical Diagram of Pain

Name_____ Date_____

Related to (circle one): Today   Past week

A = aching

B = burning

C = cramping

D = dull

E = electrical (pins and needles)

K = knots

N = numb

S = sharp

T = tender

Other = describe

On the diagram below, circle the areas where you have pain and label the areas using the key above. You may have more than one character of pain in the area; if so, include all that apply. If symptoms affect both right and left but are more predominant on one side, mark the more affected side with a +.

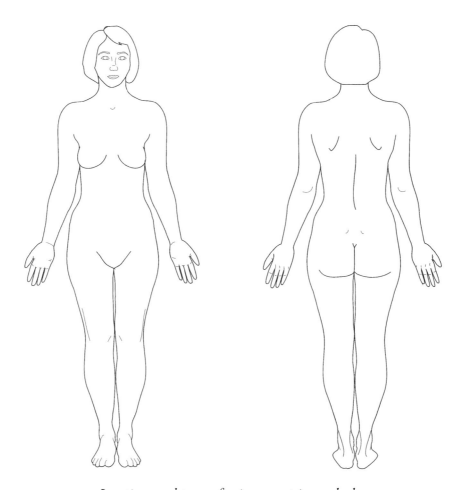

Locations and types of pain present in my body

Health History Log

For_____Date_____

Make a brief statement regarding marital status, work status, and home life adaptations.

_____

_____

_____

_____

Surgeries and Procedures

Type	Date	Results
_____	_____	_____
_____	_____	_____
_____	_____	_____
_____	_____	_____
_____	_____	_____
_____	_____	_____
_____	_____	_____
_____	_____	_____
_____	_____	_____
_____	_____	_____

Laboratory and Diagnostic Testing

Type	Date	Results
_____	_____	_____
_____	_____	_____
_____	_____	_____
_____	_____	_____
_____	_____	_____
_____	_____	_____
_____	_____	_____
_____	_____	_____
_____	_____	_____
_____	_____	_____

Reviewed with_____ on_____

3

Dialogues Within and Without

Webster's defines communication as "an act of giving or exchanging information." This chapter is devoted to learning how to share important messages that have a significant impact on your life and the lives of others around you.

After completing this chapter you should be able to:

- Organize a journal.
- Write a poem to express your feelings.
- Identify blocks to growth.
- Define the difference between external and internal communication.
- Solicit at least one person or group to give you the support you need.
- Review the significance of relationships—how you can improve them and how to get what you want from them.
- Summarize the positive key points of effective communication, including how it helps you to understand yourself and promotes a better understanding by others.
- Review tips to effective advocacy.
- Recognize resources for promoting awareness of FM, CFID, and CMP.

--------------------- ***Personal Testimony*** ---------------------

I can testify that just a few changes on my part have made a huge difference in the way others react to me and my disabilities. My friends say that previously they were afraid to share things with me because of my health problems and their unpredictability. Because I have learned how to share my experiences and how to keep the lines of effective communication open, they are no longer intimidated by me. I learned that my behavior and reactions to others only hampered smooth interactions with friends and family.

Journal Writing: An Internal Dialogue

Journaling provides immense satisfaction of self-expression, brings about growth to inner wisdom, relieves stress, blocks negative thoughts, and promotes positive action. It is a way to organize thoughts and establish a synchronized dialogue with the innermost self. Through a good understanding of what is important to your well-being, you can begin to have healthy communication. By learning to relate to others productively, you can build a unique and valuable support structure, rather than one riddled with negative thoughts and feelings.

---

internal dialogue: a dialogue with the innermost self.

Nearly every book on self-help has a section or suggestion related to journaling. This is because we know that it helps to strengthen healthy coping mechanisms, decrease stress and anxiety, and relieve depression.[1] Journaling helps us change negative energy into thoughts of encouragement, which promote the healthy coping strategies necessary to deal with the physical and emotional side effects of FM, CFID, or CMP.

In adult education the rule is: "Read it, see it, do it, teach it." You can fine-tune your skills by using this rule to work with your inner self and create an inner dialogue that builds more self-appreciation.

There are no mistakes in life—only lessons.
CHÉRIE CARTER-SCOTT, *THE RULES FOR BEING HUMAN*

Your journal should be your confidant and friend. You should be able to share your most intimate feelings and thoughts without fear of reprimand or consequences.

Select a journal that is right for you. There are many resources for learning how to start and keep a journal. You may even want to buy a notebook and build your own. Selecting what is right for you is the number one priority. It should be one you enjoy using. If it makes you feel uncomfortable, you will most likely lose interest, which will defeat the purpose of journaling. We are currently working on publishing a journal that speaks to our specific needs.

Organizing Your Journal

Include sections in your journal that you feel are important for your personal assessment and growth.

Tips for Topics

- Pictures—favorite places, people, occasions, animals, flowers, or anything that appeals to your senses.
- Letters—from others, to others, or to yourself.
- Pain chart—to chart pain and related activities, new medications, dropped medications, emotional stumbling blocks, related fatigue, weather, or diet.
- Daily issues—ones that cause you to struggle emotionally, physically, or spiritually.
- Revelations—new discoveries about yourself or your relationships with others.
- Positive acclamations—victories and accomplishments, affirmations (covered in chapter 5).
- Diary—daily, weekly, and monthly.
- Hobbies—ones you can still do or ones you would like to learn.
- Short-term tasks and goals—need specific to-do list. Prioritize in order of importance. You can include tasks such as doctors appointments or household chores.
- Long-term goals—Take an inventory of life. Make lists of what you look forward to doing. Where do you want to be six months to a year from now?
- Spiritual—goals for the soul. You might want to write down a particular excerpt from a spiritual guidance book or tape, one you don't want to forget.
- Health and fitness—long-term goals for your body, mind, and spirit.

Forty Days and Forty Nights—Tips for Content and Accomplishment Goals

- Describe your ideal place to live.
- Describe yourself and draw a self-caricature.
- Describe someone else.
- Identify your creative self, talents, personal skills, and gifts.
- Write your own prayer.
- Write your own poem. (See the Useful Tools section at the end of this chapter.)

- Describe a special moment.
- Make a calendar for tasks.
- List the best events of the day, month, and year.
- List the worst events of the day, month, and year.
- List five things to do within the next three to five days.
- Write a letter to yourself that you will read in five, ten, or twenty years. Talk about who you are now and who you hope to be.
- Write a dialogue with another person, event, or thing.
- Have a positive dialogue with a part of your body.
- Have a dialogue with a famous person.
- Do something exceptional for someone else. In other words, "Pay it forward."
- Write a story about your life.
- Photograph a special person or special moment.
- Identify blocks to spiritual growth.
- List five reasons to stay with your significant other.
- What can you do to improve friendships?
- What has been lost?
- Body improvements—make plans for exercise and diet.
- Practice mindful exercises and identify how they work for you (see chapter 4).
- Make a list of things to do when in a flare.
- Identify things you never want to do again.
- Plan an outing.
- Write down things to laugh about.
- What makes you cry?
- What makes you happy?
- What makes you sad?
- Learn to meditate.
- Reflect on your support structure. What do you see as strengths and weaknesses? Note positive contributions you can make.
- How do you feel about therapies? Think about all of them when you consider this question.
- Who are your favorite people?
- Read a self-help book or listen to a tape once a month.
- Why do you like yourself?
- What do you like about someone else?
- What do you fear?
- List your reasons for being alive.

Your journal should include topics that relate to how well you know or would like to know yourself. Often it is easy to list what we should do to improve ourselves, but listing our strengths is more difficult. We all have them; for every negative, there is a positive. Focus on the pluses in your life. How can you use your resources and talents to contribute to others? Don't be modest. Tell the truth about what you can do.

Identify Your Blocks to Growth

It isn't uncommon for people with invisible diseases to experience feelings that block personal growth, such as abandonment, absentmindedness, anxiety, avoidance, blaming, insecurity, isolation, low self-confidence, low energy, lack of trust, complaining, conflict, criticism, defensiveness, denial, depression, fears, neediness, focusing on the past, moodiness, negativity, pain, resentment, and sadness.

Once you identify obstacles to spiritual enhancement, you will be better able to connect with your subconscious. People create blocks to personal growth subconsciously as an act of self-preservation, but in reality, these unconscious coping strategies may threaten the very thing they were developed to protect.

Identify Your Defense Mechanisms

Everyone develops defensive techniques to reduce anxiety and protect the ego. However, some may actually cause you to lose touch with your inner self (soul) and block awareness into who you really are. Once you identify your defense mechanisms, you can start to unravel the ways in which they affect your life, your subconscious, and your growth as a whole person—body, mind, and spirit.

Common defensive behavior patterns we develop to protect our ego and minimize anxiety:

- Accusing or blaming
- Acting out or tantrums
- Aggressiveness
- Arguing
- Avoidance or passivity
- Compensation—for a weakness in one area by excelling in another area, rather than working on the weakness
- Compromise—in an unhealthy way
- Complaining
- Confusion

- Denial—refusal or rejection of obvious implications or consequences of a thought, deed, or situation
- Isolation
- Projection—attributing one's own thoughts or impulses to another person
- Rationalization—attempting a logical explanation for behavior
- Regression
- Suppression—intentional denial of thoughts from consciousness

The best thing about the future is that it comes only one day at a time.

ABRAHAM LINCOLN

Making Plans

Goals are nothing more than plans for plans. Learn to set goals if you wish your journal to contain an action plan. Dr. Phil—Phillip C. McGraw, Ph.D.—says, "Know your goal, make a plan, and pull the trigger."[2]

---

external dialogue: a subjective communication, with or without words, intended to share information.

Setting Goals

Remember to "keep your eye on the target." Setting unrealistic goals only adds to defeat and feelings of inadequacy. However, goals are like the tide, in perpetual motion and subject to change. If something happens to your plan and you realize it may have been unrealistic, step back, regroup, and plan a new plan. You may have been overly optimistic. On the other hand, your target may be a reasonable one, but the outcome may take longer than anticipated to achieve. Learn to be flexible with yourself.

Keep in mind the first of author Stephen Covey's *Seven Habits of Highly Successful People:* "Begin with the end in mind."

Rules

1. Set goals that are specific and measurable so you know when you have achieved them.
   - Example: "Today I will vacuum up the popcorn spilled last night."

2. Get into action and perform the task. Determine the actions needed to help you achieve your goal.

- Example A. "I will use both hands to push the vacuum."
- Example B. "I will make one sweep forward and one sweep back, parallel across the living room one time."
- Example C. "I will rest at the first sign of fatigue and resume after the given rest period."

3. Evaluate. Did you accomplish your goal?
   - Yes—Acknowledge yourself for a job well done.
   - No—Reevaluate the plan. Perhaps you expected too much of yourself. (1) Did you set a realistic goal? Maybe you are coming down with the flu and your energy level has been impaired, or you didn't sleep last night. (2) Did you follow your plan or complicate it? Maybe you overdid and made more than one sweep? (3) Did you take adequate rest periods or did you try to push yourself?

Once you identify the flaw in your plan or in its execution, you can revise it for the next time. Now you can pat yourself on the back for recognizing that although you may not be perfect, you learned something. This should make you feel good about yourself.

Journal Accomplishments

- Identify aggravating factors
- Identify alleviating elements
- Track treatment successes and failures
- Work on issues that affect your being
- Guide wellness
- Understand self and others
- Set and achieve life goals
- Record events and relationships, and improve or release
- Promote problem solving
- Develop spontaneity and positive attitude
- Understand feelings and meaning
- Explore dreams
- Pinpoint and address stressors
- Communicate effectively with self
- Identify good things and growth
- Work through feelings safely
- Learn creativity
- Reevaluate beliefs and behaviors

Dr. Bernie Siegel, who believes in using the power of the mind to help heal, believes that a drawing is worth even more than the standard thousand words. Creating a picture bypasses the conscious state of mind and verbal deceptions.[3] You might want to consider using drawings in your journal to express how you feel on any given day, and then compare your inner feelings as a milestone to your progress.

Effective Communication

I have a place in my journal where I keep a general format for meetings with members of my health care team. It includes:

- The purpose of the meeting, whether pain, distress, or flare.
- Whom the meeting is with—doctor, therapist, or counselor.
- What I hope to gain from the meeting—feel better, learn to interact better with others, get answers about medications, evaluate therapy.
- What plans are put into place to effect change or accomplish the task, such as increase therapy sessions, start a new treatment plan, or increase pain management sessions.

My journal is always with me and when I am not thinking straight, this security allows me to stay focused. When brain fog takes over, instead of becoming overwhelmed and allowing negative internal dialogue, I pull out my journal and praise myself for being armed with the tools I need for the task.

Others are merely mirrors of you. You cannot love or hate something about another person unless it reflects something you love or hate about yourself.
CHÉRIE CARTER-SCOTT

A Place for Promoting, Building, and Releasing

Relationships with others may not always be what we want them to be. Energy is precious and is wasted on those who don't wish to be mutually supportive. (Soliciting support will be discussed later in this chapter.) You can identify specific potential support structures in your journal. In these pages you can evaluate relationships you'd like to promote, devise plans for building on relationships you wish to keep, and release those that are not mutually rewarding.

"To thine own self be true" was advice written by William Shakespeare. These words relate to a particular exercise given to me by my coauthor, friend, and former therapist. I keep it in my journal and refer to it frequently, and it's been immensely helpful in building relationships. Think before responding to others . . .

> Is it true?
> Is it kind?
> Is it necessary?

Soliciting the Support You Need

A real friend is one who walks in when the rest of the world walks out.

WALTER WINCHELL

While learning to cope with FM, CFID, and CMP and all of their complications, I found I was unconsciously pushing my family and friends away. I was unaware at the time that I was using a defense mechanism called "isolating." I was walling myself off from them, and them from me. After much research and therapy, I found this reaction to chronic illness is not unusual; it's typical. This is why learning how to create and maintain a sound support structure is so critical. Your "cheering section" can play an important role in how you react to your illness(es). Ask yourself, "How does my condition affect my spouse, significant other, family, coworkers, and friends?"

Your first goal should be to work on strengthening the support structure already in place. Once you are able to do that, you can tackle the weaker associations. With these disabling disorders you need to conserve your energy for relationships with people who want to support you. In return, you need to identify ways you can help others. A healthy support system requires you to give as well as receive.

Those closest to you also grieve for your former self. They have had to make adjustments to goals and dreams too, perhaps some rather significant ones. They have lost the family member or friend you were before the illness; your role in their lives is no longer the same. They need support, too. Our bodies may be sick, but we can maintain healthy relationships.

In the following excerpt from *Finding Strength in Weakness: Help and Hope for Families Battling Chronic Fatigue Syndrome*, author Lynn Vanderzalm gives couples some useful advice on how they can support each other in the face of one partner's illness.

A healthy partner can give reassurance that:

- They **believe you** when you say you are in pain.
- They will be there to **support you**.
- They are **responsive** to your needs in times of flare.
- They see you as a **valuable** part of your relationship with them.

A sick partner can give:

- **Honesty regarding how they feel**—neither exaggerating nor hiding the way they feel.
- **Commitment** to the relationship and the needs of the "healthy" partner.
- **Understanding** for what the healthy partner is going through.
- The **gift of saving energy** for the other person and contributing what you can.[4]

An intimate relationship is one that allows you to be yourself.

DEEPAK CHOPRA, M.D.

Ten Rules for Building Supportive Relationships

1. Keep information regarding your illness basic. Don't overwhelm family and friends with information unless they are ready to receive it.
2. Avoid feelings of isolation. Fibromyalgia, CFID, and CMP are invisible disorders. No one really knows how miserable you feel. When people look at you they cannot see your pain. You may begin to feel they don't believe you, which causes you to feel alone and isolated and can lead to depression. By talking to at least one supportive person, someone identified in your inventory list (discussed later in this section), you can release these feelings of isolation.
3. Keep your support structure trustworthy. Trust is built through behavioral action. If you use your support system as a place to vent negative feelings, it's not productive for you and it will wear down your support person and potentially damage the relationship. Your supporter should, in turn, provide you with positive stimulus. Ask for it. Most of all, do not turn your back or talk negatively about the person who is taking the time to be there for you.
4. Maintain a balance of friendships with people who are healthy. Look for support from people who have other common interests, perhaps at church, in philanthropy groups, at work, or in a babysitting co-op.

5. Once you have identified a strong support system, maintain it! Maintenance requires nurturing, including planned outings.

6. Don't expect others to read your mind. Do communicate your needs, whether it is help with household chores or just needing someone to listen. Have family meetings to communicate and educate your loved ones. Be patient and keep whining to a minimum. If you must complain, counter each complaint with a positive. "But" is a powerful word; use it to your advantage.

7. Plan activities or outings. List, plan, and act on fun things to do with a family member or friend. Include activities such as seeing a movie, listening to a favorite CD, having a massage, or having lunch with a friend. Plan to feel okay that day. There is no need to make clarifying statements such as, "If I feel okay, or if I'm able." If your communication has been effective, your supporter will understand that sometimes your condition is unpredictable. Of course, if you never show up, friends may question the validity of your complaints. Everyone, even a chemotherapy patient, is able to make it sometimes.

8. Write a letter to a support member. Sometimes putting words on paper can help you identify what your needs really are. Don't be a martyr or a hero. You can expect changes in attitude, but not without action. Your body is not the same as it was before FM, CFID, or CMP took over your life, but that doesn't mean you can't be a better person than you once were. You can choose to be a victim of your disorder, or to grow from it. Soliciting support requires change.

9. Write down your needs and let your loved ones know that you are accountable. Fatigue, irritability, agitation, and forgetfulness are symptoms of your disorder. Assist your helpmate or family members in recognizing your patience may run out too quickly, regardless of how much you wish otherwise. Theirs probably will too. It is okay to acknowledge it, so that it isn't personalized. Be clear that you don't expect your partner to fix your problem (although men are wired to fix things so it may be difficult for some men to accept the non-fixer role). You need your partner to feel free of guilt, and you must do the same. Let your loved ones know there is more to you than just your illness. Other facets of your being need nurturing, and so do the people in your life.

10. Let your partner or support person know you may need a reality check from time to time, and that you are okay with that. Then be okay with that! Chronic pain can blur rational thought and you may need a little guidance from time to time. Do not see their reminders as nagging, but

as helpful reminders. Recognize you really do make more mistakes when your pain and fatigue are out of control. Own it! Let your partner or friend know there may be times when you need space because you hurt too badly. Make sure the people you care about understand that your distance is because of your illness, not because of anything they have done.

These tips will help you regain some control in your life and in your relationships. You rule the pain. Don't let the pain rule you.

Sexual Connection

Make changes in sexual behavior to accommodate your needs and feelings of intimacy, as well as your partner's. Closeness and intimacy are important basic needs. The following advice from Carol Eustice will help you make adaptations necessary to meet your partner's needs and your own.[5]

- Plan sex for the time of day you generally feel best.
- Take medications to allow the peak of the dose to occur during sex.
- Avoid extra activity that might increase your level of fatigue.
- Do gentle exercises to relax and improve your range of motion.
- Take a warm bath or shower to soothe joints and muscles.
- Try new positions that might alleviate pain during sex.

Who's on Your Team?

Take an inventory of your strongest supporters. These are people or groups who give you strength, and may include:

- Immediate family
- Extended family
- Friends
- Employer
- Coworkers
- Support groups
- Medical personnel
- Spiritual groups

Take an inventory of those you consider least supportive—people or groups you consider to be a drain on your energy.

Make a list of potentially supportive people or groups. These are people with whom you share a common interest, such as an advocacy organization for your disorder. Don't leave out other potential interest groups like a photography, camping, or sewing clubs.

When eating a fruit, think of the person who planted the tree.

VIETNAMESE PROVERB

Requirements for Giving and Receiving Support

- Your support person should have the ability to listen without judging, criticizing, or giving advice, so that you feel free to express all feelings and emotions and feel safe without fear of jeopardy.
- You should be able to say to this person, "I just need you to listen today while I vent and express my feelings. Then I want to figure it out for myself."
- You should feel comfortable saying, "Today I'd like some feedback and advice. I need a reality check."
- Support should be reciprocal.
- Your best support person will want to learn about any factor or illness that influences your life.

A good supporter is someone you like, respect, and trust, and with whom you have good rapport and share common interests. It is someone with whom you feel absolutely comfortable. Everyone has needs that require words of encouragement and someone to listen, so expect to give support in order to receive it. Once you establish this two-way support system, you will receive the help you desire and enjoy the rewards of helping others.

Do something for somebody every day for which you don't get paid.

ALBERT SCHWEITZER

Write a letter to solicit support, keeping in mind that others may be struggling with problems and feelings of their own. Following is an example of a letter you might use.

Sample Letter Soliciting Support

Date

Dear _____,

Would you be my supporter, and in return, I will be yours?

It is necessary for me to have several support people so that no one person will feel *on call*. There will be times when I get myself into a pickle and you may be unavailable because of other commitments to work, vacation, or social engagements.

I am trying to get myself as healthy as possible—mind, body, and spirit—and see this as an opportunity to build new relationships and reinforce old ones. Getting support is important, but I also *need* to give it so that I can feel useful again.

We can set aside some private, uninterrupted time to discuss our challenging issues, whether we've been able to deal with them or not. (Keep a list or we'll both forget!) Let's make dates for outings we think would be fun or just would love to do. Let's also commit to impromptu talks in times of crisis.

It would be useful to have an agenda for our structured support meeting that includes:

- A reaffirmation statement regarding our rules of support.
- Stating clearly if we want advice or just need to vent.
- A list prioritizing what we want to talk about—the one created throughout the week, be it about work, relationships, coping with illness, or not coping with any or all of these.
- A piece of educational information regarding any illness or concerns. For instance, we might share, "I read a magazine article about migraines the other day," "I saw a report on global warming, and I wanted to get your take on it," or "My physical therapist said this exercise is good for everyone and I thought of you."
- A time limit for each person. Using a timer can help keep us on schedule.
- A coin toss to see who goes first.
- A list of good things about each other.
- A list of good things that happened during the week.
- Sharing what we've learned about each other's problems and illness.
- Clarification of what the other person shared.
- Sharing a new book, song, poem, or joke.
- A statement of personal goals for the next week.
- A date for something fun to do together.

The meetings can be weekly, biweekly, monthly, or variable, depending upon need and availability. The main rule is to set a time and stick to it, and remember that scheduled meetings are for mutual benefit and sharing.

If this sounds like something you would be interested in, please let me know.

Sincerely,

_____

Relationships

Having Them, Keeping Them, and Knowing When to Let Them Go

Retreat leader Toni Packer believes we learn about ourselves through relationships with others. She says, "In married life or in living together, we make each other over in our image, but we also find out about ourselves in each other, spaciously, freely."[6]

The Face of Two
She is a woman
She is a tear of forgiveness
She is weary, yet strong
She is the face of two

He is a man
He is a provider
He is weary, yet strong
He is the face of two

She is the heart
She is the gentle touch
She is the arms that comfort
She is the face of two

He is the shoulder to lean on
He is the companion
He is the hand that fixes things
He is the face of two

CELESTE COOPER

How does FM, CFID, or CMP affect your spouse, significant other, family and/or friends?

The actions and reactions of a significant other have a profound effect on forward momentum in disease management. It is a difficult variable to compute, and the range of reactions is enormous. My thinking was significantly shifted by Leo Buscaglia's first book, *The Disabled and Their Parents*.[7] It was also altered by my connections with the Handicapper's Alliance in Michigan, during my first job in psychotherapy.

How Significant Are Significant Others?

Buscaglia looks intently at the roles parents play in the identities adopted by all family members.[8]

The responses of parents initially set the stage for the identity formation of the person experiencing the disability. In our context, the significant other often sets the stage for an expected (and sometimes met) role for the FM, CFID, and CMP patient. This role might label the patient as victim, brave hero, noble sufferer, slacker, or a variation of one of those. The significant other's perception does not set the patient's role, but the patient's view of his or her role is affected by the way the other's views are interpreted The patient might rebel, comply, or spin sideways in response to the labeling.

Secondary Losses of People Disabled by Chronic Pain

- Anger/trivialization/rejection by family, friends, and physicians
- Complicated/frustrating tasks dealing with new bureaucracies
- Agonizing pain without medication; unpleasant side effects with medication
- Denial of legally entitled disability benefits[9]

The Human Factor

To love another person is to see the face of God.

VICTOR HUGO

My association with the Handicapper Alliance, a group of people who demanded to be addressed as "handicappers"—an active term suggesting the person who sets the odds—was liberating in my own identity as a human experiencing "disabilities." These women and men were the Black Panthers of the wheelchair/prosthetic/sensory impairment brigade.* Handicappers suggest the ability to affect positive action, as opposed to disabled, impaired, handicapped, deformed, and similar terms that are bogged down in negation and passive acceptance. The Handicappers Alliance's guidelines for dealing with the Temporarily Able Bodied (TAB), who are labeled normal, were hilarious. Accepting the statistical inevitable, they declared that any human who lives long enough will become dependent on prosthetics, mobility devices, and assistance from others. Hearing aids, glasses, false teeth, mechanical hips,

---

*The Handicapper Alliance has become a funded NGO in Lansing, Michigan, with the new name Capitol Area Center for Independent Living.

hearts, larynxes, walkers, wheelchairs, and nursing aids will be their lot. Thus they are currently temporarily able bodied, but will eventually join the majority of humans who require at least one "crutch" to function.

When You Meet Temporarily Able-Bodied People
A Handout Prepared by the Michigan Handicapper Alliance[10]

- First, remember that TABs are people. They are like anyone else except for the special limitations of their attitudes and self-image.
- TABs need not be ignored or denied between friends. While your relationship is developing, show friendly interest in him/her as a person and don't act or be afraid of being seen with that person in public.
- Be yourself when you meet a TAB.
- Talk about the same things you would with anyone else.
- Help them only when they request it. A TAB who falls may wish to get up without assistance, just as many handicappers prefer to get along without assistance. So offer help but wait for approval before giving assistance.
- Be patient. Let TABs set their own pace in walking or talking.
- Don't be afraid to laugh with them. TABs are people, too, but be careful to avoid making it look as though you might be laughing at them instead of with them.
- Don't stop and stare when you see TABs you don't know. They deserve the same courtesy any person should receive.
- Don't be overprotective or oversolicitous. Don't shower TABs with kindness.
- Don't ask embarrassing questions. A TAB who wants to tell you about his or her problems will bring up the subject.
- Don't offer pity or charity. TABs want to be treated as equals. They want a chance to prove themselves.
- Don't force TABs to stand and wait. They might prefer to sit and be comfortable.
- When dining with TABs don't offer help in cutting their food or make a fuss over them; they will ask you or a waiter if they need assistance.
- Don't make up your mind ahead of time about TABs. You might be surprised how wrong you are in judging their interests and abilities.
- Enjoy your friendship with TABs. Their philosophy and good humor will give you inspiration.

My current thinking on the role of significant others in the management of these conditions is informed by the vast differences in the perception and acceptance of limitations by those with the limitations (you), and those in their close proximity (mate, family, friends, neighbors, and associates).

Some common role types for significant others are as follows:

- The Psychotherapist knows what you should do and what you should be expected to contribute. Capable of pity or advice, inspiration, or criticism, the significant other playing the role of armchair psychologist does not fully grasp the experience you are having, but has an answer anyway.
- The Drill Sergeant assumes you need a couple of swift kicks in the derriere to "get over" the condition. This person says, "Buck up" and "Don't complain." Usually this is the person who would whine first, if faced with our challenges.
- The Second Victim is drenched in woe and sadness, and complains of a life derailed by another's illness. "Look at how your illness has affected me."
- Angry Person is the flip side of Second Victim, related to Drill Sergeant. "Your illness is not my fault and I refuse to let it affect my life."
- Mr.(s) Nice Guy: A noble effort is made, but it's not quite sincere or assistive. "Oh, I feel so bad that you can't get your groceries this week. Well, off to the mall now, talk later."
- A Listening Helpmate is the ideal—an endlessly patient best friend who accepts your assessment of what today's 100 percent is and offers encouragement without enabling helplessness. This is the one who says, "I understand you had a less than terrific day today, so how can I help you have a terrific tomorrow? I understand your need to be able to accomplish things on your own, how can I assist you in that?" If you've heard Bill Murray's very sensitive reading of *The Razor's Edge* by W. Somerset Maugham (no stranger to handicaps), you'll know what I mean.

Some of us just go along . . . until that marvelous day people stop intimidating us; or, should I say, we refuse to let them intimidate us.

PEGGY LEE

The Interactive Pain/Energy Meter (see p. 159) is a very useful tool for getting needed support from your significant other. Jeff brought up an important point during my therapy. As mentioned above, spouses or significant others often do not make the best supporters. We tend to think that since they live with us, they should be able to see our pain and dysfunction. *Wrong!* Jeff gave me a helpful chart to post on the fridge. My family's is tailored to camping in the Colorado mountains, since that's something we enjoy doing, but you can tailor your chart to your interests.

Jeff suggested I denote my worst day as "semi-terrific," indicating a day with little to no energy and a lot of pain. My initial response was to think, "Are you nuts? You apparently don't understand either." But Jeff knew that using the word *bad* would make me feel even worse because there is a mind-body connection—my body would literally believe every word I said. That was several years ago. At that particular time I had been dealing with the pain and complications of CMP for some fifteen years, but had just been diagnosed with FM and was in the throes of depression as a result of my physical illnesses.

Posting your pain and energy meter where your family can access it gives everyone the information they need. It will help them in assessing the right time to approach you with help they may need, and let them know when to offer needed support. This tool helps your mate refrain from an enabling relationship and lets your family know when you are able to make contributions, which will improve your feelings of self worth. It will help you to avoid energy drains and promote positive communication among all parties involved.

You can also use this data to chart medium- and long-term trends in pain and energy level. This tool may be invaluable in assessing the impact of any treatment change if you chart it in your journal. You might surprise yourself. You could find you really are getting along better (this month) when your (immediate) perception is not so bright. I'd recommend running an average daily score over weeks and months, paying careful attention to any change in treatment or other notable conditions.

Making our needs known and being receptive to the needs of others affects productive communication and brings about constructive relationships. It is important to remember that listening is just as significant as being heard. Building an enduring support system will not only promote a better understanding by others, but for others in return.

It Takes Two to Tango—You and Your Mate

You never understand a person until you consider things from his point of view.

Harper Lee

It is very easy to blame and point fingers when you are in chronic pain. You have heard that old homily, "What goes around comes around." Negativity breeds negative reactions and positivism breeds positive responses.

So, how do you relate to your mate or significant other? If you are having difficulty, maybe the exercise "It Takes Two to Tango" on page 160 will help. Both you and your mate should complete this lesson.

The exercise is a very difficult one in terms of being able to accept criticism, own it, and do something about it. Remember, constructive criticism is beneficial. The study of human behavior—psychology—has determined we dislike in someone else things we dislike about ourselves. You, of course, do not leave the toilet seat up. But you do leave the lid up, the garage door open, or the back door unlocked. There is a shift in what, where, or when, but the category of "unwitting mistakes" is yours, too, or it wouldn't mean anything to you.

Airing your thoughts and feelings will help your relationship to grow, and if it's worth having, it's worth the work. You and your significant other can learn a great deal if you complete the lesson honestly.

The Power of Support

As Bill Withers wrote in a song, "We all need somebody to lean on." If pride comes between you and asking for help from someone, try this little exercise I call "switching shoes." How do you feel when a friend, or even a stranger, asks for your help? Are you annoyed, angered, or put upon? Do you despise the other person as weak or incompetent? Of course not! (If you answered yes, go see a therapist immediately.) You treasure the opportunity to be of service. You relish being part of a solution and you cherish that "thank you" you receive in turn. Why would you deny another person this kind of gratification? Others will leap to help you if only they hear a request, just as you would.

Advocacy—A Constructive Way to Vent

If the creator had a purpose in equipping us with a neck, he surely meant us to stick it out.

ARTHUR KOESTLER

The Foundation

The foundation of advocacy includes raising public awareness, promoting research funding, obtaining proper treatment, and asking for adequate support from family and friends.

People who survive despite illness make the best advocates. We survivors are the only ones who know what it is like to live with FM, CFID, and/or CMP. We are better prepared for the task of spreading the word, and can educate others about raising awareness for our cause.

An article on fibromyalgia published in a prominent women's magazine thrilled and appalled me at the same time. After reading the article I found it was only partially informative, which left me feeling ambivalent about the content. The article gave the impression that if you take a pill before sleep, exercise, and go to work, you will be just fine. While this is partially true for some, it neglected to detail what one endures when traditional treatments fail.

Additionally, the article did not address the feelings of isolation, the numerous medication trials, or the devastating depression that results from inadequate pain control or inappropriate responses from others. There are those of us who have a healthy diet and lifestyle, stretch daily, meditate, get massages, and develop healthy coping mechanisms through psychotherapy. Yet we are still unable to function or experience quality of life, because of chronic pain, fatigue, and other coexisting conditions. I thought the article should have included some statement for those of us with a more complicated health status.

A friend shared this article with me. She had now been misinformed, and I felt it my duty to provide her with accurate information. I wanted her to have all the facts before speaking out. Even though she does not have any of these three illnesses, she is now a staunch advocate and supporter. It is important to seize the opportunity to vent our feelings constructively when we see misinformation proliferating. By correcting inaccurate or incomplete information, we can turn negative energy into a positive force.

Great works are performed not by strength, but by perseverance.

SAMUEL JOHNSON

The Tools

- Join organizations that address your specific needs, such as your local FM, CFID, or chronic pain foundations. This not only provides a support structure, but also a collective partnership for educating those who would otherwise remain ignorant. These organizations can provide valuable information regarding our conditions and how to advocate.
- Share brochures or educational information with those who express interest in learning more, such as family, friends, health care providers, coworkers, or civic and religious associations. You would be surprised at the opportunities. I have handed out cards with my website address at restaurants, stores, the doctor's office, and even in parking lots. Organizations listed in the resource section will support you in your endeavors and provide brochures.
- Write letters to organizations that provide research for chronic pain disorders, such as the National Fibromyalgia Alliance, The CFID Foundation, or the Chronic Pain Relief Coalition. (Contact information is located

in the resource section at the end of this book.) Ask how you or your organization or support group can raise funding for research and public awareness.

- Become politically active.
  - Support lobbyist activities in Congress and the National Institutes of Health.
  - Find out who your senators and legislators are (contact information is in the resource section) and write advocacy letters to them (see an example in the useful tools section at the end of this chapter). Find out which bills they support, such as the Patients' Bill of Rights, Social Security, and where they stand on health care. Let them know how you feel about their work.
  - Familiarize yourself with your state's laws regarding disability and chronic pain.
- Write letters to health care organizations, such as the American Medical Association, the American Osteopathic Association, nursing organizations, and the National Institutes of Health (contact information is in the resource section).
- Write letters to the insurance commissioner regarding lack of provision for insurance codes.
- Create a petition, get it signed, and send it to your local representatives.
- Write letters of thanks to those who help.

During your advocacy you may meet some resistance. If this happens, remember to stay calm, stick to the facts, and don't take it personally.

Always do good. It gratifies some and mystifies the rest.

MARK TWAIN

Summary Exercise: Reaction to Interaction

1. Identify three blocks to growth that you experience. (For example, abandonment, absentmindedness, anxiety, avoidance, blaming, insecurity, isolation, low self-confidence, low energy, lack of trust, complaining, conflict, criticism, defensiveness, denial, depression, fear, feeling needy, focusing on the past, moodiness, negativity, pain, resentment, or sadness.)

_____

_____

_____

2. Define the difference between external and internal communication.

_____

_____

_____

3. Identify at least one person or group to give you the support you need, and set a goal for interacting with that person or group.

Person/group

_____

Target date for interaction

_____

4. List at least three goals for your journal that will be positive key points of effective communication for internal and external dialogue.

_____

_____

_____

5. On a separate piece of paper or in your journal, write a letter to yourself that you will read in five, ten, or twenty years. Talk about who you are now and who you hope to be at that future time.

6. Write at least five of the ten rules for building supportive relationships.

_____

_____

_____

_____

_____

7. On a separate piece of paper, write your own poem (see Useful Tools section for guidelines).

8. List at least two reactions you might have when you meet temporarily able-bodied people.

_____

_____

9. List at least two tips for effective advocacy.

_____

_____

10. The resource section at the end of this book includes listings and contact information for a wide variety of advocacy groups that promote awareness of invisible disorders. It also provides information on how to contact members of the U.S. Congress for your district and provides contact information for other government agencies and departments, such as the Social Security Administration, the U.S. Department of Health and Human Services, the U.S. Department of Education, and the U.S. Department of Labor. Take a look at the resource section and list below several resources that you could use in your advocacy campaign—include advocacy groups, lawmakers, and public servants who make public policy related to our cause.

_____

_____

_____

_____

11. Using the advocacy letter example provided in the following Useful Tools section, list four tips for planning your letter.

_____

_____

_____

_____

Useful Tools
for
Inner and Outer Self-Expression

Included here are four tools that will help you develop your skills of self-expression: tips for creating poetry to describe your feelings; handy ways of alerting your family to your fluctuating levels of pain and energy; practice exercises for honest communication with your partner; and suggestions for effectively advocating for yourself in the wider political arena.

- A Baker's Dozen—Thirteen Tips for Expressing Your Feelings through Poetry
- Interactive Pain/Energy Meter
- It Takes Two to Tango—Rules for Possibly the Most Important Date in Your Relationship
- Sample Advocacy Letter

A Baker's Dozen
Thirteen Tips for Expressing Your Feelings through Poetry

1. Imagine yourself somewhere—in a forest, on a beach, at a party—anywhere.

2. Write down sentences about two things you see, such as a pine tree, a beach ball, people, a traffic signal. Begin the lines with the words "I see."

3. Write down two things you hear, such as birds chirping, waves crashing to shore, people talking, or a siren. Begin the lines with "I hear."

4. Write down two things you smell, for example, the scent of pine, salt in the air, acrid smoke, or food cooking.

5. Write down two things you can feel—the texture of tree bark, of a rock, someone's skin, and so on.

6. Randomly pick at least two adjectives, for example, colors or shapes, to describe your nouns; and at least two adverbs—loudly, quickly (or similar)—to describe your action words.

7. Write down three pairs of rhymes, such as sun/fun, friend/lend, tree/free, tall/small, high/dry, cry/sigh, rhyme/time.

8. The last line or your poem should reflect how you feel in response to what you see, touch, smell, and hear—your emotions. Does it make you feel happy, sad, comforted, remorseful, pained, pain-free, tired, rested, anxious, calm, agitated, or serene? Use words like those you found in chapter 2 for describing your symptoms.

Spiffing It Up

9. Return to the lines you wrote and replace the "I see," "I hear," "I smell," and "I feel," with the objects, adjectives, and adverbs you wrote. For instance: green, cone-shaped prickly pine trees; loudly crashing cool waves; screeching sirens. As your poem is being born, you may decide to recreate your rhymes, adjectives, and adverbs. It's your poem, so feel free to allow your creative juices to flow.

10. Return to each line and add similes and metaphors.

    *   A simile is a figure of speech that compares two nouns that are not alike, such as trees and sun.

        "The trees are like sentries blocking access to the forest."

    *   A metaphor is a term or phrase used to suggest a likeness that is more symbolic than literal.

        "The chirping birds are balm to my soul."

11. Now personalize what you have written, using words like my, they, her, and we.

12. Add rhyme, using your pairs.

13. And lastly, create a tempo. Tempo (meter) is the rhythm (as in music) of the words. It can be regular: /// /// ///; or regularly irregular: // /// // ///.

Poetry can be a way of expressing your feelings. Feelings are an important part of who we are, and writing about them can have an impact on you, regardless of your experience at being a poet. Poetry can have an impact on both the poet and the reader.

Interactive Pain/Energy Meter

Feel free to photocopy the pain/energy meter below. Cut the black arrow out and fasten it to the black spot with a paper fastener that allows rotational movement. You can post the meter on your refrigerator and use it to communicate your day-to-day levels of pain and energy to your family.

PAIN/ENERGY METER

Danger
MODERATE
Pain is noticeable but
tolerable.
My energy level is
about 60%.

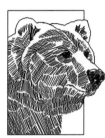
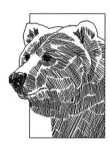

Danger
HIGH
Pain is less than
tolerable.
My energy token is
jammed in the "get up
and go" meter.

Danger
LOW
"Go for it!"

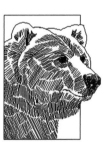

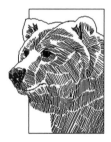

Danger
VERY HIGH
Pain level is a TEN
and I need to keep
my complaints
company today.

It Takes Two to Tango
Rules for Possibly the Most Important Date in Your Relationship

Stop! This exercise requires two people. (If you're single, no problem. You won't need to do this exercise.)

Sit down and make a list of the things your mate does that irritate you, or that provoke a response you're not proud to acknowledge. You can add to it as issues arise. There is no magic number.

Now go back to the beginning of your list and identify how your mate's behaviors make you feel inside. Do they make you feel angry, agitated, untrusting? You get the drift.

Make a date to sit down and review your lists together. Make it at a time when you know you will not be interrupted. *Do not* discuss what is on this list prior to your date.

Before your "date," sit down and prioritize your list, putting the most important issues at the top.

Set a time limit for "the date," such as fifteen minutes, an hour, or whatever works best for you. This date could get exhausting, especially if you are already fatigued and in pain.

Make a commitment not to interrupt the other person. Take turns, one item at a time from each list. *Don't interrupt!*

After presenting each item, one at a time, allow your partner a rebuttal.

Partner—when responding, focus on your mate's feelings, not the deed.

Limit your discussion to no more than the first three items on your list, depending upon the time you have set. The remaining items will wait until the next date, and by then the order of priority may have changed, depending upon what happens between now and then.

Discover what is at the "heart" of the matter.

Last but certainly not least: *Each of you should end every date with acknowledgment of at least one positive feeling about your mate.* Now, add that remark to the top of your agenda/list for the next meeting, and begin the next meeting with acknowledgment of that positive statement.

You might find your priorities changing. This doesn't mean you can't backslide; we are all human. But now you have a tool to help you work as "soul mates."

Sample Advocacy Letter

You can use the sample letter below as a model for personal advocacy letters to send to elected representatives, members of health commissions, hospital directors, health care providers, or anyone else in a position to affect health care policy.

Date

Organization name

Address

Dear Gentlemen and Gentlewomen,

[*State the purpose of your letter.*]

I see an escalating problem with treatment by managed care health organizations of patients who have fibromyalgia, chronic fatigue immunodysfunction, and chronic myofascial disease.

At a time when health care costs are skyrocketing, we are being treated inappropriately for our overwhelming pain and fatigue. Some inappropriate therapies are not only costly, they make our symptoms worse and compound our difficulty with normal activities of daily living. Many of us have been denied our rights to appropriate pain management. Awareness and education is greatly lacking in the health care community, the work place, the public arena, and among those who write the laws that affect us directly.

[*Make it personal. State your personal experience with your disorder and how it has affected your quality of life. Include the onset, your symptoms, and how you have been physically and emotionally treated. Then state what you would like in response.*]

It is my hope that you will help us make a difference by listening to our plight, speaking out, and providing education to those who hold our care in their hands.

[*Provide the opportunity for follow-up.*]

If I can provide you with further information regarding these disorders, I would be happy to do so. Please contact me at [*List your full name, address, and any other information you feel comfortable giving out, such as e-mail address, phone number, or fax.*]

Sincerely,

Signature [*Type or sign your name here.*]

Attachments: [*Name any attachments that support your letter and its content.*]

4
My Body Is Matter and It Matters

This chapter is dedicated to helping you understand what specific actions you can take to improve pain management and your quality of life. You will be able to:

- Identify elements of good sleep hygiene.
- Complete a dietary assessment.
- Identify how to make changes to accommodate your needs, and determine what therapies or treatments would be most beneficial for you.
- Review and define the differences between alternative medicine and complementary alternative medicine (CAM), and what is available in each.
- Review the importance of different treatment modalities that can help you improve the way you feel. You will be able to:
  - Select which treatments are most beneficial for your disorder(s).
  - Note dietary factors that may affect your well-being.
  - Evaluate the benefits of treatment by physiatrists (rehabilitation physicians), pain management specialists, psychologists, chiropractors, myofascial release therapists, and other health care providers.
  - Evaluate alternative therapies such as reflexology, yoga, t'ai chi, stretching, acupuncture, massage therapy, spray and stretch, bodywork, trigger point therapy, self-hypnosis, biofeedback, and other miscellaneous treatments.

Chronic pain, regardless of its origin, affects a person's whole being to some extent. Learning what you can do to be emotionally, mentally, physically, and spiritually complete will result in an amazing outcome.

Recognizing different healing methods and incorporating them into your care plan can have a positive effect on your life.

Understanding and Treating Pain

The study of pain is called *algology,* and someone who is a student, investigator, or practitioner of algology is called an *algologist*. Therefore, in a way, we are all algologists. Who makes a better student of pain than someone who lives with it every day?

Freedom from pain should be a basic human right limited only by our ability to achieve it.

ARTHUR LIPMAN, PHARM.D. (NOVEMBER 2001 AMERICAN
COLLEGE OF RHEUMATOLOGY SYMPOSIUM)

Algologists describe pain as "an unpleasant sensory or emotional experience primarily associated with tissue damage." The pain of FM and CFID is thought to be central pain associated with a messaging problem in the central nervous system. The origin of pain in chronic myofascial pain is related to trigger points in the muscles.

Pain can result from a decreased pain threshold and improper control of aggravating factors. A decrease in the pain threshold means it takes a lesser stimulus than normal to initiate the pain response for that individual. Any time one of the aggravating factors is not addressed, you are at risk for a flare. This is a period when the discomfort intensifies beyond the normal boundaries of a person's chronic pain.

---

acute pain: a pain response with rapid onset.

chronic pain: pain that has exceeded its benefit as a warning sign to an acute problem.

Pain intolerance happens when you are bombarded by painful stimuli or impulses. As a result, your other body systems start to break down. Severe pain can become so extreme that it can cause vomiting or total decompensation—losing all defense mechanisms and grasp on reality. Chronic pain can be life threatening when it reaches proportions of great magnitude. In their article "Pathological Pain," C. R. Chapman and M. Stillman say, "Moderate or severe persisting pain of long duration that disrupts sleep and normal living ceases to serve a protective function and instead degrades health and functional capacity."[1] Treatments for FM, CFID, and CMP may not totally eradicate pain, but can help decrease its severity to a tolerable level. Once you know how to identify your condition or conditions and aggravating factors, you are better able to manage your pain and take care of yourself.

Quality of life is affected by the ability to carry on activities of daily living, and people with chronic pain disorders use many adaptive strategies to cope with their pain and fatigue. This section will give you some options for improving the quality of your life.

Treatment goals are to decrease pain, improve function, diminish fatigue, and improve mental outlook and inner strength. Some treatments may overlap, just as symptoms do. Treatment should be tailored to your specific needs.

Before you continue, take an inventory of your known precipitating events, including triggers and aggravating factors. Keep in mind that some therapies may help one condition but aggravate another. It is more difficult when you have more than one of the three major disorders or several coexisting conditions. Let your body be the best gauge for your tolerance or intolerance to new therapies.

Introduce new treatments one at a time, as you do when starting new medications. You need to be able to evaluate the benefit or intolerance logically. If the intervention is beneficial, incorporate it into your treatment plan. After gaining some proficiency at your new therapy, you can look at initiating another one.

There is no universal treatment plan for managing pain and sleep disturbances, the two primary concerns for people with FM, CFID, and CMP. All therapies and treatments are aimed at relieving pain and/or sleep problems. You can learn to make changes in the way you deal with disordered sleep and fatigue, and you can learn to control pain instead of the pain controlling you. Intermittent pain happens to everyone; acute pain is a warning sign that something is wrong and you should pay attention. For those of us who experience pain every day, learning to accept it can be a difficult challenge, but achievable. What we don't have to do is allow it to negatively affect us emotionally, mentally, or spiritually. When we realize we have to accept having pain in our lives, we can be successful in minimizing our symptoms.

Improving Sleep

Sleep deprivation can affect your mental, physical, emotional, and spiritual health. The immune response is weakened, leaving you more susceptible to other diseases[2] and lowering your pain threshold.[3]

Sleep deprivation also has an effect on pain and can interfere with the therapeutic effects of pain medication. It is not known if this is due to a decrease in the quality (that is, appropriate sleep stages) or quantity of restful sleep.[4] We must do the best we can at promoting good sleep habits.

A normal sleep pattern progresses through several stages, or cycles, throughout the sleep period. We tend to traumatize soft tissue throughout the day when we overexert, and a disruption in our sleep pattern may prevent adequate healing.[5]

Sleep abnormalities include inability to fall asleep, difficulty staying asleep, and poor quality of sleep. Other sleep factors that can affect some people are physical obstructions to breathing or abnormal breathing patterns.

Treating sleep disorders starts with examining any underlying causes, which could include periodic limb movement, restless leg syndrome, sleep apnea, teeth grinding, or pain.

A study done by Gold, Dipalo, Gold, and Broderick concluded that inspiratory sleep airflow in women with fibromyalgia is limited, which may explain the effect of abnormal sleep on their somatic (physical) complaints.[6] Studies are also in progress that will help correlate sleep problems to the symptoms described by patients with CFID.[7]

---

somatic: pertaining to, or characteristic of, the body (soma).

Fibromyalgia and chronic fatigue immunodysfunction are associated with complaints of sleep disruption or not feeling rested, but they are not considered sleep disorders.[8] Studies show head and neck myofascial pain patients and patients with FM experience sleep disruption,[9] as do those with temporomandibular dysfunction and chronic daily headaches.[10] One would conclude that people with disorders that cause pain have difficulty with sleep. This doesn't mean that if you have a sleep disorder, such as sleep apnea, you will get FM, CFID, or CMP. Drs. Millott and Berlin suggest that a "combination of pharmacotherapy, physical therapy, and patient education, along with positive sleep hygiene habits, play an important role" in helping with sleep disruption.[11]

Sleep retraining may be indicated when your internal clock (circadian rhythm) is off kilter. Melatonin is a brain chemical produced when the brain receives a signal from the eye that daylight is ending. In contrast, when your brain perceives the light impulse, melatonin production shuts down and allows you to awaken. This is why it is important to maintain regular sleep habits. Shift workers often experience adverse symptoms from disruption to the body's normal circadian rhythm.[12]

Following are some suggestions to help you maintain your internal clock:

Preparing for Bed

- Avoid alcohol or nicotine near bedtime.
- Keep caffeine use to a minimum. Limit intake after mid-morning.
- Be aware that prescription and over-the-counter preparations may include stimulants that can interfere with sleep.
- Sleep in a comfortable bed, one that will help decrease pressure on the oversensitive tissue of FM, decrease pressure on the trigger points of CMP, and promote sleep for those who suffer CFID. This may include a firm or semi-firm mattress, free of lumps and bumps. The use of a lamb's wool pad, a heated waterbed, a foam rubber pad, or an air mattress can help with pressure points.
- Sleep in a bedroom that is at a comfortable temperature.
- Keep a routine bedtime ritual. This could include drinking a soothing bedtime tea (being careful not to overconsume and prompt unwanted nighttime trips to the bathroom), reading a book, taking a warm bath, meditating, listening to soothing music, or using guided relaxation imagery CDs.
- Avoid using too many pillows. A cervical pillow may help support your neck and decrease unwanted stress on your neck muscles; just make sure it is the right size for your body type.
- Sleep in a quiet place. Use earplugs if needed to obscure any sounds that interfere with relaxation, including a snoring bed partner, whether feline, canine, or human.
- Reduce external stimuli.
- Keep a sleep schedule. This includes retiring at the same time each evening and awakening at the same time each morning.
- Avoid late evening conversation or thoughts that are known to cause stress.
- Journal any activities planned for the next day or week so your mind can be clear of any tasks you think you might forget.
- Reserve the last hour before bedtime to do nothing. Activities should be only those that aid in relaxation. Relaxation activities not only calm the muscles, they also promote sleep by decreasing emotional stress.

- Avoid large evening meals, especially two to three hours before bedtime. Digestion can prevent sleep and increase risk of reflux of digestive enzymes into the esophagus, causing indigestion and other unwanted gastrointestinal symptoms.
- If you sleep with an electric blanket, turn it on thirty minutes before going to bed to avoid muscle chill.
- Avoid any exercise or activities that increase heart rate for four hours before bedtime. While exercise increases our body's own painkillers (endorphins), it also stimulates the nervous system.
- Maintain proper body alignment for the night by not lying on your stomach, and using proper body posture. The idea is to keep your spine straight. While lying on your side, keep your knees slightly bent and together. Your body should not look like a pretzel. If you can, use a body pillow that will also keep your shoulders and hips in alignment. Your neck should be in a neutral position, so make sure your pillow doesn't kink your neck. If you lie on your back to sleep, keep the same principles in mind. You can keep your spine straight with a cervical pillow under your neck and another pillow under your knees. Avoid holding your arms close to your sides or clenching your fists. These interventions help eliminate overstretching or shortening of muscles during sleep.
- Practice abdominal breathing exercises or just concentrate on the act of breathing.
- Think boring thoughts or focus on the inhale and exhale of your breath.

A HELPFUL ACRONYM FOR SLEEP HYGIENE

Schedule bedtime
Limit physical activity
Use comfort measures
Meditate
Breathe
Eliminate stress and food
Remember nothing—clear your mind

It is important to understand that although good sleep hygiene increases the likelihood of achieving sleep, sleep will not resolve your other symptoms.[13] Studies indicate imbalanced melatonin regulation and alpha-delta sleep disturbances are not clinical indications in disorders such as FM and CFID, respectively.[14] This is why just treating your sleep problems will not make all your other symptoms, mainly pain, go away. However, getting the proper amount of rest will make your other symptoms more manageable.

Medication and Supplements

We are all complex individuals with different coexisting conditions and may require medications not normally used to treat one condition alone. We may need pharmacology that treats coexisting conditions. Because new pharmaceutical products are developed almost weekly, the list would be too exhaustive to include here. That is why I have listed them according to their drug category. Your physician or pharmacist should be knowledgeable regarding individual responses to each class of drug. It may take a while to find the right combination of medications for you. From time to time you may need to adjust your individualized medication plan. Following are the drug categories (classes) you might use, depending on your diagnosis.

- Allergy drugs (for treatment of coexisting symptoms in FM and CFID)
- Analgesics (FM, CFID, CMP)
- Antianxiety medications (FM, CFID)
- Anticonvulsants (FM)
- Antidepressants (FM, CFID)
- Antihypotensives (FM, CFID)
- Anti-microbial (CFID)
- Antivirals (CFID)
- Muscle relaxants (FM, CFID, CMP)
- Nonsteroidal anti-inflammatory drugs (CFID)
- Sleep agents (FM, CFID, CMP)

analgesia: the absence of a pain response to a type of stimulation that would normally be painful, particularly without loss of consciousness.

Take your prescription medications as directed and do not share your medications with others, or take other medications without your physician's knowledge. Certain medications have potentially lethal interactions with one another. This includes over-the-counter (OTC) medications, herbs, and vitamins. The quantity of a medication isn't the only thing that can cause unwanted side effects; negative interactions between medications and sup-plements can also occur. Some therapeutic doses of medications become life threatening when used in combination with certain other medications. If you have any questions regarding the safety of your medication combinations, please discuss them with your doctor or pharmacist.

It is also important to remember not to crush or cut your medication unless specifically told to do so. Some may release dangerous or toxic amounts into your body if their time-release properties are manipulated.

Educate yourself regarding the side effects of your medications and know which ones you should report to your doctor. With prescription costs sky-rocketing, pharmacy shopping may save you money. Just be sure each phar-macist has your complete, up-to-date medication list, including medication allergies.

If you feel you need a dosage change, talk it over with your doctor first. *Do not* stop or increase the dose of your medications. The chemical structure of some medications can make abrupt withdrawal serious, and possibly life threatening.

Pay close attention here. Educate yourself on the use of drug combi-nations. Over-the-counter and prescription medications can have more than one active ingredient in the same tablet or capsule. Because of their analgesic qualities, acetaminophen (the active ingredient in Tylenol), non-steroidal anti-inflammatories, and aspirin are commonly used in combina-tion preparations for headaches, colds, and allergy symptoms. For example, Tylenol #3 is acetaminophen with codeine. Acetaminophen and codeine are both active ingredients. Nighttime "sleep and don't wake up with a headache medicine" is Tylenol (acetaminophen) with Benadryl (diphen-hydramine), also both active ingredients. Why is this important to you? The same active ingredient in one medication (in this case, acetaminophen) may also be present as an active ingredient in another. You could be tak-ing regular Tylenol for pain, a cold remedy that includes acetaminophen, an antihistamine with acetaminophen, and decongestant with acetamino-phen. You could potentially overdose on acetaminophen without realizing it. The damage does not have to be immediately life threatening. Organ damage from too much of something can occur gradually. You might not even know it is happening until that organ ceases to function properly, if at all. Serious interactions can occur with medications, supplements, and herbal remedies. There are so many medications on the market that you are at risk unless you understand what your medications are, what they are for, and what they contain. Your pharmacist needs to know the names of *all* your medications, so that those databases can be checked. Your motto should be, "When in doubt, check it out."

The only pain that is tolerable is somebody else's.

DAVID SHERRY, M.D. (PEDIATRIC RHEUMATOLOGIST)

Opioids

Opioids are considered narcotics and can be either synthetic or naturally occurring chemicals that reduce pain and produce a sedative effect. Because the use of opioids for treatment of chronic pain is controversial, there needs to be a more in-depth study of its use in nonmalignant pain disorders, such as FM, CFID, and CMP.

Opioids are stringently regulated by the Drug Enforcement Agency (DEA). Because of federal regulations, the DEA functions as a watchdog over physicians and their prescribing practices. Doctors can get into serious legal trouble, even to the point of losing their licences, for prescribing opioids to people who don't really need them, that is, to people who want to use them as recreational drugs. This makes some doctors hesitant to prescribe narcotic medications for pain, even when they think their patient can benefit from them. However, the Joint Commission on Accreditation of Healthcare Organizations (JCAHO), the largest hospital-credentialing agency in the United States, has set new standards. Their emphasis is on the evaluation and management of pain and the patient's rights to appropriate assessment.[15]

To some extent, your physician may feel caught in this struggle between undertreatment of pain and DEA regulations. Doctors do have recourse in dealing with the DEA, if they document their prescribing practices correctly.[16] Because of lawsuits regarding undertreatment of pain and the threat of DEA scrutiny, some doctors have backed away from any pain treatment at all by outsourcing patients to pain management specialists. Problems arise when the patient does not have financial resources or the patient's insurance coverage restricts primary doctor referrals.

One more reason physicians are reluctant to treat pain with narcotic pain medication is their invalidated fear of patients' becoming "addicted."[17] Very few receive extensive medical education on pain management. If they did, they would realize that tolerance is not addiction.

Our bodies learn to tolerate many medications. The big drive for chronic pain management is to prescribe antiseizure or other central nervous system disorder medications.[18] Even though the new drug Lyrica (pregabalin), an antiseizure medication, has passed clinical trials, has been approved, and has been shown to be beneficial for treatment in some FM patients,[19] not all patients tolerate the side effects. As we all know, many new FDA approved drugs don't get the real test until the public starts using them. If they work for you, I'm glad, but please be aware that some of these medications can have serious side effects, more serious than constipation or euphoria. Psychotropic drugs, for example, have the ability to interact with many other medications, yet they are liberally prescribed for pain without consideration of the consequences. Pharmaceutical companies are encouraging their use to treat some conditions that may not have not been proven in clinical trials, which makes me wonder if they are exploiting the public for financial gain. I will probably have stones thrown at me for saying this, but when this is allowed to happen it makes me doubtful whether "the big boys," the FDA, are really worried about the safety of medications coming from other countries. These new psychotropic drugs have the potential to induce euphoria, as do opioids, until the body learns to tolerate them, yet in the case of psychotropic drugs, the euphoric effect may never go away. Care must also be taken not to discontinue them abruptly. While this class of medication is beneficial for some, it doesn't meet the needs of all patients. Many anticonvulsants and psychotropic drugs have not been proven for use as pain medication,[20] yet there is never hesitation to prescribe them over opioids, which have been used for hundreds of years. Many antidepressants used to treat sleep disruption also have the propensity to cause side effects. Sometimes your body learns to tolerate them, sometimes it does not. Does taking these medications that can cause withdrawal symptoms make you a drug addict? Somehow, I think not. If you do not have a drug addiction history, you should not be denied pain control with the use of opioids because of someone else's fear that you will become addicted. After all, medication that targets pain should be the first line drug for treating pain.[21]

Addictive behavior is not a common finding in chronic pain patients,[22] and unlike the patient who struggles with chemical dependency, the use of opioids and other medications for treatment of chronic pain actually improves the patient's ability to function.[23]

The Pain Patient (Pseudo-addiction)
- Medications improve their quality of life. They are in control of their medications.
- The pain patient will want to decrease the medication if side effects are present.

- The pain patient is concerned about physical problems.
- The pain patient follows the contract for the use of opioids. (Pain specialists will most likely have you sign a contract with them stating that you will follow their prescribing instructions.)
- The pain patient will have medication left over.

The Addict

- The medications cause a decreased quality of life. An addict is out of control with medication.
- The addict will want to continue medication regardless of side effects.
- The addict is in denial.
- The addict doesn't follow the contract for the use of opioids.
- The addict doesn't have medication left over. Addicts lose prescriptions and always have a story.

The preceding lists are an excerpt from Fibromyalgia Network, April, 2001, based on Dr. Heit's work at the Georgetown University School of Medicine (2001) and Dr. Heit's presentation, "Opioid Prescribing: An Update on Clinical, Ethical and Legal Guidelines" from the *Journal of Law, Medicine & Ethics,* 22(3) 252–56, (Fall) 1994.[24]

Risks and Benefits

Even chronic pain patients with a history of addiction can be successfully managed with opiate analgesia.[25] Remember, improving function is the goal of all treatment, and this includes the medications you use to control pain. If your medication is not helping you improve function, regardless of the drug class (antidepressant, antiseizure, or narcotic), then you should not take it for pain.

Narcotics also come with unwanted baggage. Opioid analgesics may interfere with restorative sleep and cause constipation, and some types may cause rebound headaches. This is why they are reserved as the medication of last resort. However, most leading authorities in pain management recognize the need for their use to control chronic pain in patients resistant to other therapies.[26]

The dose of opioids may also vary from individual to individual and does not correlate with disability or depression;[27] and chronic use does not significantly impair perception, cognition, coordination, or behavior.[28] It has been shown that narcotics used for nonmalignant chronic pain are not as likely to increase tolerance and require escalated dosing.[29] Garvil Pasternak,

M.D., Ph.D., of Cornell University in New York City, believes opioid therapy should be individualized to each patient because each person's response to mu opioids (opioids such as morphine, codeine, and fentanyl activated at a certain type of opioid receptor in the brain and spinal cord), is likely due to genetics;[30] positron emission tomography (PET scan) verifies this in FM patients.[31] This would explain why some people respond better to different types of opioids and different doses.

Not everybody responds favorably to patients who need opioids to help control their pain. Some health care providers, caregivers, coworkers, friends, and even family members still have preconceived notions regarding the use of pain medication,[32] despite a better understanding in the medical and scientific community of the underlying mechanisms of chronic pain. These rigid, "zero-tolerance" attitudes are often exaggerated by people pursuing personal gain, whether financially, emotionally, or politically. With all this documented evidence, patients are still not receiving adequate pain management. There are many in my support group who still deal with stigma associated with opioids. It should be our right to have our pain properly managed without political involvement.

Opioid use for pain management is the treatment option of last resort. We do not expect our medication to resolve our pain completely. However, we do expect opioids to allow us the ability to have some function, which will improve our quality of life and allow us to work on other important life achievements. The goal of treatment with narcotic pain relievers is to give the patient the ability to participate in therapy that will improve body, mind, and spirit. The use of an opioid analgesic can result in better management of pain with minimal adverse effects.[33] If a person has a physician who implies the patient is at fault for having a chronic pain disease, it is time for a referral to a doctor who offers respect and dignity.

Everything constantly shifts with these illnesses. A periodic review and adjustment of medications may be indicated if your "usual" medications are no longer effective. As your body changes, your needs and chemical reactions change.

The Federation of State Medical Boards of the United States, Inc., has developed "Model Guidelines for the Use of Controlled Substances for the Treatment of Pain," which has been adopted by most states. Their efforts should be recognized because the guidelines are geared to meeting patient needs and protecting the physician. I hope that models such as this will encourage physicians to treat intractable chronic pain by prescribing appropriate pain management technique without fear of prosecution.

MODEL POLICY FOR THE USE OF CONTROLLED SUBSTANCES FOR THE TREATMENT OF PAIN

Section II—Guidelines*

1. Complete medical history and exam

2. Treatment plan

3. Informed consent

4. Agreement for treatment

5. Periodic review

6. Consultation (willing to refer)

7. Medical records (file must include documentation of items 1–6)

8. Compliance with laws and regulations (physician with license to prescribe)

*From the Federation of State Medical Boards of the United States, Inc., Pain Policy Resource Center

The bottom line is that if you are taking any medication, regardless of its composition, for any reason other than to be more functional in everyday life, you are abusing the substance.

NMDA

Untreated or undertreated pain activates the NMDA (N-methyl-D-aspartate) receptors in the spinal cord. Activation of NMDA causes widespread pain and the brain disproportionately processes the pain as extreme, even when a mild pain stimulus is exerted.[34]

Research is showing that the addition of NMDA receptor antagonists, such as dextromethorphan,[35] to opioid therapy may enhance the pain-relieving effects. However, dextromethorphan can cause serious side effects, such as mental confusion, sexual dysfunction, temporary decrease in bowel motility, and sleep disturbance. These side effects are because this NMDA antagonist targets all NMDA receptors. If medications are developed that target specific NMDA receptors, this could minimize the unwanted side effects seen in current NMDA receptor antagonist medications. Studies on selective NMDA receptors are being conducted.[36] If NMDA receptor antagonists are proven effective as an agonist (helper) to narcotics, this could be a breakthrough. Activation of the NMDA-receptor increases the cell's response to pain stimuli. Therefore, if NMDA receptors are inhibited specifically, the response to pain may be diminished without causing other side effects. NMDA receptors also decrease nerve cell sensitivity to opioid receptor helpers. In addition to preventing central sensitization, coadministration of NMDA-receptor antagonists with an opioid may prevent tolerance to opioid analgesia.[37] What does this mean? In a nutshell, the development of a target specific NMDA antagonist could result in lesser amounts of narcotic being needed to achieve the same pain relief, and would decrease recurrence of unwanted side effects.

---

antagonist: counteracts, works against.

agonist: helper, works with.

Medicinal Marijuana

This is a very controversial issue because of its political implications. The ability to study the medical benefits of marijuana (cannabis) will increase as a result of legalization in different parts of the country and the world.

The active ingredient in marijuana, THC, has been used successfully in treatment of nausea associated with chemotherapy treatment and pain in the terminally ill, and is being studied for use in treatment of migraine, fibromyalgia, painful eyelid twitching, and irritable bowel syndrome.[38] Patients from states that have legalized medicinal marijuana testify to its benefits for treatment of chronic pain. Synthetic marijuana, Nabilone, has been shown to be of great benefit.[39] Current studies include the benefits of marijuana for appetite stimulation,[40] nausea and vomiting following anticancer therapy, neurological and movement disorders, analgesia, glaucoma,[41] gastrointestinal diseases,[42] Parkinson's, arthritis,[43] and multiple sclerosis.[44] The studies showing potential usefulness as an anti-inflammatory agent[45] could be groundbreaking, because the anti-inflammatory drugs currently available have the potential to create more problems than they solve.

The information regarding cannaboid medical use is staggering. As I noted in my literature review, studies have been proposed on the risk/benefit ratio of smoking marijuana versus ingesting it in pill form, and separating the biophysical properties from psychotropic (mind-altering) properties. Battle lines have been drawn.

Supplements, Herbs, and Vitamins

Buyer beware! There are many claims that supplements can cure FM and CFID. If this were the case, those two disorders would not be in this book. Experimenting with supplements can be a very costly venture; however, there are some reported benefits from their use. Therefore, as long as people claim a benefit from supplements, herbs, and vitamins, others will try them as well. We tend to listen to anyone reporting good news on treating chronic pain.

There are some "dos and don'ts" for trying OTC herbs and supplements. Avoid combination remedies so that you can assess each exact ingredient. Be alert—these remedies are not regulated by the FDA and safe doses and interactions have not been studied sufficiently. They may have unwanted side effects or could be potentially dangerous for you. Many herbal remedy users are not as knowledgeable about these products as they should be. I would suggest speaking with your physician and pharmacist first. In my personal experience, only one has been beneficial, and it has helped me with one of my coexisting conditions, rather than FM, CFID, or CMP. I have, however, heard enthusiastic testimony from some of my online support friends. Remember, we are all unique and have different reactions to different medications, and have different coexisting conditions.

There have been an amazing number of studies in the past few years on the drawbacks and benefits of various herbs and supplements. We are grateful and may find some benefits that we have been missing. Scientific studies will help us understand which are good or bad for what conditions, how much is enough, and how much is too much. Nature's way is generally the best way when possible, but we should not randomly consume nature's remedies.

Hints for Safe Use of Supplements, Herbs, and Vitamins

- Read labels for content, storage, guidelines, and dosage.
- Research and ask questions regarding purity and potency. Also, keep in mind that dosages commonly suggested have not necessarily been tested. Manufacturers are not required to meet FDA guidelines.
- As with any medication, get immediate medical help if you develop hives or wheezing after taking any herbs or supplements.
- Don't take unnecessary risks. If you are pregnant, breast-feeding, on chemotherapy, undergoing surgical procedures, have other underlying health issues, or take other medications, discuss your use of over-the-counter medications, herbs, and supplements with everyone who needs to know. Make sure your pharmacist has a complete, up-to-date list of all your medications, including any OTC preparations you use.

The following supplements are not suggested substitutes for sound medical care, and should only be considered as possible additive therapy.

Acidophilus

The digestive tract's primary purpose is to capture nutrients from what we eat so our bodies can utilize the food for energy. The bowel is host to many types of bacteria and yeast, among them Lactobacillus acidophilus. Acidophilus is a friendly bacteria that acts as a natural killer of potentially harmful organisms in the digestive tract. Taking acidophilus as a nutritional supplement may restore the normal balance in the intestines and vagina. This is especially true when taking antibiotics, which deplete beneficial bacteria along with the harmful strains. Because acidophilus helps maintain normal flora, it may be helpful to people with the coexisting condition of leaky gut syndrome. Probiotics like acidophilus are being studied for their health benefits in the gastrointestinal tract.[46]

Yogurt is a well-known food source for acidophilus, but read the label carefully to make sure it contains live, or "active," lactobacillus acidophilus. Because lactobacillus acidophilus is a live culture, it should be stored in a cool, dry place—usually the refrigerator—even in capsule form, unless otherwise indicated on the bottle.

Antioxidants

Antioxidants are substances that prevent oxidation of cellular membranes and protect them from damage by free radicals, which are highly destructive, reactive, unpaired (free) molecules. Because of this, many believe they boost the immune system.[47] Anecdotally, I can tell you that since I started taking antioxidants approximately five years ago, I have noted a strengthening in my immune system. Prior to that I succumbed to every virus that came my way.

Vitamin E, in particular, has received a lot of attention in the news media. However, you and your doctor or naturopath should make a risk/benefit assessment. A moderate amount of less than 1600 IU per day is safe for most adults.[48] Labels list the recommended daily allowance.

Antioxidant supplements are best taken in the form of combination products, because regardless of dose, multiple antioxidants appear to work together more effectively than when taken alone. The antioxidant formula is one of the exceptions to the avoidance of combination remedies. The most common combination antioxidant supplements contain vitamins A (usually as beta-carotene), C, and E. Sometimes minerals, such as zinc, copper, and selenium, are added, because they are thought to help strengthen the body's own antioxidant protection system.

Bioflavonoids

Flavonoids found in plants help maintain blood vessel walls.[49] Bioflavonoids—flavonoids for the human body—are found in many sources including beets, grape seed extract, gingko biloba, green tea, apples, onions, citrus fruit, berries, and red wine. The naturally occurring chemicals found in flavonoids—proanthocyanidins, polyphenols, silymarin, and quercetin—are thought to help the body metabolize antioxidants and decrease damage from free radicals.

Chromium Picolinate

Chromium is an essential trace mineral that helps regulate the body's blood sugar. Chromium picolinate is a patented synthetic form of chromium.

Because of conflicting evidence regarding safety and effectiveness, the Federal Trade Commission has limited claims that can be made about chromium picolinate. More studies are indicated to determine its benefits and risks. Most people don't need chromium supplements because this mineral is readily accessible in a balanced diet; however, it is believed by some that people with FM, who also have confirmed insulin resistance, may benefit from its use.[50]

As stated previously, check with your doctor before taking any supplement. High levels of this mineral can cause serious organ damage and the benefit may not outweigh the risk.

Coenzyme Q10 (CoQ10)

Coenzyme Q10 is a natural compound produced by the body. In addition to a staggering number of proposed benefits, there are anecdotal reports that it helps with brain fog.

On a cellular chemistry level, this antioxidant helps convert food into energy. Doctors who emphasize nutritional complementary medicine believe that supplemental use of CoQ10 may play a role in keeping cholesterol-lowering statin drugs from depleting natural CoQ10. Studies are underway regarding its effect as a supplement and its usefulness in tandem with cholesterol lowering drugs.

A recent study suggests that both vitamin E and CoQ10 could improve free radical ability to clean and protect basic cellular oxidative reactions. Such reactions include the process that makes energy in food available for cellular metabolism.[51] Beneficial effects, prolonged use, and appropriate dosing are questions that still need to be answered.

DHEA

Manufacturers of DHEA claim it can help improve stamina and rejuvenate libido. Most likely this suggestion is because DHEA turns into estrogen (a female hormone) and testosterone (a male hormone) in your body.

Because your body naturally produces DHEA and overdosing on hormones can be life threatening,[52] it should only be taken if your doctor determines that your own blood levels are low or believes the benefits outweigh the risks.

Digestive Enzymes

Digestive enzymes aid in utilization of nutrients and improve gut environment and function. Natural supplemental enzymes may help your digestive tract break down food for use by the body.

Glucosamine and Chondroitin

Glucosamine and chondroitin have similar actions of benefiting joint health. They are often combined, so for the sake of ease are both discussed under this heading.

Glucosamine supplements are primarily for people with degenerative osteoarthritis, but may not be indicated for people who also have CMP. Glucosamine is said to decrease pain and improve mobility. Studies show that glucosamine has been as effective as NSAIDS, such as ibuprofen, and may help repair damaged cartilage (the gel-like material that cushion joints).[53]

Glucosamine forms a substrate on which hyaluronic acid builds. Hyaluronic acid helps form part of what Dr. Starlanyl terms "geloid masses."[54] See the box on page 180.[55]

More groundbreaking experiments are needed regarding geloid masses and their relationship to glucose metabolic dysfunction, such as diabetes or insulin resistance, and resistant TrPs.

There have been studies regarding the benefits of glucosamine in relationship to joint disease. However, since glucosamine helps hyaluronic acid form more easily (a good thing for some), it is still to be determined if the benefits for arthritis outweigh the risks for people with additional disorders, such as ours. What we know about supplements in general is largely dependent upon a historical (anecdotal) account from those who use them.

I have written my congressman regarding how unfair I think it is for the government to punish those of us who seek prescription medications from other countries for a lower cost. His response was that the United States can not verify their safety. Seriously? Not all the medications you buy at your local pharmacy are even manufactured in the United States. Believe me, I responded to his response and he earned a place on my do not re-elect list. I have strong opinions about government regulation of out-of-country medications and pharmaceutical exploitation, but the downside of the FDA's not being involved in regulation of herbs and supplements is a lack of government funding for needed studies. This is one place where we welcome "big brother" involvement.

GELOID MASSES

Geloid masses are like gelatin, but often very firm. They are clearly defined and measurable masses that overlie resistant myofascial trigger points. They are found in some patients who have long-standing, resistant TrPs in the patient who has both CMP and FM, or with glucose metabolic dysfunction. Transdermal (topical, on the skin) T3, a naturally occurring thyroid hormone that can trigger enzymes effecting hyaluronic acid, has shown it can affect geloid masses. Results from patients studied in 2001–2002 found topical T3 softened geloid masses. It does not eradicate TrPs, however, transdermal T3 allows the TrPs and taut bands to become more accessible and treatable. Some patients in the study reported reduced pain, reduced medication use, increased function, and/or improved mood and cognitive skills.

There are some general interactions and cautions between glucosamine and other medications, so check with your doctor before taking.

Chondroitin sulfate is a compound that appears to block the enzymes that destroy cartilage tissue. The body uses glucosamine to help make chondroitin. Therefore, it may also increase joint mobility and slow cartilage loss in people who suffer from arthritis.

Like glucosamine, chondroitin has some contraindications that may warrant careful consideration before taking it.

Grape Seed Extract

Grape seed extract comes from ground red grape seeds and, sometimes, skins. It contains powerful antioxidants called proanthocyanidins (PCOs), which are also found in pine bark extract (pycnogenol). Like other antioxidants, PCOs taken long term may help protect muscle cells from damage, by controlling free radicals.

PCOs also inhibit enzymes that are destructive to collagen, elastin, and hyaluronic acid around blood vessels; and may be beneficial to vascular structures and skin.[56]

No adverse reactions have been reported; however, research on grape seed extract is limited. Resveratrol, found in the skin of red grapes has shown some anti-cancer, blood-sugar-lowering, and anti-inflammatory affects in rats, but this finding has not been completely duplicated in humans. Like so many other supplements, the purity varies among manufacturers, and is affected by processing. It is rapidly metabolized by humans, so the properties we are looking for may not be utilized before they are excreted. More research and development on the polyphenolic compound resveratrol is indicated.

Human Growth Hormone (Somatotropin)

Human Growth Hormone (HGH) is an endocrine hormone produced by the pituitary during sleep, which decreases with age. Supplementation may be beneficial in a certain subset of patients with FM who have decreased insulin-like growth factor-1 (IGF-1).[57]

Over-the-counter use is strictly inadvisable because of dangerous effects. Appropriate testing by your treating physician to determine if you are in the subset of FM patients who have *documented* low HGH is absolutely necessary.

5-Hydroxytryptophan (5-HTP)

A form of tryptophan (an amino acid), 5-HTP is converted by the body into serotonin. Because serotonin easily crosses the blood brain barrier, it eases depression, modulates pain, and improves sleep.

---

serotonin: a vasoconstrictor present in the blood, central nervous system, and other tissues. Produced enzymatically from tryptophan, it also stimulates smooth muscle and serves as a central neurotransmitter. It's also known as hydroxytriptamine.

amino acids: the building blocks of protein.

Deficiency in 5-HTP has been seen in FM[58] and CFID patients. Fifty FM patients were given 5-HTP (100 mg) or a placebo three times a day in a double blind study. The group that received 5-HTP showed significant improvement in their symptoms, compared to the placebo group.[59]

It is best absorbed on an empty stomach, which is the exception to the "taking medications and supplements with food" rule. Good results from 5-HTP use are usually seen within thirty days, but better results are reported after ninety days.[60]

A combination of 5-HTP with St. John's wort, and St. John's wort with magnesium may render better results. (See St. John's wort in conjunction with 5-HTP and magnesium.)

As with many supplements, 5-HTP should be used with caution and discussed with your doctor and pharmacist. It does adversely interact with certain medications and alcohol, escalate the effects of certain medications, and its use is contraindicated in certain medical conditions.

Kava or Kava Kava

Kava is a popular herb that produces a relaxed feeling. The active compound is kavalactone, or kava alphapyrones, and is found in the root of the kava plant.

There is a consumer advisory alert for possible liver damage from kava use, while claims are being investigated. Toxic reactions can develop and high doses can depress breathing or cause general health problems.

Kava not only has hypnotic qualities, it is also thought to enhance quality of sleep.[61] However, its effectiveness as an herbal medicine for treatment of insomnia and anxiety needs to be further studied in relationship to proper dosage and long-term effects in humans.

Magnesium

Low levels of magnesium can cause muscle weakness and other problems. Thus, it should come as no surprise that magnesium deficiency is common in FM and CFID,[62] and may play a role in tension migraine and muscle tension.[63] Because of this, it may be beneficial for FM, CFID, and CMP.

Magnesium is critical to cellular function, including energy production, protein formation, and cellular replication. It participates in more than three hundred enzymatic reactions, especially those that produce cellular energy (adenosine triphospate),[64] so it is crucial for many metabolic functions in the body. The rationale for treatment of FM with magnesium and malic acid is that sleep deprivation decreases utilization of magnesium.[65] Because of cellular metabolism, magnesium citrate is better utilized than magnesium oxide.[66]

Although magnesium has been infrequently studied, new findings indicate it may affect many metabolic reactions in the body's soft tissue. Paired with calcium, it helps stabilize metabolism, regulate nerves and muscles, and stabilize heart rhythm. We are now recognizing that its role in healthy body function is more important than previously thought.

Low and high levels of magnesium result in unwanted side effects. Therefore, you should consult with your doctor regarding its potential use. Monitoring of magnesium levels may be indicated.

Malic Acid

Malic acid produces chemical energy at the cellular level and is thought to aid metabolism of carbohydrates. Magnesium and vitamin B6 must be present in order for malic acid to be utilized. A study of twenty-four patients at the University of Texas Health Science Center in San Antonio found that two months of treatment with this combination reduced pain and tenderness.[67] However, a review showed limited evidence of helping the body-wide pain of FM.[68] Combination use may be the key here. (See magnesium.)

Melatonin

Melatonin is a hormone secreted by the pineal gland. The pineal gland is located at the base of the brain and secretes melatonin when daylight ends, peaks in early morning hours, and falls off again at dawn. The body changes melatonin into serotonin.

Supplements are proposed to treat insomnia, ease sleep problems caused by pain or stress, and help fight jet lag.

It is believed that patients with FM and CFID may have low melatonin secretion, which could explain the lack of restorative sleep and pain modulation impairments;[69] however, a study done in the United Kingdom by Williams, Waterhouse, Mugarza, Minors, and Hayden does not support this belief.[70] To the contrary, they found treatment with melatonin and phototherapy to be ineffective.[71]

Questions regarding potency and purity have been raised, and as with all hormone supplements, safety concerns are valid.

It may be more important to find a medication that will encourage use of the melatonin manufactured by the body. Some of these melatonin "helpers," agonists, are now being used in clinical trials for treatment of insomnia or circadian rhythm sleep disorders.[72]

NADH (ENADA)

NADH, or nicotinamide adenine dinucleotide, is a coenzyme compound found naturally in food that plays a central role in the process by which cells convert food into energy. It is believed that the chemical jump-starts the production of ATP, the basic cycle of cellular metabolism, in muscles. It may enhance energy levels and improve cognitive performance.[73] A study of chronic fatigue patients found NADH might help increase energy levels in patients with CFID.[74]

Omega-3

Omega-3, also known as omega-3 fatty acid, is thought to reduce pain, stabilize mood, and possibly reduce cholesterol.[75] It may also play a role in reducing production of cytokines, indicating possible benefits of supplemental use in treatment of chronic fatigue syndrome.[76] Studies regarding omega-3 and FM are limited and may be indicated for future investigation, because it does appear to reduce cytokines[77] and oxidative stress, which are thought to play a role in FM.

I cannot give you the formula for success, but I can give you the formula for failure, which is: Try to please everybody.

HERBERT BAYARD SWOPE, JOURNALIST

SAM-e

SAM-e (S-adenosyl-methionine) is a naturally occurring chemical compound produced by our bodies from the amino acid methionine. Methionine is found in protein-rich foods.

One study involving HIV/AIDs patients showed SAM-e might reduce symptoms of depression.[78]

According to the *Arthritis Today,* on-line supplement guide, accessed in August of 2009, SAM-e allegedly helps with joint swelling, lack of mobility, FM, bursitis, tendonitis, chronic low back pain, and depression. It may even help rebuild cartilage. It has a known anti-inflammatory and pain-relieving effect for people with osteoarthritis, and its anti-inflammatory effects are equal to nonsteroidal anti-inflammatory (NSAIDS) medications in clinical studies. It may interact with certain medications, so check with your doctor or pharmacist before using.[79]

St. John's Wort

St. John's wort, the common name for Hypericum perforatum, refers to John the Baptist. A medicinal herb that was once believed to have magical powers, this common, shrub-like perennial has been used for centuries to treat anxiety; depression; insomnia; stomach, bladder, bowel, kidney, and lung problems; and even cancer. According to the National Institute of Health there is strong scientific evidence for its use as a treatment for mild to moderate depression.[80]

Though benefits of using St. John's wort in depression, which can be a coexisting condition in FM, CFID, and CMP, have been noted, there is potential for an adverse reaction in people with chronic illness and compromised immune systems,[81] so use caution if you are in a certain subset of patients. It does interact with certain medications.[82]

St. John's Wort in Conjunction with 5-HTP: Research indicates that taking 5-HTP in conjunction with St. John's wort produces significantly better results.[83]

Keep in mind that any substance that alters the body's physiology is a drug. This includes supplements, whether under the regulation of the FDA or not. Supplements and herbs may have side effects or toxic reactions when combined with prescription drugs, over-the-counter preparations, or foods. Discuss your wish to try them with your doctor before introducing them into your medication regimen.

Over-the-Counter Medications
Benadryl (Diphenhydramine)

Benadryl is an antihistamine used in allergy medications. Since it has the side effect of drowsiness, it is also found in most OTC sleep aids. It can be used safely; however, there may be contraindications to its use in certain cases, so check with your physician. As with all sleep medications, take them only when you are preparing for bed, unless instructed otherwise. Because of its side effects, it could increase the risk of falling.

Diphenhydramine also has the propensity to cause confusion,[84] just like the psychotropic drugs discussed earlier. So pay attention to the warning labels on all medications. Be alert to the possibility of an opposite effect from diphenhydramine. Amytriptyline, an antidepressant often used to treat insomnia and sleep disruption in FM, kept me up for days. It took a while to identify the cause because this is an unusual reaction. How did I recognize the culprit? One day, after I'd been sobbing and begging for sleep for hours, my husband said to me, "I believe this manic mode began when you started that new medication." Guess what! When I stopped it, the mania, agitation, and depression from "severe sleep deprivation" ended. This is an example of why you should introduce only one new medication at a time, including over-the-counter preparations. You need to be able to evaluate each reaction independently.

Guaifenesin

"I will consider changing my medications, my physical therapies, and my exercise routines, but I will not consider going without guaifenesin." This is an anecdotal remark made by Devin J. Starlanyl in her book, *Fibromyalgia and Chronic Myofascial Pain Syndrome: A Survival Manual.*

Dr. R. Paul St. Amand developed guaifenesin (also called guai) therapy. He theorized that it helps FM patients rid muscles of toxins. Dr. Amand conducted a study using massive doses of guai; however, skeptics claim the study was flawed, and guai's use is still considered experimental.

Guaifenesin is found in OTC cold preparations at 100 mg per teaspoon, and is the active ingredient in the medications Humibid and Mucinex. It can also be found in combination with pseudoephedrin, as guaifed. Some Internet sites offer large-dose pills, but the treatment protocol is very specific.

Anecdotal evidence and the flawed study suggest it may be beneficial for some. However, as with all treatments, *do no harm*. The protocol must be followed precisely. Investigate it, research it, and discuss it with your doctor before determining whether or not to try this treatment option.

NSAIDS (Nonsteroidal Anti-inflammatories)

NSAIDS are used to treat various inflammatory musculoskeletal problems. NSAIDS are anti-inflammatory medications, and although FM and CMP are not inflammatory conditions,[85] NSAIDS provide an analgesic quality. In CFID patients whose symptoms are from an inflammatory response, they may be particularly beneficial.

Topical Agents

Topical agents such as Aspercreme, menthol products, numbing agents (such as those containing lidocaine), or capsaicin may bring temporary relief of symptoms. Capsaicin's active ingredient is a derivative of hot peppers. Because the heat from the menthol and capsaicin products can be significant, some patients with FM or CFID may not tolerate them well, particularly if there are multiple chemical sensitivities.

While medications help us gain some control over our symptoms, we should not expect them to be the only form of pain and symptom control. It is important that we recognize there is no quick fix to these disorders. It takes a multidisciplined health care team and a multimodal treatment plan to reach an acceptable comfort zone.

An excellent resource for checking doses, interactions, and safety for the use of herbs, vitamins, and other supplements is noted in the resources section at the end of the book in the "Medications, Herbs, and Supplements" section.

Pain Management Therapies

There are two important questions to ask regarding therapies: How you do them, and which one is the right fit for you? A valuable therapy is one that fits your personality and individual needs. If it feels right, you are more likely to stick to it and thereby reap the benefits.

Acutherapy

Acutherapy is a general term for any therapy that stimulates acupoints of the body. A preliminary study showed a correlation between specific areas of the brain and ancient practices of acupoint stimulation using a functional MRI.[86] This experiment confirmed the scientific validity of a very ancient Asian form of medicine.

---

dermatome: the segment of skin or subcutaneous tissue supplied with sensory (afferent) nerve fibers.

Acutherapists study the body's acupoints and/or meridians, which are pathways of energy called *chi* (or *qi*). For our purposes, acutherapy includes acupuncture, acupressure, and shiatsu.

Acupuncture

Acupuncture is an ancient Chinese therapeutic approach using strategically inserted needles to unblock healing energy. This energy circulates throughout the body in predetermined meridians, different from dermatomes. Acupuncture points are believed to stimulate release of chemicals into the muscles, spinal cord, and brain. These chemicals either change the perception of pain or release other chemicals, such as hormones, which influence the body's ability to create a system of checks and balances. The ancient practitioners of acupuncture believed it caused a shift in flow, or distribution, of the body's chi to correct imbalances. Success has been reported in the use of acupuncture for treatment of illness, chronic disorders, and pain.

True acupuncture using meridians may not benefit people with CMP; however, if the technique is used to treat trigger points specifically, acupuncture may be beneficial.[87] Western scientists who support the use of acupuncture do so on the basis of scientific evidence.[88] Electromagnetic signals are relayed faster with acupuncture and are believed to initiate the flow of painkilling body chemicals, called endorphins. They also believe the signal calls for a faster response from the immune system when cells are damaged due to injury or disease. Studies have shown that acupuncture changes brain chemistry, and that the release of neurotransmitters and neurohormones triggers sensation and involuntary bodily functions. It has the potential to affect immune reactions, blood pressure, blood flow, and body temperature, and has been helpful in treating some patients with FM.[89] Its success in treating chronic pain may be related to the neuro-chemical activity it initiates. One study using a SPECT scan, single-photon emission computed tomography, detected changes in cerebral blood flow associated with pain. The scan also recorded that acupuncture analgesia is associated with changes in the activity of the frontal lobes, brain stem, and thalami.[90] The results of studies like this are promising.

More and more studies are showing the benefits of acupuncture; however, further scientific evidence is indicated before it will become mainstream. Once the benefits are proven and accepted, those of us who suffer from chronic pain can reap the rewards.

Finding the right acupuncturist should start with a referral from someone you know. You want to make sure you see a skilled therapist. If your state does not require certification, check with professional organizations, such as those listed in the resource section in the back of this book. Interview an acupuncturist as you would any new doctor or therapist.

Acupressure

Acupressure is like acupuncture, but uses touch instead of needles, with moderate to firm pressure. You will want a bodywork therapist who specializes in acupressure.

Shiatsu

Shiatsu is Japanese acupressure massage. The term actually means "finger pressure." Practitioners use a technique of press and release, applying pressure to acupoints for three to five seconds with thumbs, fingers, and elbows. Shiatsu practitioners treat specific points and wider areas. Stimulating acupoints helps redistribute and rebalance energy blocks caused by stress. This form of meditation massage awakens the body's natural gravitation toward balance by improving lymph and blood flow, and increasing energy.

We have writing and teaching, science and power; we have tamed the beasts and schooled the lightning . . . but we have still to tame ourselves.

H. G. WELLS

Aqua Therapy

Exercise in warm water has great benefits for arthritis because it decreases stress on the joints, but allows the exercise needed to help strengthen the supporting joint structures. Studies show it can help FM patients with pain and cognitive deficits.[91] By improving the pain threshold, cognition improves.

Biofeedback

Biofeedback is a form of neurotherapy that teaches patients to voluntarily relax specific muscles, improve concentration and sleep, and control chronic pain. It provides the technologist with ways to monitor a patient's body response, including brainwave activity, muscle tension, breathing, heart rate, and blood pressure in relationship to the patient's relaxation efforts.

There are several types of biofeedback, including muscle/EMG, which measures the electricity between nerve and muscle; thermal/PST, which helps patients learn to control body temperature reflecting relaxation; sweating response/EDR (electro-galvanic response), which monitors skin perspiration indicating anxiousness; and EEG-biofeedback, which monitors brain waves and helps retrain the brain.

EEG Biofeedback—Neuro-electrotherapy

Neuro-electrotherapy, also known as EEG biofeedback, is a noninvasive procedure, meaning you are not prodded with needles or anything that pierces the skin. It is used to treat chronic muscle pain conditions,[92] muscle pain related to FM,[93] and fatigue and confusion associated with CFID.[94]

Diaphragmatic Breathing

Any restriction to the chest such as pain, injury, tender points, or trigger points can result in a decreased ability to breathe.

Biofeedback devices have proven the benefits of diaphragmatic breathing for relaxation. It helps calm the body, lower heart rate, and decrease blood pressure.

Improper breathing is easy to correct. The act of breathing allows our lungs to take in oxygen from the air surrounding us. When we inhale, our lungs expand and increase their capacity for oxygen rich air. Oxygen is used by every cell in the body to create energy; therefore, when lung capacity is diminished or breathing is too shallow, so is cellular energy. Proper breathing can have a positive effect on how we feel.

Diaphragmatic breathing, or belly breathing, increases your breath or inspiratory volume. When you breathe with your diaphragm you allow the diaphragm (which keeps your lungs from dropping down to your knees) to increase the chest space (thoracic cavity), and thereby increase your lung capacity. This gives the lungs room to expand and fill with air. Have you ever noticed how much more difficult it is to breathe when you overeat? This is because you constrict the diaphragm. Tight clothing also decreases the amount of room your lungs have to inflate. See "Breathing Meditation for People with FM, CFID and CMP" in the Useful Tools section at the end of this chapter.

To make sure you are breathing from your diaphragm, lie on the floor with a paper towel on your belly and another on your chest. Practice breathing in through your nose and expanding your lungs, making the piece of paper on your belly go up as you inhale and letting it drop as you exhale. If the one on your belly isn't rising as you take in air (inspiration), you aren't breathing from your diaphragm. Your belly should expand on inspiration, not as you exhale.

Diaphragmatic breathing has the power to help the healing process, calm the body, and rejuvenate the mind. Not only does this deep breathing encourage relaxation, it also provides a gentle stretch to the painful muscles between the ribs that become so contracted from both FM and CMP, and increases energy reserves for FM and CFID. Live healthy by breathing healthy.

Managing Your Diet

Diet includes what we eat, how we prepare what we eat, and how we eat it.

There are no specific nutritional guidelines for the treatment of FM, CFID, or CMP; however, there are nutritional goals that focus on nutrient therapy for minimizing symptoms.

Basic goals for healthy eating are to maintain a healthy weight, avoid excessive caffeine and alcohol intake, and limit foods known to cause gastrointestinal distress or aggravate symptoms. Unless specifically contraindicated because of other health issues, we should eat plenty of low density, complex carbohydrates, including raw fruits and vegetables; and low-fat proteins, such as fish. Diet should be supplemented with a daily multivitamin.[95]

As the lungs provide oxygen that is processed for cellular energy, food provides energy for body and mind. The digestive tract converts nutrients into fuel and conserves what isn't needed immediately.

The way food is converted, used, and stored depends upon the body's metabolism. Sugar and complex carbohydrates trigger insulin release from the pancreas into the blood. Insulin plays a major role in carbohydrate metabolism and helps regulate the way our bodies utilize carbohydrates, lipids (fats), and amino acids (protein element) for cellular energy.

THE SICKENING SIX

In their book *Arthritis Survival,* Robert S. Ivker and Todd Nelson list the six categories of food and drink that, consumed in excess, contribute most often to poor health.[96]

Fats

Sugar

Refined carbohydrates

Alcohol

Caffeine

Salt

What We Eat

A balanced diet is important to everybody's health, but crucial for people with FM, CFID, CMP, and coexisting conditions. Certain foods and nutritional deficiencies can be major perpetuating factors, and we all have specific needs. For instance, small amounts of caffeine are often indicated for migraine and may stimulate you when you are fatigued; however, too much caffeine intensifies symptoms of the gastrointestinal system, causes headaches, puts stress on the heart by chemically increasing heart rate and blood pressure, and interferes with sleep in some people.

I used to consume large amounts of carbohydrates, and as if it were something to be proud of, I deemed myself a carbo junky. My body craved these demons of desire, and I was literally making myself sick. Of course, our bodies do require some carbohydrates, but I found by limiting the ratio of carbohydrates in my diet and being selective of what types I consumed, I began to feel less fatigued. Now, I am no saint and I do "treat" myself periodically, but you will no longer find me sitting in my recliner stuffing my face with potato chips and dip. Well, maybe a little bit on the first Saturday of every month, but here again, it becomes the "pay if you play" game. Once I realized what an impact bad carbohydrates had on my body, it became much easier to resist temptation and set limits.

Learning how certain foods correlate with your symptoms will help you learn how to adjust your diet to eliminate aggravating foods. Minimizing use of sugar and saturated fat will help you feel better. Sugar is known to stimulate the growth of microflora in the digestive tract, such as the dreaded candida (yeast). It also generates free radicals and raises insulin production. And fat? Well . . . fat is difficult to digest! It clings to the inside of blood vessels and the outside of hips.

Before you make any blanket decisions regarding your food intake, be sure to clear it with your doctor. Certain blood tests may be needed to verify the safety of a particular diet for you. Some FMers tend to have weight gain, either from a less physically active lifestyle or from a coexisting condition, such as reactive hypoglycemia. Fad diets are tempting, but some can be life threatening for people with serious health problems.

A study done by Iris Bell, M.D., Ph.D., and others at the University of Arizona-Tucson showed that FM patients have significantly low resting blood sugar.[97] The ramifications of this study suggest that at least some of the symptoms of these patients may be eradicated by addressing that coexisting condition.

Diets that are higher in monounsaturated fatty acids, fiber, and low glycemic index foods appear to have advantages in insulin resistance, blood glucose control, and circulating lipids (fats).[98]

As previously noted, insulin, a protein hormone, is important to cellular metabolism. It helps the body regulate energy. Insulin resistance happens when your body no longer responds appropriately to insulin. Changes in your diet may help with the side effects of brain fog, the aggravated TrPs of CMP,[99] fatigue, tremors, palpitations, anxiety, sweating, and hunger. Paresthesias and more serious symptoms, like seizure or coma, may result from insufficient brain glucose (sugar). Excessive insulin production prevents carbohydrates from being utilized for cellular energy, and some people can tolerate very low levels of blood sugar without the usual warning symptoms.[100] In some cases, insulin resistance can lead to RHG.[101]

According to Dr. Starlanyl, RHG is a type of hypoglycemia "that is specific to low blood sugar and occurs in response to a high carbohydrate intake." This is not the same as hypoglycemia (low blood sugar) from not eating. In the case of RHG, the body overreacts two to three hours after a high carbohydrate meal, causing excessive insulin production that significantly lowers the blood sugar.[102]

Routine tests for checking blood sugar levels are not specific to detecting RHG. People with RHG may have normal findings from standard tests. Researchers are finding that a hyperglucidic (high sugar) breakfast test is more specific for detecting RHG. This is a food challenge that is different from the typical postprandial test. Doctors Brun, Fedou, and Mercier from the Department of Exploration and Readaptation of Metabolic and Muscular Abnormalities at Lapeyronie Hospital in Montpellier, France, suggest this type of food challenge will give a more accurate diagnosis. They also suggest that the problem is worsened by a high-carbohydrate/low-fat diet, and alcohol.[103] In that case, the treatment is *diet modification.*

RHG may be a coexisting condition for you. Metabolic disorders like hypoglycemia in association with CMP may make treatment of the TrPs of CMP more difficult.[104]

Glucose intolerance has also been linked to TMJ/TMD,[105] which suggests, at least to me, that in these cases TMJ/TMD may be due to untreated TrPs.

If you have reactive hypoglycemia, you may benefit from the Zone diet, because of its balance of protein and fat with carbohydrates.[106] Developed by Berry Sears, Ph.D., the Zone diet calls for 30 percent of dietary calories from protein, 30 percent from fat, and 40 percent from carbohydrates.[107]

Diets with a high glycemic index (high carbohydrate) can cause the following:

- Fatigue and brain fog
- Fluctuating energy levels and mood swings
- Increased risk of developing other chronic diseases

The glycemic index measures how quickly a food raises your blood sugar and how rapidly your body responds. The higher the glycemic index, the greater the likelihood a food will raise blood sugar. As carbohydrate consumption goes up, there is an increase in insulin production. This increase in insulin production increases fat stores. Low-density carbohydrates, such as most fruits and vegetables, are nutritionally sound and provide vitamins and fiber. Higher-density carbohydrates, such as pasta, bread, bagels, cornflakes, cookies, cakes, and all the foods most carb junkies enjoy, raise the glycemic index. High density, high glycemic carbs break down into sugar quickly, which causes a surge in insulin and fat production. Fat is actually a way of storing carbohydrates for future energy needs resulting from restricted calories or increased activity. Protein and fat lower the glycemic index and take longer to be utilized by the body. When you add a protein to every meal or snack, you decrease the risk of surges in blood sugar and insulin production. This can be particularly helpful in relieving symptoms of hypoglycemia.

What Is a Balanced Diet?

The answer to that question varies depending upon the organization that publishes it, the data substantiating it, the year the balanced diet criteria were printed, and perhaps even financial interests of certain food production lobbies.

In the early 1990s the USDA (United States Department of Agriculture) issued the food pyramid, which suggested the daily diet should include the following balance of foods:[108]

- 6–11 servings of bread, cereal, rice, or pasta
- 3–5 servings of vegetables
- 2–4 servings of fruit
- 2–3 servings of milk, yogurt, or cheese
- 2–3 servings of meat, poultry, fish, beans, eggs, and nuts
- Sparse servings of fats, oils, and sweets

We heralded this recommended diet as if it were the Great Pyramid of Egypt.

The 2005 USDA recommendations, scheduled to be revised sometime in 2010, recommended that we increase our daily intake of fruits, vegetables, whole grain, and low-fat milk and milk products. They said Americans were already getting enough protein, equaling 10–35 percent of total caloric intake, so "go lean" with protein and choose leaner meats and poultry and vary protein intake with more fish. For a 2000 calorie/day diet they recommended two cups of fruit; two and a half cups of vegetables, consisting of dark green veggies, such as broccoli, kale, and other dark leafy greens; orange veggies, such as carrots, sweet potatoes, pumpkin, and winter squash; and beans and peas, such as pinto beans, kidney beans, black beans, garbanzo beans, split peas, and lentils; make half of your grain intake whole, three or more ounce-equivalents, and the other 50 percent from enriched grain products; and three cups of non-fat or low-fat milk, or an equivalent amount of low-fat yogurt and/or low-fat cheese (1½ ounces of cheese equals 1 cup of milk). They also suggest that you vary your vegetable and fruit intake.[109]

Although the RDA (recommended daily allowance) may vary slightly among organizations, the World Health Organization offers the general recommendations below.[110]

- Achieve energy balance and healthy weight.
- Limit energy intake from total fats, eliminate trans-fatty acids, and shift consumptions from saturated to unsaturated fats.
- Increase consumption of fruits, vegetables, legumes, whole grains, and nuts.
- Limit intake of free sugars, such as simple sugar and refined sugars from cane, beet and corn (high fructose corn syrup), and sugars found naturally in honey, syrups, and fruit juices.
- Limit salt intake from all sources and make sure salt in diet is iodized.

The USDA RDAs are quite different from the ones suggested by the popular Zone and Atkins diets. There is controversy in diet recommendations and opinions vary widely, which leads to confusion on what is nutritionally sound. However, all newer dietary recommendations suggest lower glycemic index carbohydrates. That is why you should always check with your physician before starting any new diet.

Some people have touchy stomachs and are intolerant of raw, spicy, or fried foods. Some of us aggravate coexisting conditions when we eat gas-forming foods. If you have IBS (irritable bowel syndrome) or LGS (leaky gut syndrome), poor nutrition can magnify the symptoms. By identifying foods that aggravate existing conditions, you diminish the likelihood of triggering a flare. If you have known food intolerances, it is wise to avoid those foods. For example, if cabbage puts you in a flare, avoid it, regardless of how much weight your friend lost on the cabbage soup diet.

As a rule, it is extremely important for people with FM, CFID, or CMP to limit intake of processed meals (generally high in salt), foods with high preservative content, saturated fats, and foods with excessive artificial coloring or flavoring. Moderate your use of "the sickening six" listed on page 191—unhealthy fats, sugar, refined carbohydrates, alcohol, caffeine, and salt. If you can commit this to memory and apply it, you may see a difference in the way you feel. Finding the diet that's right for you may be a challenge, but keeping a diary will help you to determine what foods aggravate your symptoms.

"You are what you eat" was an expression popularized in the 1960s when people became more aware of natural foods, but you are also what you drink. Unless you have a medical condition that requires limiting fluid intake, the best drink is water and plenty of it. Try to avoid liquids that are sweetened with artificial sweeteners and dyed with artificial coloring. There is still a great deal of controversy regarding caffeine found in coffee, tea, and colas. We know the effects of caffeine on heart rate and blood pressure, so if you have problems in these areas, be careful. On the flip side, small amounts of caffeine help with such disorders as migraine headaches, attention deficit disorder, and "small to moderate amounts of caffeine may help to minimize TrPs by increasing vaso-dilatation in the skeletal musculature."[111] If you are in doubt, keep a diary and track your responses to caffeine to determine whether it is a good thing for you or something you should avoid. There are said to be antioxidants in both tea and coffee, but the caffeine might outweigh that benefit for you. If you are sensitive to chemicals, you may even want to drink only purified or natural spring water; just make sure it isn't bottled tap water.

How We Prepare Food

Cooking requires time and energy, often in short supply for people with chronic pain disorders. Preparation requires learning about the diet, planning and shopping for ingredients, and organizing and putting groceries away, all before you even start cooking. Did I mention planning? As with everything else we do, we must also organize and plan our daily meals. Once you find the right diet, the following guidelines will help you manage your nutritional needs.

Pep Up Your Pooped-out Culinary Skills

- Avoid elaborate diets. Your menu doesn't have to be complicated to meet basic nutritional needs.
- Heed warning signs—today may not be the best day to try out that new recipe. On "semi-terrific" days try to delegate meal preparation or order food to be delivered.
- Use recipes that have simple directions and ingredients.
- Plan your shopping excursion at a high-energy time of day. For most of us that is between 10 a.m. and 2 p.m.
- Shop where there is a sacker and a grocery pick-up service. For groceries you are able to carry, bring your own cloth bags or ask for paper bags; plastic ones can cause undue stress on your hands and easily activate a latent TrP. Be sure the contents are weighted evenly, and carry the bag with both hands.
- Double or triple easy-to-reheat recipes so that leftovers can be popped in the freezer for another meal.

- Make meal preparation easier by washing and spinning all of your salad greens at a time of day when your symptoms are least severe. Prepare enough for several dinners or healthy snacks. They keep well stored in zip-lock bags and it's wonderful to have that detail out of the way when preparing the rest of a meal.
- Use a deli or catering service when planning meals for large gatherings, so that you'll have time to add your own special little touches without becoming overwhelmed and fatigued.
- Learn to use frozen mixed vegetables instead of preparing each vegetable for casseroles, stews, and soups.
- Use nonstick vegetable or olive oil sprays, foil, and disposable containers to lessen clean-up when you know you aren't able to do more.
- Organize your favorite cooking utensils for ease of use.
- Use appliances that minimize repetitive or fine motor movement, such as food processors for chopping, jar grabbers for removing lids, scissors for opening packages, and large-grip utensils for cooking.
- Bring your workload to you. Sit when you can while preparing food, or lower your work area when standing by placing mixing bowls in the sink or on nonskid material on a tabletop.
- Use a utility gripper to reach hard-to-get items and avoid improper stretching. When this is not possible, think before you move and use proper, well-balanced body mechanics.
- Do controlled stretching and deep breathing between tasks.
- If you live alone or are frequently home alone, use a utility cart to aid in putting groceries and other items away.
- Hang dishtowels in drawer handles for easy opening.
- Limit entertaining as the primary host or hostess.
- Encourage and teach others in the household the art of culinary design, then utilize their skills. Hint! Act like cooking is the best thing since sliced bread, or they will easily lose their interest in learning.
- If you find comfort in your cooking skills and the reward is therapeutic, don't give it up. Just learn to make modifications.
- Learn to cook from the soul. By bringing awareness into food preparation you can improve feelings of love and joy. You may also find that your food tastes better.

Hint! Many of these principles are basic and can be easily applied to other household and outside chores.

The Way We Eat

The way we eat and the kinds of food we eat can make a difference in how we feel. Remember when your parents said to chew your food slowly? This was actually very good advice. When we chew we release digestive enzymes that break down food so that it can be properly utilized. Taking small bites and chewing slowly aids in digestion of food nutrients and also decreases the risk of choking. You'll also tend to eat less, and this "mindful" eating is a great way to decrease calorie intake without sacrifice.

Smaller and less complex frequent meals help us avoid overstressing the body's fuel needs. Running on empty has been shown to add to mental confusion and cause fatigue. The brain needs fuel to process thoughts. Eating five small meals per day or three meals with a mid-morning and mid-afternoon snack is really "food for thought." A good way to identify eating patterns is to keep a food intake diary, such as the diet assessment guide in the useful tools section of this chapter. It is important to try to keep your meals on a regular schedule. You probably don't wait until your car runs out of gas before refueling, do you?

There are some vitamins we cannot get enough of by diet alone. However, eating the right combination of carbohydrates, dietary fat, and protein, and taking a multivitamin puts you in the driver's seat for controlling symptoms that otherwise might stem from an improper diet.

Exercise—Use It or Lose It

Fear of movement is a significant concern for chronic pain sufferers, but the very thing we are afraid of—movement—is what we need. The improvement of symptoms may or may not be directly linked to FM, CFID, or CMP, but it is directly linked to mental and emotional balance, which is imperative to feelings of self-esteem and self-worth.

When done appropriately, exercise is therapeutic for restoring muscle function, preventing bone loss, and creating well-being. It increases oxygen to the tissues, which in turn helps rid muscles of unwanted toxic waste. According to a study done by Robert Swezey, M.D., patients with FM have an increased chance of accelerated bone loss (osteoporosis) in the hip and spine. As a result of the study, he advocates the benefits of resistive (isometric) and weight bearing exercise.[112]

Benefits of Exercise

Exercise is known to boost the release of endorphins, our natural painkillers, and other neurotransmitters (brain chemicals) that give us a feeling of well-being. It increases bone mass (helping to prevent or repair osteoporosis) and lowers blood glucose levels (especially important for diabetics). Exercise has also been shown to reduce dependence on alcohol and drugs, alleviate insomnia, improve concentration and memory, increase self esteem,[113] burn calories, improve flexibility, improve balance, and build strength.

Many of the stretching exercises you'll find in the Useful Tools section of this chapter are modified or basic yoga asanas. Also, to help you achieve your exercise goals, we have included a source for yoga props in the resource section at the end of this book, as well as a reference to a book and CD on therapeutic yoga, which offer a wide range of modified postures for people with physical challenges.

exercise: performance of physical exertion for improvement of health or correction of physical deformity. To improve or maintain mobility of joints and soft tissue, maintain muscle fiber, improve strength and endurance, and relieve tension.

isometric: sustained contraction with equal opposing force, such as putting your palms together and pushing to create contraction of the pectoral (chest) muscles.

weight bearing: exercise with weights to cause contraction of specific muscles.

"Dos" of Exercise

- Recognize the need for exercise when you are not experiencing a flare of FM, CFID, or CMP symptoms.
- Start slowly and carefully.
- Address aggravating factors before starting, such as poor posture, metabolic upset, stress, pain, active TrPs, and so forth. (See the resource section for information on Kinesio taping, which might help with posture and holding proper alignment of muscles without strain while exercising. While allowing full range of motion, Kinesio tape helps to support muscles that have become overstressed or overstretched during exercise, preventing them from going into painful spasm.)

- Perform daily gentle stretching. If you have CMP, treat TrPs prior to stretching, not after.
- Address strengthening exercises carefully. Build tolerance over time. Try to do your routine three to five times per week, or every other day, to prevent muscles from tightening.
- Vary your type of exercise. Work different muscle groups and avoid boredom.
- Modify your exercise plan to meet any special needs you have. Any exercise is better than no exercise.
- Warm up before starting—bathe in warm water or do gentle, active ROM (range of motion) to warm up muscles.
- Provide a cool-down period by gently stretching your muscles and being aware of your breathing. Relax slowly to decrease the risk of rebound cramping.
- Wear comfortable, nonrestrictive clothing.
- Wear appropriate footwear for the type of exercise.
- Exercise at a time of day when you have the least amount of pain and stiffness. Morning exercise is discouraged because the muscles have not had a chance to warm up, and late evening exercise is discouraged because it may interfere with sleep.
- Provide yourself with adequate rest periods when doing tasks that require repetitive movement, such as vacuuming, raking leaves, or working on a computer.
- Breathe regularly and practice abdominal breathing and relaxation during exercise. Increased oxygen demands are put on the body during physical activity.
- Increase the minutes of each session to tolerance. If your endurance is low you may want to increase the number of sessions and decrease the number of minutes.
- Try low-impact aerobic exercise, such as aquatic therapy, biking, or walking. Most chronic pain patients generally tolerate these forms of exercise.
- Drink plenty of water after exercising to aid the body in flushing toxins released into the blood stream from the tissue.
- Wait at least one hour after eating before exercising.
- Modify your exercise program if the perpetuating factors are out of control.

"Don'ts" of Exercise

- Don't exercise to exhaustion. If the exercise causes more pain than you started with, you overdid it. Allow the muscle to return to its pre-exercise state before continuing.

- Don't try to do repetitive or strengthening exercise before treating trigger points. (Repetitive motion aggravates them.) Your muscles must be free of trigger points, lengthened, and relaxed.

- Don't exercise before trying to go to sleep. Exercise stimulates the release of adrenaline to increase heart rate, which helps the body compensate for the increased oxygen demand. The release of adrenaline may help with pain; however, increased adrenaline also interferes with sleep.

- Don't try to keep up with your otherwise healthy friends or neighbors. High-impact exercise is contraindicated for people with FM, CFID, and CMP.

- Stop exercising if you become symptomatic. Symptoms may include light-headedness, chest pain, profuse perspiration, nausea, or sharp pain. Your body is letting you know you are placing too much stress on it. Use common sense. If symptoms don't stop with rest, consult a medical specialist immediately.

---

angina: acute pain resulting from a strangulation of the blood supply to the heart muscle.

- Don't give up daily stretching and breathing exercises. If time doesn't permit, eliminate strengthening exercise, but not stretching, even if you have only two minutes to devote to it.

- If exercise for FM and CFID aggravates trigger points of CMP, reevaluate your routine. Do not continue to exercise with active trigger points. Treat them, then return to it.

- Don't give up if you experience pain. Reassess and reset the goal-setting plan laid out in your journal until you get it right for you.

- Don't try to make up for lost time.

- Don't exercise right after consuming a large meal. During digestion blood is diverted away from your heart and other parts of your body to your gut to aid in digestion. Exercise places stress on the heart by raising heart rate to meet the oxygen demands of your muscles. Placing undue stress by exercising right after eating could have harmful effects on your health, and in some cases could be life threatening.

Why does my blood thus muster to my heart, making both it unable for itself, and dispossessing all my other parts of necessary fitness?

WILLIAM SHAKESPEARE

A technique called post-isometric relaxation, studied by Drs. Lewit and Simons, is very effective in relieving pain and prolonging relief after treatments to the muscles of CMP patients.[114] It involves placing the muscle in a stretched position, then performing a minimal resistance isometric contraction, followed by relaxation and then a gentle stretch as the muscle releases. I found this technique to be very significant in my rehabilitation from shoulder reconstruction surgery. You can achieve a better stretch with a minimal amount of discomfort by using this technique, so I incorporate it into my regular stretching and exercising routine. As the study suggests, patients who practice this technique at home are more likely to have lasting results.

Movement may be difficult for people with the painful conditions of FM, CFID, and CMP, but when done properly, it can yield many benefits. A sedentary lifestyle causes decreases in blood flow to muscles, organs, and tissues. One study done on FM patients found that progressive strengthening and aerobic exercise can be safe; well tolerated; and effective for improving muscle strength, cardiovascular endurance, and functional status, without aggravating symptoms.[115] Some CFID patients report increased fatigue with graded exercise, exercise that starts slowly and increases in small increments, and some researchers believe it may weaken the CFID patient's immune system.[116] Another study showed that CFID patients were able to do graduated exercise, but the researchers did not see exercise as a cure, because the participants did not report an improvement in their symptoms.[117] Nevertheless, these patients were able to exercise and despite the lack of improvement in their CFID symptoms, one would hope they continued because of the general health benefits.

The goal of exercise for CMP patients is to decrease pain and improve muscle function, but first the TrPs area must be treated successfully. The taut band will only rebel and become tighter, causing more symptoms, if you try to do strengthening or repetitive exercises while TrPs are active. You must first rid the muscle of the TrP, then follow with gentle, nonrepetitive lengthening exercises. You may be able to prevent recurrence of the TrP, but this can be difficult when TrPs are extensive. Despite due diligence, we may miss some. Before you begin any type of exercise, your muscles must be free of trigger points, lengthened, and relaxed.

The important thing to remember regarding exercise and FM, CFID, or CMP is that we are more than our illness. The rest of the body needs help in working efficiently so it can sustain us through the trials of our disorders.

Some types of exercise may require prudent consideration on your part. For instance, stretching is helpful to nearly everyone, but especially if you have FM. However, although stretching is beneficial for central trigger points in CMP patients, it may worsen attachment TrPs,[118] and you should not try to strengthen a taut band of muscle riddled with TrPs. If you have any combination of the three—FM, CFID, or CMP—what you do for one may aggravate the other. So take care and be aware of the risks involved so you can make appropriate modifications. Let your body be your guide and pay attention to what it is telling you. You may want to note any new exercise routines in your journal and keep track of your symptoms. This will help you decipher which movements and exercise types are best for you. It may take some fine-tuning, but you will get there.

Anaerobic training such as isometrics, light weight-lifting, and stretching helps preserve muscle tone and strength, and eliminate toxins, but should be practiced with caution and proper assessment.

anaerobic exercise: exercise in which the task does not cause a significant increase in heart rate.

Giving up a particular physical activity you used to enjoy may not be necessary, but you may have to modify it. If you are capable of making the adaptations necessary to live a better life, the reward is an immense feeling of accomplishment.

_____ *Personal Testimony* _____

Because any body movement can aggravate my CMP, I learned several years ago that the risk of pain from playing golf, skiing, and bowling was just not worth it. My hands are no longer the helpmates they once were. I've given up the treadmill, and stairs are difficult because of hip bursitis, knee problems, meralgia paresthetica, and piriformis syndrome. However, I refuse to give up walking. Hiking is my ultimate favorite exercise and the views are fantastic. At one time I navigated the moderate to difficult trails of Colorado with ease. I have always felt one with nature in the mountains, skiing in winter and hiking in summer. Why should I have to give this up? The answer is, I don't! With careful planning and modification, new goals can be met.

My brother-in-law, a stroke survivor, used to stay with us in Colorado, and we made a pact to exercise. We took only easy trails because we both had to use customized assistive devices. We rested frequently, took plenty of water, and limited the hike to no more than two miles, which generally took us around two-and-a-half hours. We have aged now, so readjustments to our plan have been improvised once again. We do no more hiking on uneven surfaces, but we do still walk, and that is what is important.

Because of physical difficulties, I've traded snow skiing for amateur photography. For me it is an equal exchange. My camera goes everywhere I go.

You just haven't seen the world until you've seen it through the lens of a camera. Capturing the essence of a mountain view, a wild animal performing its daily antics, a waterfall, or an aspen grove starting to turn colors in the early fall is something that wakes up my soul.

We don't have to spend an arm and a leg (literally!) to stay active. The world is right there for us. All we have to do is reach out and grab it.

range of motion (ROM): ROM exercises move each joint through its full range of motion, its greatest degree of motion capability.

active exercise: motion that involves voluntary contraction and relaxation of controlling muscles. It's the kind of exercise you do when lifting weights or doing jumping jacks.

passive exercise: motion imparted to a segment of the body by another person, machine, or other outside force. Passive motion may also be achieved by voluntary effort of another segment of your own body. An example is raising your left arm with your right arm, without any assistance from the left arm muscles. In this instance the left arm would be experiencing passive exercise, and the right arm would be doing active exercise.

Exercise targets the three major disorders in different ways. The goal for FM is to stretch the connective tissue surrounding the muscle so it can move freely, and to maintain tone by strengthening. The goal of exercise for CFID patients is to maintain muscle health and avoid the deterioration that comes with disuse. Most agree active participation in low-level exercise is necessary. The overall goal of exercise for CMP patients is to improve range of motion and function. Find the type of exercise you like and enjoy, one that you tolerate well. Find your limits and stay within the boundaries.

Types of Exercise

Aerobic

Aerobic exercise is any sustained activity that increases oxygen demand and heart rate, such as bicycling, swimming, jogging, or walking. The energy force is reliant on the presence of oxygen supplied by breathing or inspiration in aerobic exercise. This type of exercise is categorized as low impact, moderate impact, or high impact. Generally, lower impact aerobic exercise is the best place to start. Studies of high intensity aerobic activity for FM patients do not necessarily show positive results when compared to low intensity aerobic activity.[119] The levels of aerobic exercise are expressed by calculating your "target" heart rate, which is the maximum number of heartbeats per minute. You can assess your heart rate by checking your pulse manually or with a heart rate monitor, which is a gadget that generally fits on your fingertip or ear. Aerobic training should not be attempted until you are certain of your limitations.

CAUTION

Exercise increases oxygen demand, so if you have a known heart condition, clear your proposed exercise routine with your physician before beginning.

To checking your pulse: Place your index and middle fingers of your right hand side by side on your opposite wrist, in this case the left wrist, just at the base of your thumb. Making sure those two fingers are parallel with your arm bone, slide them to the palm side of your wrist just a little, until you feel a groove. You should now be able to feel your pulse with your fingertips. Don't be discouraged if you don't feel it at first; it takes practice.

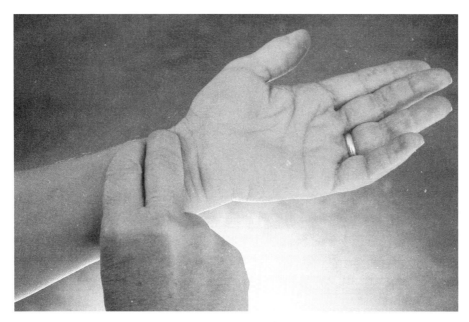

Taking your pulse

The important thing to remember is to use common sense when performing aerobic exercise. If you are so short of breath that you cannot speak while exercising, you are doing too much. Stop and rest. The goal of aerobic exercise is to benefit the body, not put it under undue strain.

TARGET HEART RATE (THR)

Low impact

220 - (minus) age x (times) 60% = THR

    Example:

    If your age is 50, your aerobic exercise THR is:

    220 - 50 = 170; 170 x 60% = 102 beats per minute

Moderate impact

220 - (minus) age x (times) 70–80% = THR

    Example:

    If your age is 40, your aerobic exercise THR is:

    220 – 40 = 180; 180 x 70% = 126 beats per minute

    to 220 – 40 = 180; 180 x 80% = 136 beats per minute

High-impact exercise is strenuous and should be reserved for athletes with properly conditioned bodies.

Aston Patterning

Founded by former dancer Judith Aston, Aston Patterning is an integrated system of movement education, bodywork, and environmental evaluation. In specifically designed sessions, teacher and client work together to reveal and define the body's individual posture and movement patterns while training the body to move more efficiently and effortlessly. Sessions can include any one or a combination of movement education tools. These tools include learning about alternatives that are right for you, identifying stressful habits, using massage-like bodywork for chronic physical and mental stress, and identifying environmental hazards. The environmental consultation assesses how the individual can modify surroundings to reduce unnecessary stress and promote ease of movement.

Bounce Back Chair or Large Exercise Balls

Dysfunction of the autonomic nervous system, or dysautonomia, in astronauts has been studied by N.A.S.A. Bouncing may be beneficial for helping correct this dysfunction. When compared to running, this form of exercise provides maximum gain for minimal effort.[120] Take care, it is easy to become enthralled with childhood memories. It's easy to be too aggressive because it requires minimal effort, but your body still responds to the activity. Remember to protect your central nervous system and those TrPs.

---

dysautonomia: a disruption in the autonomic nervous system.

Chi Kung or Qi Gong

Qi gong is a Chinese restorative-meditative form of specific exercises used to relieve stress and promote health through rhythmic movement, balance, breathing, and focusing.

---

chi = qi = ki = prana: Traditional Chinese medicine refers to our vital life-force energy as *chi* or *qi*. Japanese call it *ki,* and it is known as *prana* in the ayurvedic medical tradition of India.

According to Roger Jahnke in the January-February 1991 issue of the

Townsend Letter for Doctors, qi gong initiates the "relaxation response,"[121] which reduces stress, decreases heart rate, lowers blood pressure, and promotes tissue regeneration.

Qi gong is not the same as t'ai chi or any traditional meditation. *Qi* means "air" or "breath," and *gong* means "work," so it is air work, or breath work. No wonder it is so good for so many conditions! Good breathing has many glorious benefits for health, happiness, and feelings of well-being.

You may need to let go of preconceived notions or biases to begin to understand how qi gong can direct healing qi to a certain body organ or area of pain.[122] Qi gong can be easily practiced at home, and studies done on FM[123] and CFID[124] patients have documented specific benefits.

CAUTION

People with TrPs should avoid holding postures or doing repetition type exercise until their TrPs have been addressed. Immobility and repetition can both set the stage for activating TrPs.

Feldenkrais (Movement Therapy)

As part of his recovery from a sports-related injury, nuclear physicist Moshe Feldenkrais devoted his life to the study of the nervous system and human behavior. He developed what he called a "method of somatic education" for moving the body with less effort. His technique combines subtle exercise, movement training, gentle touch, and verbal dialogue. Feldenkrais encompasses two forms of training. The first, Functional Integration, involves an individual, tailored session wherein the practitioner touches and guides the student with gentle manipulation and movement exercises to improve breathing and body alignment. The second form involves a series of classes, called Awareness through Movement. The lessons teach slow, nonaerobic motions through which the subject achieves a greater awareness of movement patterns and learns ways to move more efficiently. The method helps reduce stress and tension, alleviate chronic pain, and improve balance and coordination. This is a good exercise to help control related aggravating factors.

Counseling has to do with intuition, with work on oneself, with the quietness of one's mind, and the openness of one's heart.

RAM DASS

Hellerwork

Developed by former aerospace engineer Joseph Heller, this technique combines deep-tissue muscle therapy with movement that minimizes effort. It also incorporates counseling on emotional issues that may have an impact on physical posture. Emphasis by practitioners is on the connection between mind and body. For example, Hellerwork practitioners believe stooped shoulders may be a physical manifestation of feelings of insecurity. Participants usually engage in several hourly sessions. Hellerwork is considered helpful in chronic pain conditions and in otherwise healthy people. Its goal is to help people learn to minimize mechanical stress by encouraging a personal physical and emotional balance.

Rocking Chair Exercise

When we rock in a rocking chair, we are actually doing a low impact exercise that is beneficial for circulation. If you are able to be more physically active, rocking is not the only exercise you should do. However, it is one way to exercise without having to put forth a lot of effort. The movement of the feet on the floor is very similar to a type of exercise given to patients who suffer from leg cramping due to poor circulation in the lower extremities. It is very important that you maintain correct body positioning and use a chair that is the right size for your body. Your buttocks should be to the back of the chair and the back of your knees should be at least an inch beyond the seat. You should be able to put your feet flat on the floor and the arm rests should be at the level of your elbows so that you can rest them comfortably. A comfortable chair is important no matter what your activity. What kind of chair are you sitting in right now?

Stretching

Benefits of stretching have been discussed exhaustively, but it is extremely important for people with FM, CFID, and CMP. Stretch as part of your exercise warm up, and continue to stretch throughout the day. It is important to get enough stretch to reap the benefits without aggravating another condition. Don't attempt to stretch immediately after coming in from the cold or after you have used ice. Just as old Betsy tends to clench and stutter on a cold day, so will you.

A good rule of thumb is to briefly stretch to a point of maximum tension, and then ease off to a level somewhere between feeling the stretch and mild discomfort. Hold the stretch for three to thirty seconds, depending upon your tolerance. Here again, start with a low number of repetitions and build slowly. The length of the hold and the number of repetitions may vary among practitioners, so the important thing to remember is that you assess your own tolerance. Remember to breathe through your stretch, stretch each muscle group individually, and if a particular muscle group balks, don't press it. Try not to be too aggressive. The goal is to keep the muscles supple, not cause rebound tenderness or activate trigger points that lurk in waiting.

CAUTION

General repetitive or bounce stretching exercise is not indicated if you have TrPs in a taut band of muscle fiber. Treat them first. Please see "Trigger Point Therapies—Treating the TrPs of CMP" and "Stretching the Muscle during TrP Treatment" on pages 224–25.

Visualize, if you will, every muscle in your body. You will note that some are tense and some are more flaccid (weak, limp, floppy). The goal is to have tone without tension. Can't you just imagine how good you would feel if every muscle were supple and toned?

Stretching daily may be easier to do routinely if you learn how to incorporate an adequate stretch into nearly everything you do. Examples would be to stretch as you apply lotion to your legs, or as you dry yourself off after your bath or shower. Use the lotion or towel to help you glide down the front of your legs as you bend at the waist. Feel the stretch through the back of your legs and your back. Take a nice, deep breath while holding the stretch and feel the stretch between your back ribs. Then slowly bring your hands back up, remembering to always bring your head up last, and take a deep abdominal breath, lifting your arms over your head. Modify, if you need to, by placing one foot on the commode cover. Like a modified yoga lunge (see the Useful Tools section at the end of this chaper).

Find a stretching routine that is easily modified to meet your needs. Aggressive exercise treatment of FM, CFID, and CMP consists of nonaggressive exercise.

Doorway Stretch

This stretch is one you can do anywhere there is a door that accommodates your "wing span." It is a comprehensive exercise that stretches muscles in the chest, around your shoulder girth, calves, hamstrings, and hips.

Place your forearms up against each side of the doorway, with one foot behind the other, and begin to lean forward. You can control the amount of stretch by the distance you move the front leg forward. As you lean forward, you will feel the stretch in your shoulder muscles and in the pectoral muscles of your chest. You will also feel the stretch in your calves, hamstrings, and hip flexors.

Now turn to one side as you lean forward. This helps stretch the muscles above the rib cage (serratus anterior). Put your other foot forward and repeat the exercise. Visualize relaxing and lengthening the muscle fiber as you stretch.

T'ai Chi

T'ai chi is a Chinese system of rhythmic moving meditation that promotes flexibility and strength. This therapeutic exercise involves graceful, dance-like, nonstraining movements performed in synchrony with slow, controlled, effortless breathing and mental focus. T'ai chi promotes tranquillity while developing mind and body strength.

Daily yoga or t'ai chi is beneficial for FM[125] and CFID,[126] and helps maintain muscle health of well-tended TrPs. Because of the focused movement, it not only helps physically, it also helps the mind focus away from pain. Stretching tender, contracted muscles helps the FM patient maintain flexibility and minimizes any coexisting tendonitis and bursitis. Even CFID patients should be able to tolerate this low level of activity without triggering a flare. Of course, if you are in a flare, any activity should be minimized until your body has a chance to regroup.

T'ai chi aids emotional stability, increases flexibility, strengthens the heart, reduces mental stress, alleviates physical stress, boosts the immune system, and is gentle on bones, muscles, and joints." Not only does it do all this, it promotes healing, expands the mind, creates lightheartedness, and enhances life.[127]

Avoid strengthening and repetitive exercise of any kind if you have active trigger points.

Weight Lifting

Weight lifting is best attempted after you have established a successful stretching program and aerobic routine. Weight lifting is a strengthening exercise, and if you have CMP, it should not be attempted until all TrPs are completely gone. Even then, weight lifting should be started at a very low level. A low level consists of lifting one to ten pounds using small muscle groups. Great modification is needed. For us, even low-level weight lifting requires the guidance of someone with a strong knowledge base, particularly regarding our disorders.

As with all exercise, there is a right way and a wrong way of lifting weights. Inappropriate weight or technique can cause muscle trauma. Your body worker, physical therapist, or qualified trainer should be able to help you in determining what is best for you, and how to proceed with the proper weight lifting exercises for your condition.

Yoga

Yoga was originally a Hindu philosophy and the physical poses were intended to promote spiritual growth. Modern yoga is practiced to bring about harmony and relieve stress. The most familiar forms of yoga involve gentle movement and regular breathing exercises. Some yoga practices also include visualization, progressive relaxation, and meditation. By assuming various yoga positions (asanas) and practicing controlled breathing, it's possible to achieve an altered state of mind and increase oxygen and blood flow to the body's organs. Yoga also promotes alignment of the spine by improving flexibility. Many practitioners believe it purifies the body of impurities by harmonious regulation of the endocrine and nervous systems.

Many of the stretching exercises you'll find in the Useful Tools section of this chapter are modified or basic yoga asanas.

Laughter

You don't stop laughing because you grow old; you grow old because you stop laughing.

AUTHOR UNKNOWN

Laughter flexes the diaphragm, chest, and abdominal muscles, causing deep breathing. It helps relax the shoulders, neck, and facial muscles; and aids digestion, stimulates the heart, and increases the production of endorphins, which help relieve pain. A hearty laugh can burn up as many calories per hour as a brisk walk.[128]

Laughter removes us from the self-absorbed ego and releases negative thoughts. It helps us to balance our perspective on painful experiences and deal with difficulties in a healthy way.

A cheerful heart is good medicine, but a downcast spirit dries up the bones.

PROVERBS 17:22

Concluding Thoughts on Exercise

No matter the type of exercise, muscles that are well cared for can help reduce chronic pain. Regular exercise, when done within your limits, is known to increase endorphins, our natural painkilling chemicals. Properly done routine exercise plays a role in increasing natural killer cells, the frontline of immune system defense.[129] This indicates that exercise improves our immune system and helps us fight off unwanted microorganisms and diseases.

The important thing to remember when choosing a type of exercise is to choose one that keeps you FIT—Fun, Intelligent, and Therapeutic.

Bodywork—Toiling over the Anatomy

Bodywork is helpful because it helps rid the body of unwanted cellular waste. The following are different types of bodywork techniques. In our case, you may find modifications to certain therapies are needed. Modification—there's that word again.

Massage Therapy

Massage therapy is usually manual manipulation of muscles, but a mechanical or electrical device developed for treatment of soft tissue may also be used. The goal of therapeutic massage is to promote deep muscle relaxation and thereby relieve the pain caused by tight muscles. Massage is extremely beneficial for people with musculoskeletal disorders. Properly done massage techniques can help alleviate pain, relieve muscle tension, decrease soreness, ease spasm, enhance muscle and joint function, improve circulation of blood and lymph, and promote the release of painkilling endorphins.

There are many types and forms of massage, including lymphatic, Swedish, traditional, deep tissue, hot stone, and shiatsu. The type is just as important as the massage itself. What works well for one person may not necessarily be the type that works best for you, and people with disorders involving the muscles are at risk of easy injury. Even micro-trauma that can be insignificant to others can be devastating to people with FM, CFID, or CMP.

Massage therapy is based on the concept that everything in the body is connected and that soft tissue responds to touch. Unlike a healthy, resilient muscle that is designed to keep the body performing like a well-oiled machine, a shortened muscle cannot execute the workload.

It is important to choose a therapist who understands the implications of your disorder.

Alexander Technique

Alexander Technique is a movement therapy named for the actor who created it. After concluding that bad posture and poor physical habits were responsible for his chronic voice loss, he developed a method of physical retraining using a series of simple movements to put the body into relaxed balance. Practitioners teach simple, efficient physical movements designed to improve balance, posture, and coordination, and to relieve pain. Instructors offer gentle, hands-on guidance and verbal instruction to retrain students in the optimal use of their bodies. A session may focus on movements as basic as getting up from a chair properly.

Craniosacral Therapy (Cranial Osteopathy)

Osteopathic physician William Garner Sutherland developed craniosacral therapy and wrote a book about it, *Cranial Bowl,* in 1939. This form of manipulative therapy pays particular attention to structural alterations in the head and sacrum (tailbone). The practitioner is usually an osteopathic physician, medical doctor, dentist, chiropractor, naturopathic doctor, acupuncturist, or licensed body worker. Their trained hands can feel restriction in movement of the cranial bones, scalp, and neck. Once imbalances are detected, the therapist targets manipulation of the affected area. Structural alterations in the head and sacrum are thought to inhibit motion of the brain and spinal cord and cause disruption in the fluctuation of the cerebrospinal fluid. Techniques for the head include gentle manipulation inside the mouth, as well as treating the cranium.

"Your hand bone's connected to your arm bone, your arm bone's connected to your shoulder bone . . ." and your head is connected, by the way.

Myofascial Release

Myofascial release (MFR) is a hands-on manipulation of the muscles, their covering (fascia), and the surrounding soft tissue. Myofascia surrounds the muscle fibers and the bundles of fibers that make up the muscle. The goal of myofascial release is to help free restrictive fascia from the muscle, the fibers, or the bundles of fibers. Over time, the covering of the muscle (myofascia) may adhere to muscle fibers, causing a type of restriction, like that found with adhesions and scarring. Releasing the muscle tissue from the surrounding myofascia facilitates easier movement. Note how on a chicken breast the skin slides freely but is still attached. This is how healthy myofascia "should be." Many physical therapists are trained in this mild and gentle form of stretching. Health insurance companies sometimes cover MFR when it's done by a licensed health care provider.

Research shoes that abnormal "active scars" can cause myofascial pain, and if left untreated, these scars can block therapeutic results. Micro- or macro-adhesions (scars) need to be properly released through manipulative therapy in order to restore movement and function, promote blood and lymphatic flow, and provide muscle symmetry.

Aggressive MFR can accelerate the release of toxins, which can cause longer-lasting effects in people with FM and CFID. Rest and drink plenty of water after treatment to help the body flush out these unwanted chemicals.

Reflexology

Reflexology is massage at corresponding pressure points on the hands and feet to relieve disruptive symptoms produced by the body's disequilibria. People who use this form of treatment believe that acupressure-type therapy on particular points of the extremities will help relieve certain symptoms in other areas of the body.

Rolfing

As with myofascial release, Rolfing works on the connective tissue, or fascia. A complete Rolfing treatment consists of ten one-hour sessions of deep massage, each session building on the previous, with total body alignment as the goal. Biochemist Ida Rolf (1896–1979) was ahead of her time. She realized that deep manipulation and stretching of the fascia could help restore the body's natural alignment, which may have become rigid through protecting or compensating for an injury, disease, emotional trauma, or inefficient movement habits. Our bodies get "out of whack" from walking, sleeping, physical activity, poor posture, and injuries. We have already discussed how improper body alignment, for any reason, can affect our pain. Each session of Rolfing is focused on releasing tension in an individual body part and resolving overall vulnerability in the body's structure. Misalignment can compromise body function. Rolfing was once thought to be too aggressive for patients with FM; however, when the practitioner has a patient-focused approach, it may be used successfully.[130] Rolf practitioners are certified through the Rolf Institute in Boulder, Colorado.

Rosen Method

Developed by former physical therapist Marion Rosen, this method uses gentle touch therapy and verbal communication to evoke relaxation and self-awareness. The work is sometimes used in conjunction with counseling, and can bring up buried feelings and emotions that have an effect on total well-being. This method may be particularly helpful to FM patients.[131]

Spray and Stretch

Spray and stretch in conjunction with other therapies is beneficial for all types of muscle restriction. The technique involves manipulation of muscles after application of a spray coolant. The coolant deadens the pain sensation while the affected muscle is being stretched, and is particularly beneficial during times of flare. Spray and stretch is not limited to trained professionals. You or your family members can also learn this technique. It is important to note, however, that proper timing, correct application of the vapocoolant, proper muscle re-warming, and range of motion stretches within the muscle's limits can make the difference between a good outcome and a poor one. If you stretch the taut band of muscle of CMP too far, you can actually cause further trauma to supporting structures.

Trager Work

Trager is a form of gentle, rhythmic touch and passive movement developed by Milton Trager, M.D., a specialist in neuromuscular conditions and a former boxer, acrobat, and dancer.

Trager believed in the power of the mind to bypass the state of consciousness and access the unconscious. His method focuses on learning effective movement and good posture to release tension caused by emotional stress. The practitioner perceives the energy flow of the client through the meditative state.

The purpose of Trager work is to raise awareness of body positioning and move beyond old patterns of restriction. When the body has greater flexibility, blood flow to painful areas improves. All these "side effects" are ones that we would welcome with open arms.

Trigger Point Therapy

Certain massage techniques that are used as part of trigger point therapy are specific to TrPs, so they will be covered in greater lengths in "Myofascial Trigger Point Therapy," "Trigger Point Therapy: Treating the TrPs of CMP," and "Stretching the Muscle during TrP Treatment." Clair Davies has a separate chapter in his 2004, second edition of *The Trigger Point Therapy Workbook* devoted specifically to "showing your massage therapist how to effectively treat trigger points."[132]

Vodder Manual Lymphatic Massage/Drainage

It is normal for lymph fluid to accumulate in the lymph system. If you remember from chapter 1, this is where noxious agents such as damaged cells, bacteria, and toxins collect. The cellular garbage is cleaned up by lymphocyte and macrophage cells, and is then returned to circulation as plasma. Sometimes this system requires encouragement due to certain factors.

There are three types of swelling. Diffuse swelling occurs with interstitial edema, localized swelling takes place around a lymph node from chronic infection, and there is swelling from myofascial entrapment of lymph and blood vessels.

Let's talk about diffuse swelling first. Idiopathic edema, a form of fluid retention found in FM, occurs more frequently in women.[133] Interstitial edema is caused by abnormal biochemicals that cause fluid to be retained in the spaces between tissues. These spaces, called interstitial spaces, are part of the ground substance in the myofascia. In Dr. Starlanyl's view, interstitial edema is extremely difficult to treat because it requires moving the excess fluid from the interstitial spaces to the lymph vessels so that it can be removed from the body. There is no easy way to do this. You have to figure out why the edema is building up in the interstitial spaces, and remedy that perpetuating factor. "Treating the cause is the best way to treat the effect."[134]

---

idiopathic: self-originating, occurring without known cause.

The second type of swelling is that caused by obstructed lymph flow. Swelling that occurs around a lymph node is the result of accumulated dead cellular matter and bacteria in the node as a response to chronic infection. Lymph nodes act like filters. The filter—the lymph node—can get stopped up from excessive accumulation of unwanted organisms, like a shower drain clogs with hair. When this happens, the lymph fluid backs up in the lymph vessels causing localized swelling. People with FM, CFID, and CMP can have this kind of swelling; however, it is more commonly seen in CFID patients.

We have talked about two types of swelling: diffuse idiopathic edema seen in FM patients, and local swelling seen predominantly in CFID patients because of clogged lymph nodes. The third kind of swelling is that seen in CMP patients. This is swelling caused by blood or lymph vessel entrapment by taut bands of muscle fiber, as discussed in chapter 1. Trigger points that occur near lymph nodes may be mistaken for swollen nodes when they are actually TrPs.

Lymph fluid, unlike blood, which is moved along by specific vessel mechanics, requires modalities such as exercise, deep breathing, body movement, and properly functioning organ activity to keep it moving. When any of these are disrupted, excessive lymph accumulates in the lymph system and causes swelling.

Vodder Manual Lymphatic Massage/Drainage is a technique aimed at opening lymphatic ducts and removing blockages, which aids in reducing generalized swelling. This technique sometimes involves the manipulation of lymph glands located close to genitalia and breasts, so you may want to request a gender specific therapist.

Easy Does It

The benefits of exercise and bodywork abound. Otherwise healthy people tolerate these activities with little more than reported soreness. Unlike us, their symptoms do not persist or require further treatment as the result of a workout.

Because of the detoxification caused by bodywork, it is necessary to rid your body of cellular waste gradually. If your workouts are too varied, too aggressive, too frequent, or too lengthy, you can significantly intensify your symptoms. As with every other treatment, start new bodywork techniques one at a time. It is important to identify which type you will benefit from, and how it needs to be modified to meet your individual needs.

Finding the Right Body Worker or Therapist

The goal of bodywork is to keep all body parts in motion with the least amount of stress. That is why finding the right massage therapist is just as important as finding the right doctor. A qualified massage therapist should:

1. Be licensed in the state of practice. (Most states require specific standards of performance for massage therapists.)
2. Be a member of the American Massage Therapy Association.
3. Be certified by the National Certification Board for Therapeutic Massage and Bodywork.
4. Be a graduate or student of a school accredited by the Commission on Massage Therapy Accreditation.

Some massage therapists receive advanced training. If you need a therapist to meet certain needs, it is important to make sure the therapist you work with has this advanced training. For example, if you have CMP you would want a therapist who is knowledgeable in Travell and Simons work. This means your therapist should know the difference between a tender point of FM and a trigger point of CMP, and have a basic understand of all three—FM, CFID, and CMP.

Although massage can be of great benefit, remember to use caution, regardless of the type of massage therapy you seek. Massage techniques may need to be modified in patients with coexisting FM, CFID, and/or CMP. Also, some medical problems—skin problems, certain forms of cancer, heart disease, and seizure disorders—could actually become worse with any type of massage. Some types of massage may help one problem, yet cause additional symptoms of another. Be sure to check with your doctor before you seek out a massage professional, or ask for a referral from someone who has problems similar to yours. Your support group is a good place to start.

Medical Specialists and Therapists

Ayurvedic Medicine

Ayurveda is an ancient, traditional system of medicine that originated in India and is quite possibly the most complete medical system ever created. It focuses on the relationship of body, mind, and spirit, and includes the use of herbs, food, exercise, breathing, meditation, yoga, massage, and lifestyle change to restore balance. Recommendations are based on your specific combination of doshas (mind/body types).

Chiropractic Medicine

Chiropractic medicine was developed by David Daniel Palmer more than one hundred years ago. It focuses on maintaining the health of the nervous system by therapeutic manipulation of the skeletal bones and joints. The principles of chiropractic medicine are based on the necessity of proper spinal alignment for delivery of nerve impulses and the flow of vital energy. Therefore, adjustments of the spine aid in restoring wellness. Many chiropractors augment their care by using kinesiology and providing nutritional counseling.

> **kinesiology:** a diagnostic system based on the premise that individual muscle functions provide information about a patient's overall health. Practitioners test the strength and mobility of certain muscles, analyze a patient's posture and gait, and inquire about lifestyle factors that may be contributing to an illness. Nutrition, muscle and joint manipulation, diet, and exercise are included as part of a treatment plan. Kinesiology is practiced by licensed professionals, including chiropractors, dentists, medical doctors, and osteopaths.

Infectious Disease Specialist

An infectious disease specialist is a licensed physician who specializes in treatment of diseases caused by infection. If you have chronic fatigue immunodysfunction, you might expect to be referred to an infectious disease specialist.

Naturopathic Medicine

Coined by Dr. John Scheel in 1895, the term naturopathic medicine is used to describe a combination of nontoxic therapies, including clinical nutrition, herbal medicine, homeopathy, spinal manipulation, exercise therapy, hydrotherapy, electrotherapy, stress reduction, and natural cures. The philosophy is that health is not the absence of symptoms, but absence of the cause. Naturopathy is based on the concept that the body is a self-healing organism, and places a strong emphasis on prevention. It promotes a healthy lifestyle through the integration of exercise, stress reduction, and a proper diet of natural, organic foods.

Osteopathic Medicine

Following are the holistic principles upon which osteopathic medicine was founded.

1. A person is a complete, dynamic unit of function embodied by the physical, the mental, and the spiritual.
2. Lifestyle and community have an effect on the health of each individual.
3. The body possesses self-regulatory mechanisms that are self-healing in nature.
4. The person should be considered as a whole person; that is, if there is a problem in one part of the body's structure and function, other areas may be affected.
5. The body has the ability to self-regulate. Many of osteopathic medicine's manipulative techniques are aimed at reducing or eliminating impediments to proper structure and function, to enable self-healing and restore health.

However, in a survey done by Johnson and Kurtz, only 41 percent of three thousand U.S. doctors of osteopathy responding to the survey indicated they take this holistic approach. I questioned this seemingly ambiguous term with my physician, who is a doctor of osteopathy. He indicated that the term "holistic" could also refer to other types of alternative medicine and did not reflect the fact that osteopathic physicians are medically licensed physicians like their M.D. counterparts. However, 59 percent of those surveyed believe their practice is different from allopathic doctors. A wide majority, 72 percent, confirmed that osteopathic manipulation treatment is a distinguishing feature of osteopathy; but 19 percent of those surveyed do not practice OMT because it would not be appropriate for their specialty. In the final analysis, the consensus of the survey reflects the osteopathic belief that a "caring doctor-patient relationship and a hands-on style" is of primary importance in their health care delivery.[135] Osteopaths practice in all the same specialties as M.D.s, with the greatest percentage in the primary care specialties of family practice, pediatrics, and internal medicine.[136]

---

allopathic: a system for treating disease with remedies that produce effects different from those created by the disease itself; Western medicine as commonly practiced.

Pain Management Specialist

A pain management specialist is a licensed physician whose specialty is diagnosing and treating people with acute pain due to chronic conditions or to events such as surgery, childbirth, or injury.

It is important that you have someone knowledgeable in pain management treating you for your pain. A pain management specialist is expected to care for pain patients on a regular basis and is trained specifically in pain management; however, not all of them understand FM, CFID, and CMP.

Physiatrist

A physiatrist is a licensed physician who studies and treats physical dysfunction. Physiatrists help people learn to adapt to their limitations and work with patients to restore the highest quality of function.

---

physiotherapy: therapeutic modalities that produce benefits to the body, such as touch, exercise, electrical stimulation, massage, and myofascial release.

Psychotherapy and Supportive Counseling

Having a positive attitude and learning healthy coping behaviors is of great importance in treating chronic pain. The benefits of cognitive-behavioral therapy as adjunctive treatment of chronic pain are well known. Learning how to reduce stress and improve coping mechanisms can help to alleviate symptoms.[137] Sometimes we are too close to our pain and fatigue. Someone knowledgeable in the study of human behavior can provide mental, physical, emotional, and spiritual balance that helps us focus on priorities.

Psychiatrist

A psychiatrist is a licensed physician who studies and treats mental illness. A psychiatrist can also help a patient to avert a breakdown. See chapter 5 for more information about the difference between a psychiatrist and a psychotherapist.

Rheumatologist

A rheumatologist is a physician licensed in internal medicine. This specialty involves advanced study in treatment of abnormal conditions of the muscles, tendons, joints, and bones that cause pain and/or limit movement. Rheumatologists treat such disorders as arthritis, lupus, Sjogren's syndrome, FM, CFID, scleroderma, and other chronic disorders of the soft tissue. Not all rheumatologist treat FM and CFID.

Sports Medicine

A sports medicine doctor is one who specializes in preventing, diagnosing, and treating injuries related to physical activity. They treat joint and muscle injury in patients of all ages. Although many injuries are sports related, you need not have had a sports related injury to benefit from seeing a sports medicine specialist.

Sports medicine is a subspeciality that focuses on the musculoskeletal system. Physicians are board certified doctors in family practice, internal medicine, emergency medicine, pediatrics, or physiatry and have advanced training in sports medicine through an accredited fellowship program. A doctor who practices sports medicine can be your "team leader," coordinating care with physical trainers, physical therapists, personal physicians, medical and surgical specialists, and other practitioners of specialty and rehabilitative care.

Health and Functionality Therapists

Occupational Therapy

Occupational therapists work with chronic disorders affecting the upper body. Therapy includes stretching and strengthening, and spray and stretch. The focus of occupational therapy (OT) is to help you make adjustments in your activities of daily living. OTs teach self-help therapies, as well as how to use helpful equipment, adapt to limitations, and change your environment to meet your needs.

Physical Therapy

The goal of physical therapy (PT) is to help alleviate, reverse, or manage pain, fatigue, deconditioning, muscle weakness, urinary incontinence, sleep disturbances, and other diseases or chronic disorders.

A physical therapist uses a variety of physiotherapy methods to help improve function, including active or passive exercise, stretching and strengthening, postural assessment and correction, biofeedback, electrical stimulation, massage, myofascial release, spray and stretch, and other physical methods. The purpose of these treatments is to strengthen the body and correct dysfunction due to disease or injury.

A good PT knows that proper body alignment allows the body to move with ease and efficiency. Beware if your therapist suggests starting a work hardening/conditioning program or exercising for twenty to thirty minutes per day. This would indicate someone who may be great at rehabilitation for other physical dysfunction, but is not proficient in treating our disorders.

If you have difficulty finding a therapist who knows much about FM, CFID, or CMP, your next best bet is to find someone who is familiar with treatment for rheumatoid conditions.

Myofascial Trigger Point Therapy

Therapists who are board certified in myofascial trigger point therapy (CMTPT) or have graduated from an approved school may join the National Association of Myofascial Trigger Point Therapists (NAMTPT). NAMTPT establishes and promotes standards of CMTPTs, provides opportunities for advanced training, and offers resources and supportive services. These therapists are specifically trained to treat trigger points.

Trigger Point Therapy—Treating the TrPs of CMP

We now know that a trigger point is a hypersensitive area of shortened muscle fiber within a taut band of muscle. The goal of trigger point therapy is to restore these fibers to their normal length, and thereby improve function.

As previously discussed, TrPs can be aggravated or perpetuated by factors you can help control, such as getting the proper amount of rest, addressing body misalignment, improving posture habits, improving bodywork strategies, not smoking, avoiding excessive alcohol intake, learning to breathe properly, and eating healthful foods.

The first treatment suggestion is to identify and correct perpetuating factors and adapt trigger point therapies that calm the hypersensitive areas in the myofascia.

Trigger points can breed faster than rabbits if left untended. If you suffer from CMP, it took a long time to get into this condition, so it's not reasonable to expect immediate improvement. However, due diligence can pay off. Although your problem has become chronic, it can be controlled and you can get at least temporary relief, which is something any one of us welcomes.

You can learn to treat TrPs on your own. To be successful you should anticipate learning more about your body than you ever thought possible. Some TrPs may not permanently respond to therapy, no matter how hard you try, but you can learn where and how to treat them. Continued identification and effective treatment will help you develop a sixth sense and increase the likelihood of your spending significant amounts of time TrP free. Self-treatment initially needs to be guided by an experienced therapist. You need to have confidence your technique is done properly. If you are able to learn a home treatment program, you will be more likely to achieve continuing, effective results.[138]

Releasing trigger points by massage techniques can reduce or alleviate pain generated by an active trigger point. However, it is important to remember that if you also have FM or CFID, the usual trigger-point massage techniques may need to be modified significantly. The release of TrP waste byproducts can instigate a flare of FM or CFID symptoms. If bodywork is too deep, too aggressive, too lengthy, or too frequent, the body may not be able to detoxify.

Trigger points do not respond to positive thinking, biofeedback, meditation, or progressive relaxation. They respond only to physical intervention. However, positive thinking, biofeedback, meditation, and progressive relaxation can help prevent the stress that is thought to aggravate chronic myofascial pain. In my opinion, they all should be practiced as preventive measures.

Conventional stretching exercises, like those recommended for FM and CFID, are not sufficiently specific to affect a trigger point, but keeping healthy muscle fibers supple serves as a preventive measure. Be careful, though, because overdoing stretching and strengthening can activate and exacerbate trigger points. This is why people who have FM and/or CFID along with CMP have such a difficult time finding a happy medium. Often the treatment for one disorder becomes an aggravating factor for the other. Generalized stretching should be done cautiously; however, direct therapy to trigger points must be accompanied by stretching of the area.[139] Remember, stagnant muscles build toxins and stretching helps release them.

Stretching the Muscle during TrP Treatment

A sarcomere is a tiny unit of muscle fiber. Many of them lined up end to end form myofibrils, and thousands of myofibrils make up the skeletal muscle. The sarcomere's job is to contract the muscle. Each one goes through three phases—resting, contracted, and stretched (see figure on p. 226)—and the impulse from one to the other is transmitted in a domino effect. Have you ever seen a Chinese finger trap? You put a finger in each end (this is the relaxed phase, normal length) and pull the fingers away from each other. This movement imprisons your fingers as the trap stretches, lengthens, and tightens. A sarcomere functions similarly. The finger trap contracts and shortens when you push your fingers together, thus enabling you to remove your fingers. This is the way a muscle should work: stretching to full length and contracting, or shortening, when the muscle is performing a job, putting all that energy into accomplishing the movement. Myofascial trigger points are an area of unnaturally shortened, thickened, sarcomeres in knotted, ineffective muscle fiber. These bound-up sarcomeres contract and stay that way. When this happens it weakens the rest of the myofibril (chain of sarcomeres) during a full-length stretch. This makes the muscle weak and unable to function properly. Think of it this way: Imagine a large shooter marble in the middle of that Chinese finger trap, then put a finger in each end and try to stretch it as far as it would stretch if it didn't have a marble in the middle. This demands increased force and puts stress on the part being stretched. Over time, this will weaken the finger trap, it will fray and break, and so will a muscle with untreated TrPs. It is extremely important to treat that myofascial trigger point so the sarcomeres can lengthen and contract normally. This is why applying gentle, passive range of motion to the muscle while treating TrPs improves the outcome of the treatment. It will help the knotted up fiber to relax and lengthen. This stretch is different from the daily stretching exercise of supple and TrP-free muscles, discussed previously.[140] Once you have successfully treated TrPs, you should

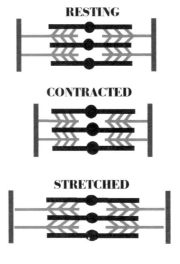

Sarcomere

maintain a routine that can keep the muscles supple and strong and prevent the redevelopment of TrPs.

Tennis Ball Therapy and Acutherapy

Tennis ball therapy is a form of self-massage using a tennis ball to treat trigger points. You can identify your own TrPs and referred pain. Scan your body by moving your hands and fingers over it to identify problem areas.

Devin Starlanyl covers this topic very thoroughly in her book, *Fibromyalgia & Chronic Myofascial Pain: A Survival Manual,* and on her website. You'll find the link in the resource section at the end of the book. Much of the following information is from her references.

CAUTION

Tennis ball therapy should not be used if you have had a stroke, a head injury, or anything that might increase your intracranial (inside your head) pressure.

Balls of different sizes can be used on different parts of the body, depending upon the shape, location, and size of the taut band of muscle fiber that contains the TrP(s).

Devin Starlanyl suggests placing two tennis balls together in a knee sock, with a knot on either side of the balls, which should be pressed tightly together. Then you can roll them down the sides of your spine, starting about the middle of the back of your head. Lean against a wall or lie on the floor using care to keep one ball on either side of the spine. This technique seems to work well because you are able to move the balls centrally over the spine, kneading the supporting muscles as you go and locating TrPs that need specific attention.

An alternative is to use a twenty-four-inch length of a hard-sponge swimming noodle. It is less specific, but it does provide a good pre-treatment massage by loosening and stimulating the entire area. There is a drawback to this particular type of treatment: Squatting and straightening as you roll the balls or noodle up and down your back may put stress on your legs. If you have untreated trigger points in your legs, you may cause a flare; however, your lower extremities can benefit from the strengthening exercise if all is well in the "south forty."

You can also do the wall or floor technique using one ball, depending on the anatomical location of the TrP(s). Move bony structures out of the way as much as possible to ensure direct TrP pressure. This decreases the risk of bruising and makes the exposed area easier to treat. For instance, if TrPs are located in the upper back, hug yourself to open up the shoulder blades. For the buttocks area, you may find treatment easier by sitting, rather than lying, on the ball. Roll the ball to cover all surfaces of the upper and lower back, finding and treating trigger points as you go. You can reach much of your sides as well. Don't neglect the sides of your ribs and hips. If you have many TrPs in the rib area, check for paradoxical breathing. You don't have to use a tennis ball; you may find that lacrosse balls are better for the back and hip areas.

The smaller the ball, the harder the ball, and the more weight you place on the ball, the firmer the pressure. Take care to continue to follow the massage guidelines above.

To work the belly, lie on the floor on the tennis ball, or a larger massage ball, and roll slowly up and down, covering the area from your sides to your rib cage. You might find some "screamers" that will take a while to work out. Be sure to treat the pubic arch, the pelvic floor, the thighs, and the groin. Do not use this form of physical therapy if you have abdominal or pelvic disease.

Continue to work the low back, the buttocks, the back of the legs, and your feet. If you are able to pinpoint a TrP you were previously unaware of, it is probably a "latent" TrP and needs to be treated.

A latent TrP is what I like to call a "latent in waiting," not to be confused with a "lady in waiting." There is nothing ladylike about a trigger point just waiting to get angry. Treating latent TrPs is just as important as treating active TrPs. As the old saying goes, "An ounce of prevention is worth a pound of cure."

One ball in the end of an old pantyhose leg is of the greatest benefit to me. It allows me to single out specific trigger points. In addition, I tend to place too much pressure on the trigger point if I use it on a hard surface, so I manipulate the ball by holding on to the end of the panty hose and throwing the ball end over my shoulder while sitting in my recliner. The soft chair provides cushioning so there is less likelihood of too much pressure on the tissue. It also makes it easier to treat TrPs in the buttocks area, because I can sit on the ball. To treat TrPs located on the sides of my body, I use the tennis ball and lie on the sofa or bed. I prefer to use ping-pong balls taped together to treat trigger points in my neck area. Devin Starlanyl suggests that softer surfaces for tennis ball compression may also be indicated if you have extremely sore TrPs. Start by sitting in a chair or sofa.[141]

Whether you find the discomfort of a latent TrP while rolling around on your ball or go directly to an active TrP, your goal is to treat the area until you get some relief. Once you locate the area, you need to apply pressure until the TrP releases. It is important to remember, however, not to apply too much pressure or maintain pressure for too long. If you are too aggressive you can bruise yourself, cause rebound pain (especially if you also have FM), or block blood and lymphatic flow to the area, trapping the toxins instead of releasing them. You can also intensify fatigue or joint pain if you have CFID. If you do it correctly, you should be able to feel the release of the trigger point and the pain should diminish, or totally vanish. For really difficult and resistant TrPs, or TrPs that are in layers, start with enough pressure to get resistance and press until you get a release. Then press a little harder until you get another release. Keep going until the TrP releases totally.[142] If there is no release, take care; you may not be on the right spot and could do more harm if you continue. Leave the area alone for a while and come back to it later. You don't want your treatment to activate yet another latent TrP, because an active TrP causes pain all the time and a latent TrP only hurts when you touch it. Active or latent, all TrPs cause shortening of muscle fiber and decreased function that restricts motion.

The Trigger Point Therapy Workbook, second edition, by Clair Davies is an excellent reference. He does a wonderful job mapping out specific trigger points by pain referral patterns, and the visual aids are useful for lay people. The book also includes information for your massage therapist and instructions for dealing with habitual muscle tension. Another good book is *Art of Body Maintenance: The Winner's Guide to Pain Relief,* by Hal Blatman, M.D., and Brad Ekvall, B.F.A., which includes an integrated program of trigger point location, referral patterns, pain control, stretching, proper breathing, and ball acupressure. All the information found in these books (details in the resource section) is valuable to the CMP patient.

Remember that the TrP site may not be located directly over the painful area. Working the wrong spot, improper technique, or incomplete treatment can result in treatment failure, so take care to locate each specific trigger point and review treatment technique suggestions. Make a map of your TrPs on the anatomical diagram if that will help you remember where you need to continue treatment. Massage of the hard tissue may be needed to loosen the fibers enough to locate the TrP. If it is resistant, meaning it will not release within the maximum treatment time of about one minute, the TrP needs to be readdressed later. You must allow time for blood and lymphatic flow to be restored to the area. When TrPs are extremely resistant, direct massage is better than treating a trigger point too hard or for too long.

Healthy people who get intermittent muscle trigger points from isolated muscle stress and injury can use acupressure therapy, too. The difference between these people and people with CMP is that their TrPs are related to a specific insult, whereas ours can be aggravated simply by movements of daily living. Nevertheless, everybody deserves to know what trigger points are and how to treat them. Don't you wish someone had told you? Believe me, when you can convince a friend or family member to try tennis ball therapy for treatment of their own intermittent TrPs, they develop trust in what you are telling them about aspects of your condition.

Additional Information on TrP Treatment

You can choose spray and stretch, ultrasonography, manipulative therapy, or injections to treat trigger points, but the goal is the same. You want to release the hyperirritable spots in the muscle band and prevent or treat accompanying problems, such as headache, ringing in the ears, jaw pain, poor posture, eye twitches, or the many other side effects. Your goal is to return the contorted muscle to a healthy state, thereby improving function of both muscles and joints.

Theracane

A Theracane is a cane-shaped apparatus with knobs of different lengths extending from the cane in various spots. The outermost bars are easy to

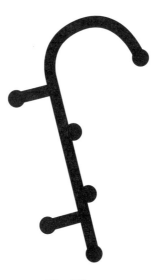

The Theracane

grasp and enable you to treat your own trigger point areas on the backside of your body.

This tool can be used to address TrPs in the muscles that cause local and referred pain, and to reduce the stress put on your hands and fingers. You will find it particularly helpful in reaching normally inaccessible sore points. Life without my Theracane would be unbearable. It's portable and can go anywhere I go. See the assistive devices part of the resource section for Theracane ordering information.

The MA Roller

There are some other effective massage tools available for purchase in the marketplace. One that is especially good for massaging the muscles that run along either side of the spine is the MA Roller. But take care with this tool; it is made of hardwood, so the pressure it exerts would be too intense for someone with FM if used on a hard floor. Using it on a softer surface would help to ease the pressure. We have listed a source for the MA Roller in the resource section.

Trigger Point Injections

According to a leading authority in treatment of myofascial pain, Professor David Simons, trigger point injections for treatment of CMP are used when conservative, non-invasive forms of therapy have been unsuccessful. Finding someone experienced in treatment of CMP versus acute trigger points is a must. Injections for TrPs must be administered in the proper manner, regardless of whether TrPs are latent, active, or any other kind. After proper identification by palpation, or, in the case of hidden TrPs, located by the pain or symptom referral pattern, the patient should be properly positioned for each specific muscle being treated, and trigger point injections should be performed along with bodywork, such as spray and stretch or stretch and heat.[143] If your specialist is not well-versed in the differences among treatments, uses steroids to treat you, or is not experienced in treating patients with multiple trigger points found in CMP, then you are less likely to obtain the results you desire. Before you make your appointment, ask what treatment the doctor uses.

Dry needling, which is somewhat akin to acupuncture, is sometimes used,[144] but if anesthesia is injected, procaine or lidocaine is usually the local anesthetic of choice. This is because it is less likely to cause destruction and toxicity of the tissue being infiltrated.[145]

Pre-treatment

Vitamin C is recommended before and during treatment. Pre-treatment analgesia has been proven effective,[146] but avoid aspirin or blood thinning (anticoagulant) medications or herbs to decrease the likelihood of bruising.

Post-treatment

It is just as important to care for your trigger points after treatment. Your physician should apply local pressure and "individual muscles from the functional unit must always be stretched to their full passive range of motion."[147] Post–trigger point treatment also includes getting plenty of rest and water. Dr. John Whiteside, fellow, Australasian College of Nutritional and Environmental Medicine (www.myomed.com.au), is a leading authority in treatment of trigger points. He suggests that treatment be delayed if you have been fasting or have recently been ill, because those conditions decrease the likelihood of successful treatment.[148]

Botox has been used in treatment of trigger points and various other conditions involving neuromuscular dysfunction, such as difficulty in swallowing. Even though botulinum toxin treatment may prove useful in treatment of trigger point pain and dysfunction,[149] its use in treatment of trigger points is still experimental and there is insufficient clinical evidence of its effectiveness in treating non-neurologic, chronic, musculoskeletal pain conditions.[150] My pain management doctor suggested that I try botox as a treatment of last resort for a particularly resistant trigger point but the treatment exacerbated my CFID and FM symptoms, so I advise caution in using it for CMP if you have coexisting conditions.

Miscellaneous Treatments

Electronic Stimulation Devices

Electronic stimulation devices, such as micro-current stimulators, interferential stimulation devices, NMES (neuromuscular electrical simulation), interferential therapy, galvanic stimulation, ATOIMS (automated twitch-obtaining intramuscular stimulation), ETOIMS (electrical twitch-obtaining intramuscular stimulation), and TENS (transmuscular electro-neuro stimulation) units may be helpful for FM, CFID, and CMP, because they may help block pain impulses.[151] They are often used by physical therapists to induce healing at an injured area, and the NMES may help with interstitial edema problems.[152] Some devices are the size of a small pager, with probes and wires that connect the unit to a gel pad that is placed on the pain site.

TENS units have been found effective in reducing the pain caused by trigger points without altering the signals in the muscle fiber. They may also help improve range of motion that has been impeded by chronic myofascial pain.[153] As TrPs are treated and muscles soften, more underlying TrPs may become apparent. Aggressive treatment with electrical units may cause the same symptoms as aggressive manual treatment, such as nausea and increased fatigue. Take care not to overdo, to rest, and to drink plenty of water.

Depending on your coexisting conditions you may find electrical stimulation (E-stim) devices helpful or harmful. I have found that treatment of my CMP pain with E-stim benefits me. However, it can aggravate my FM and CFID symptoms. You must make the choice of treating the greatest problem.

As you can see there are several types of electrical stimulation devices, and you can usually find them on the Internet at the links listed under the Physical Therapy and Medical Equipment Suppliers heading in the resource section near the back of the book. In some instances a physician's prescription is required. If you believe that E-stim may be an option for you, discuss it with your doctor or physical therapist. Someone knowledgeable should train you in proper placement, safe handling, and therapeutic use. These units should not be used around people with pacemakers; in the lower trunk of pregnant women; if you have certain heart problems, seizure disorder, or cancer; or around the heart or carotid arteries in the neck. Always read the manufacturers' information regarding safe handling and use. Heed all warnings to avoid potential injury.

As with all treatments, you are most likely to be successful in treating CMP once you identify and eliminate the aggravating factors. You are probably saying, "Yes, yes, I get that." If you are, then I have accomplished what I set out to do.

Neuro-electrotherapy—EEG Biofeedback

Neuro-electrotherapy, also known as EEG biofeedback, is a noninvasive procedure used to treat chronic muscle pain conditions. It is important to remember that TrPs respond to direct treatment. However, additional treatment methods, such as EEG biofeedback, can be beneficial if they help to identify preventive measures. Muscle tension alone can perpetuate activation of latent TrPs and exacerbate symptoms of FM and CFID.

Topical Agents

There are many topical agents, such as capsaicin cream or topical lidocaine, that may bring some relief when applied to localized areas of pain, but take care with capsaicin and similar products. They may not be well tolerated by some FM and CFID patients.

It is a good sign to have one's feet grow cold when he is writing.
A great writer and speaker once told me that he often wrote with his feet in hot water; but for this, all his blood would have run into his head, as the mercury sometimes withdraws into the ball of a thermometer.

OLIVER WENDELL HOLMES, *THE AUTOCRAT OF THE BREAKFAST TABLE*

Effectiveness of Alternative and Complementary Therapies

According to the National Institutes of Health (NIH), complementary medicine is a "group of diverse medical and health care systems, practices, and products that are not presently considered to be part of conventional medicine."[154]

There are no magic bullets for treatment of chronic pain. This may be why nearly 50 percent of adults living in the United States seek medical treatment outside conventional medical methodology. The move toward complementary treatments has been so great since early 1990 that in 1998, NIH reorganized their office of complementary medicine into a "full strength agency," called the National Center for Complementary and Alternative Medicine.[155]

---

alternative medicine: medicine used in place of conventional medicine.

complementary medicine: alternative medicine used in combination with conventional medicine.

Ebell and Beck have reviewed past studies on complementary alternative medicine (CAM) in treatment of FM and found evidence-based answers. "Acupuncture, biofeedback, and SAM-e have shown some efficacy in treatment of FM in randomized controlled trials. Spa treatments, hypnotherapy, massage, and meditation may be the inexpensive and safe approach." They also found that bright light, lasers, selenium, chiropractic medicine, musical tones, and malic acid/magnesium were not effective.[156] However, there is anecdotal evidence that some of these treatments are quite effective for certain people.

Chronic fatigue immunodysfunction patients frequently use alternative medical treatments, yet rarely communicate this use to their medical doctors.[157]

In a questionnaire that collected information from FM patients regarding complementary treatments and their effectiveness, aromatherapy, support groups, heat, and massage were rated most effective.[158] This strongly suggests that patients seeking symptom relief look elsewhere to supplement traditional medicine. If people were not reaping the benefits, there would not be a surge in unconventional medicine and treatments.

Unfortunately, there are people who would like to capitalize on the needs of others and make outrageous claims for their own financial gain. The Internet is full of miraculous claims for weight loss, rejuvenation, and even miracle cures for FM and CFID. Do not be tempted by preposterous assertions.

There are many useful tips on "how not to get duped." Following are a few.

Beware of the Dragon

- If an advertising claim suggests it is a "miracle cure." (If there were a cure, people would not have the disorder.)
- If the ad suggests a treatment that is not backed by scientific evidence.
- If a vitamin or other preparation does not have a contact name listed on the label. (If the manufacturer is reputable, it will be there.)
- If it is a steroid or other hormonal preparation. (Remember that your doctor should always check your hormone levels to determine need. If necessary, a medication will be prescribed, not an over-the-counter drug.)
- If the practitioner claims to be able to cure an illness that no one else can.
- If the practitioner has no credentials or avoids showing them. (Most of us like to show off our achievements. Look for those diplomas on the wall and read what they say.)
- If a practitioner demands a signed financial contract for services, instead of listening to your complaint.
- If a practitioner intimidates you or tries to put you on the defensive.

Once an alternative medicine treatment shows scientific merit, the health care system incorporates the alternative approach into conventional treatment plans. For instance, acupuncture, once considered "alternative," is strongly moving into medical mainstream. This makes it a complementary medicine approach.

The usefulness and safety of many alternative treatments are now being acknowledged by the medical community. Complementary approaches to conventional medicine will gain recognition as you share your experience with your health care provider. If you have found an alternative treatment that works for you, share it. You can make a difference.

Chapter Conclusion

Keep your health care team, family, and friends informed about your progress. Also let them know about any changes you have made in your treatment plan so that they can detect any outward signs of intolerance.

You will learn which plan is right for you and how to make it meet your body's needs on any given day. "Based on current evidence, a step-wise program emphasizing education, certain medications, exercise, cognitive therapy, or all four should be recommended."[159]

Chronic pain sufferers feel others judge them as being weak. In actuality, it is quite the contrary. People who suffer chronic pain learn over time to endure a great deal of suffering. When people treat us as if we are freaks or drug addicts, it only compounds feelings of guilt. However, the only guilty party here is the person who believes we are somehow responsible for our disorder.

Richard Gracely, Ph.D., and Daniel Clauw, M.D., have preliminary data from their functional MRI (fMRI) study. The fMRI measures neurological activity in the brain and evidence shows "altered physiologic processing in FM" to pressure stimulus. Other findings suggest there is "an adaptive mechanism in FM patients that doesn't evoke the same emotional response observed in people unaccustomed to such pain."[160] Similar study results were reported in 2008,[161] giving further evidence for a physiological explanation for FM pain. More studies are in progress using the fMRI to investigate serotonin metabolism and the 5-HT3 receptor's role in FM. It appears that the HPA (hyopthalmus-pituitary-adrenal) axis may also be altered in late CFID. "These HPA axis changes may be treated by raising levels of cortisol pharmacologically, which may temporarily alleviate symptoms of fatigue and can be reversed by addressing behavioral features of the illness, such as inactivity, deconditioning, and sleep disturbance."[162]

The most difficult part of dealing with chronic myofascial pain is that there is poor understanding of the condition, which results in underdiagnosis and inadequate management. Compounding the problem, when CMP coexists with FM, CFID, or other disorders, treatments for coexisting conditions can make trigger points worse. But we know that trigger points are the source of the pain, which can be localized to the trigger point or to a referred zone, and CMP is treatable when you find the right health care team.

Don't be discouraged if you experience a relapse or flare despite your active role in your treatment plan. Relapses or flares in chronic conditions such as ours may be experienced regardless of how diligently we try to deal with them. Fibromyalgia and CFID, by their nature, have unforeseeable setbacks that are independent of other factors. You may have to ride out the period and pick up where you left off, but the good times will be better.

Decreasing pain, improving sleep quality, improving function, becoming balanced, and learning a successful self-management program are important goals to achieve. Integrative healing practices, such as breathing right, eating a healthy diet, sleeping well, exercising routinely and correctly, getting out in fresh air and natural light, practicing routine relaxation techniques, participating in beneficial therapies, doing things you love, and being with people you admire will improve your body, mind, and spirit. My grandmother always told me, "Anything in life worth having doesn't come easy." If we take control, set reasonable goals, and actively participate in pain management, we can look forward to the many rewards life has to offer.

Still, there is no denying that not every physical illness can be cured. We can, however, make use of all illness to help us redirect our lives.

BERNIE SIEGEL, M.D.

Summary Exercise: Exercising Your Options

1. Select two treatments you feel might be beneficial for you.

_____

_____

2. What improvements can you make in your diet? Complete the dietary assessment. (See the Useful Tools section at the end of this chapter.)

_____

_____

3. Write down at least three tips for finding a therapist.

_____

_____

_____

4. List some benefits you might find from treatment by physiatrists, pain management specialists, chiropractors, and myofascial release therapists.

   _____

   _____

   _____

5. Briefly describe alternative therapies such as reflexology, yoga, t'ai chi, stretching, acupuncture, massage therapy, spray and stretch, body work, trigger point therapy, self-hypnosis, meditation, biofeedback, and other miscellaneous treatments.

   _____

   _____

   _____

6. Take an inventory of your known precipitating events, triggers, and aggravating factors.

   _____

   _____

   _____

7. If you have trouble sleeping because of pain, what have you tried to help you sleep?

   _____

   _____

8. Have you stopped any medications because of their side effects?

   _____

   _____

9. List any known stressors to your pain or sleep, such as emotional stress, treatments, or weather pattern changes.

   _____

   _____

10. What past treatments/therapies have been most helpful?

   _____

   _____

11. Does pain or lack of sleep keep you from work or relationships with family and friends? If so, how?

_____

_____

_____

12. Do you have other side effects from pain, such as loss of appetite or nausea? If so, what have you tried to alleviate them?

_____

_____

_____

13. List at least two exercise therapies you haven't done that you think you might find beneficial.

_____

_____

14. List at least two types of massage.

_____

_____

15. Name three ways to pep up your "pooped out" culinary skills.

_____

_____

_____

16. Describe the difference between alternative and complementary medicine.

_____

_____

_____

17. Name at least two things you can change or improve to prepare for sleep.

_____

_____

Useful Tools
for a
Healthy Lifestyle

The useful tools in this chapter are designed to address two areas of health we are repeatedly encouraged to pay attention to: diet and exercise. The diet assessment guide will help you figure out what you're really eating, how you're eating it, and how your diet might be affecting your health. The stretches offered in the second tool will help you to improve your range of motion and overall flexibility.

- Diet Assessment Guide
- Stretches for Every Part of Your Body

Diet Assessment Guide

1. List foods known to cause unwanted symptoms.

FOOD OR DRINK   SYMPTOM

_____   _____

_____   _____

_____   _____

_____   _____

2. Keep track of your dietary intake for seven consecutive days.

	TIME	TIME	TIME	TIME	TIME
Mon	_____	_____	_____	_____	_____
Tues	_____	_____	_____	_____	_____
Wed	_____	_____	_____	_____	_____
Thurs	_____	_____	_____	_____	_____
Fri	_____	_____	_____	_____	_____
Sat	_____	_____	_____	_____	_____
Sun	_____	_____	_____	_____	_____

3. Use a calorie-counting reference guide that lists calories from protein, fat, and carbohydrates in various foods. Calculate total calories for category, then calculate the percentage. For example, to find your percentage of calories from protein, divide protein calories by total calories. This will give you a general idea of what you need to eliminate or increase in your routine diet.

	CALORIES FROM:					PERCENTAGE FROM:			
	Protein	Fat	Sugar	Carbs	Total	Protein	Fat	Sugar	Carbs
Mon	____	____	____	____	____	____	____	____	____
Tues	____	____	____	____	____	____	____	____	____
Wed	____	____	____	____	____	____	____	____	____
Thurs	____	____	____	____	____	____	____	____	____
Fri	____	____	____	____	____	____	____	____	____
Sat	____	____	____	____	____	____	____	____	____
Sun	____	____	____	____	____	____	____	____	____

4. List identified problem areas, such as reasons for eating, time of day, amount, nutritional value, and unwanted symptoms.

_____

_____

_____

_____

_____

Make special notes if you ate your meal or snack for reasons other than nutrition. This would include symptoms, boredom, depression, anxiety, anger, or habit.

5. Formulate your plan for diet improvement if you identified any problems. Set goals. Be specific.

_____

_____

_____

_____

_____

Reviewed with (doctor or dietician) _____Date _____

Stretches for Every Part of Your Body

You may need to modify some of these stretches. Talk it over with your therapist. The number of repetitions is up to you and your specific tolerance. Select a routine that your condition can take and that you will keep.

CAUTION

Be careful not to overdo. If you have active trigger points,
remember to work on them first.

Exercise 1—Fingers and Wrists

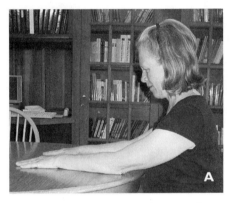 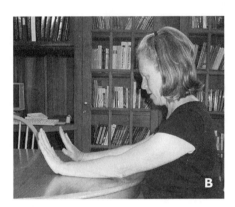

1. Sit in a chair and place your forearms flat on a table in front of you.
2. Extend your forearms forward, still flat on the table with palms down (A).
3. Lift up your fingers and feel a stretch through your palm, fingers, and wrist (B).

Exercise 2—Fingers

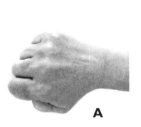 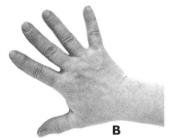 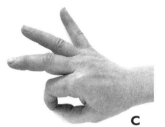

1. Make a fist with your fingers and thumb (A).
2. Open your hand and extend your fingers straight out, stretching them wide in five directions (B).
3. Now bring the tip of each finger, one at a time, over to touch your thumb (C).

Exercise 3—Shoulders and Neck

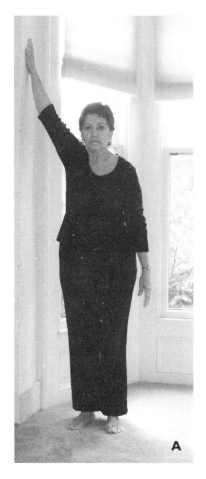
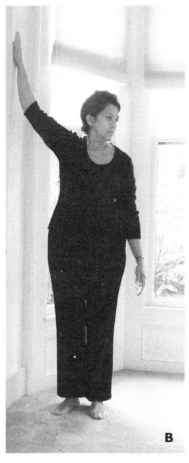
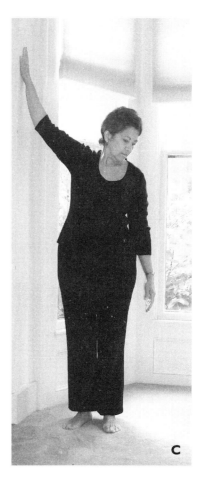

1. Stand on a firm surface with your side toward the wall, twelve inches away from the wall.

2. Place the palm of your hand that is closest to the wall as high up on the wall as you can, until a hard stretch is felt (A). Then ease back to a moderate or mild stretch.

3. Keeping your feet and hand in place, twist your upper body away from the wall, looking over your outer shoulder until you feel a good stretch (about thirty seconds) (B), then dip your chin down to stretch the back and side of your neck (thirty seconds) (C).

4. Come back to center, and then turn your entire body (a 180-degree turn) so that your other side is now toward the wall. Repeat the exercise to get the same stretch for this side of your body.

Exercise 4—Legs and Trunk (Yoga: Standing Side Stretch)

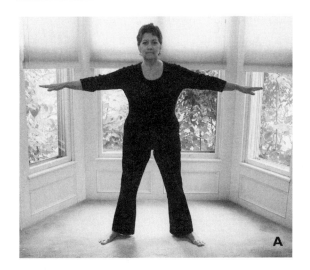

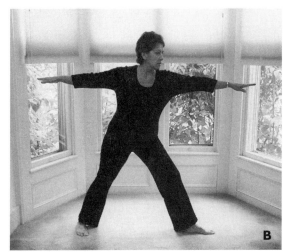

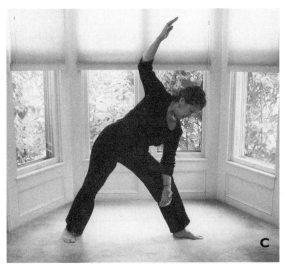

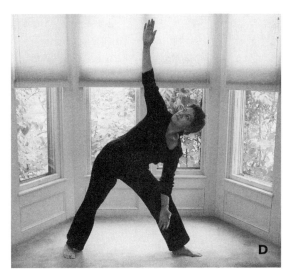

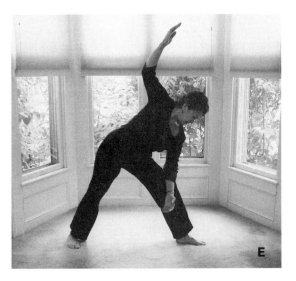

1. Assume a wide stance with plenty of space around you. Extend your arms and hands straight out to the sides, palms facing down (A).

2. Rotate your left leg out, pointing your left toes outward and bending your knee (B).

3. Place your left elbow on your left knee. This will require leaning over, but keep your body facing forward as much as possible (C). As you do this, turn your right arm palm up, lengthening and extending it over your head (D) so that you feel a stretch along the

right side of your body. Be sure to keep your left foot under your left knee. Your foot and knee should be aligned, so if your foot is turned out more than your knee, bring it back into alignment directly beneath your knee.

4. As you inhale, look upward over your right shoulder toward your right hand expanding your ribs and relaxing all the way out through your fingertips (D).

5. As you exhale, return your gaze to the floor, tuck your tailbone under, gently pulling your right shoulder back and pushing your left knee into the floor (E). Be sure to continue to keep your left knee and foot aligned so that you have a stable base.

6. Come slowly back to center and then repeat on the other side.

Exercise 5—Legs, Groin, Shoulders, and Arms

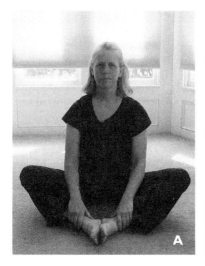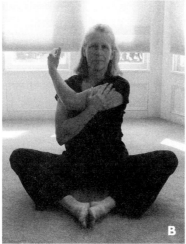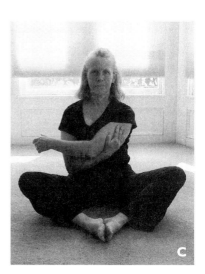

1. Sit on the floor or a firm surface with your knees bent and your feet together (A). Use support if needed.

2. Bring your left arm across your body, gently pushing your upper arm toward your right shoulder (B). Relax your hand and hold the stretch for thirty seconds.

3. Now drop your left arm, stretch it gently across your lower chest and hold it for thirty seconds (C).

4. Relax your left arm, then perform both stretches with your right arm.

Exercise 6—Legs, Upper Arms, and Back Ribs (Yoga: Child's Pose)

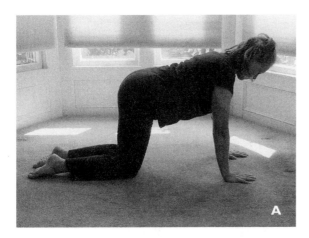

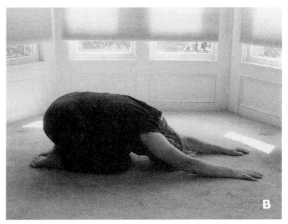

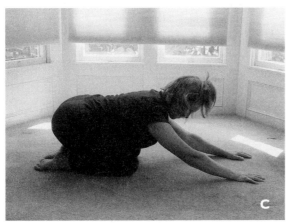

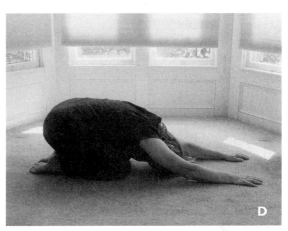

1. Position yourself on the floor on all fours. Keep your hands in line under your shoulders and facing forward, hips over your knees (A).
2. Lean back, pushing your hips toward your calves until your buttocks rest on your heels. Keep your arms outstretched forward (B).
3. Inhale into your lower back ribs, reaching your head straight forward (not back, which could strain your neck) (C).
4. Exhale, let your neck relax and your forehead drop to the floor, still keeping your arms and hands stretched forward (D).

Exercise 7—Upper Legs and Balance (Yoga: Lunge)

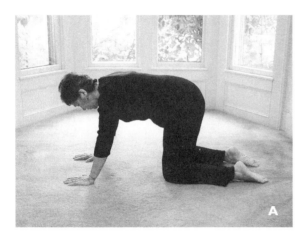

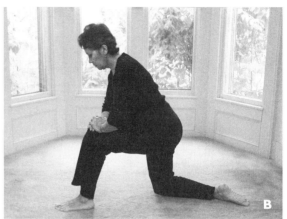

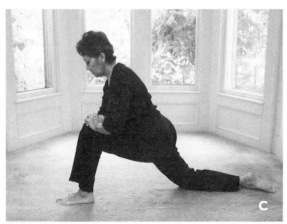

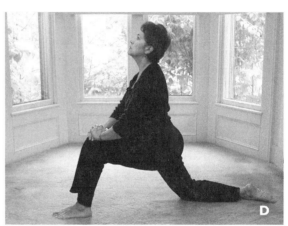

1. Start by kneeling on all fours (A).
2. Bring your left knee up so that your left foot is flat on the floor, and place both hands on that knee (B).
3. Extend your left foot back, resting your knee and the top of your foot on the floor (C). You should feel a stretch in the upper thigh of the extended leg.
4. Inhale, lifting your chest and bringing your head up (D).

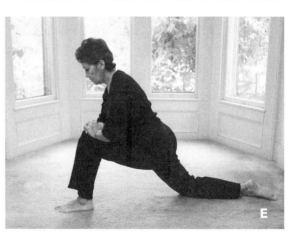

5. Exhale, push your hips down, and lean forward into the stretch (E). You will feel your extended leg glide backward and forward as you breath in and out. Breathing in brings oxygen rich air to the tissues and energizes your exhale, allowing a greater stretch.
6. Repeat on the other side.

Exercise 8—Legs and Waist

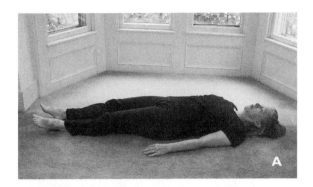 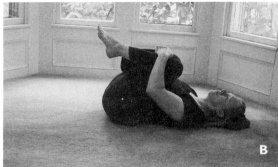

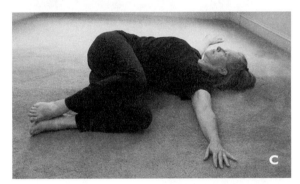 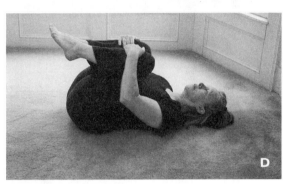

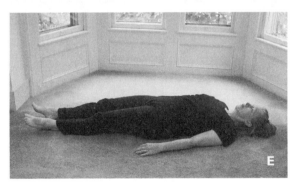

1. Lie on your back on the floor or a firm surface (A).
2. Bring both knees to your chest (B).
3. Twist your body so that your knees are stacked on top of each other, lying to one side, and hold for thirty seconds (C).
4. Using the muscles in your abdomen, return to the neutral knees-to-chest position by bringing the top bent leg back to the center, then following with the other leg (D).
5. Now twist to other side and hold for thirty seconds.
6. Come back to neutral one bent knee at a time, as before, then lower legs flat to the floor, one at a time (E).

**Exercise 9—Hips, Lower Legs, Ankles, and Feet
(Yoga inversion: Downward Facing Dog)**

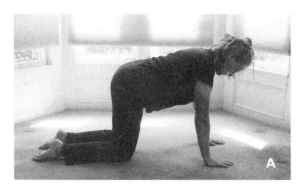
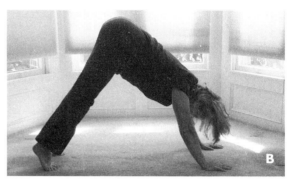

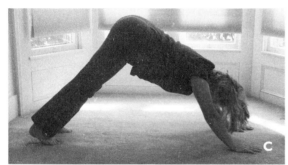
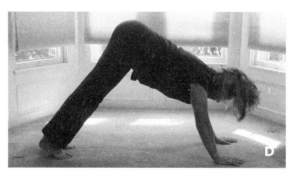

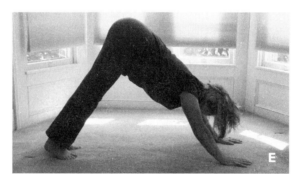

1. Start on all fours (A).
2. Push your hips toward the ceiling, being careful not to overstretch behind your knees (B).
3. Move your feet backward until you feel maximum stretch in the backs of your legs (C), then back off until you feel a moderate or mild stretch.
4. Inhale to lengthen the spine, keeping your neck in a neutral position (D).
5. As you exhale, keep your hands flat on the floor, arms straight, and push back into your heels, pushing your buttocks toward the ceiling to stretch the back of your legs and feet (E). Keep your neck in a relaxed position to avoid strain. By drawing in your abdomen and pressing your sternum toward the floor you can also provide a nice stretch to your underarms, rib cage, and thoracic spine.

Exercise 10—Buttocks (Piriformis stretch)

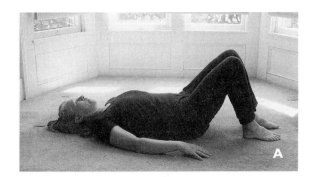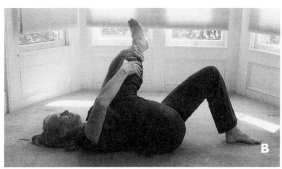
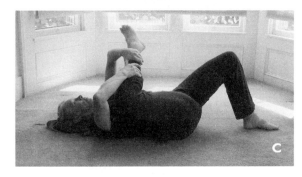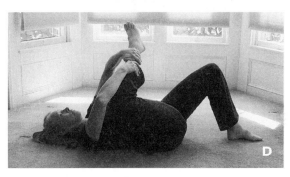

1. Lie on your back and slightly bend both knees (A).
2. Lift your right foot off the floor, bringing your right knee to your chest, and place the palms of both hands against your outer shin above the ankle. Beginning gently, press your right foot across your body toward your left shoulder (B).
3. Bring you right hip and thigh to its maximum stretch toward the shoulder, with your right foot as high as possible on your body (C). You should feel the stretch in your buttock.
4. Then back off to a moderate or mild stretch and hold it for thirty seconds (D).
5. Repeat on the other side.

Exercise 11—Yoga Relaxation Pose

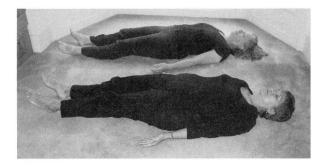

1. Lie on your back, arms stretched to the side.
2. Take some deep abdominal breaths and relax. You deserve it!

5

The Power of Mind, Body, and Spirit

Chronic pain disrupts the harmony of our overall well-being, not just physically, but spiritually, mentally, and emotionally. When being treated for pain, a person should be treated as a whole, not merely a collection of symptoms. Treatment goals should include preservation of functional capacity, as well as emotional, mental, and spiritual soundness.

A qualitative study done in 2004 at the Division of Rehabilitation Medicine, Karolinska Institute in Stockholm, Sweden, on patients who suffer widespread musculoskeletal pain concluded that a rehabilitation program can improve self-image, communication, and inter-social relationships.[1] The study noted that the program and semi-structured interviews helped participants shift from "shame to respect." They learned new ways of dealing with their pain and coexisting symptoms by balancing their entire being.

This chapter will help you:

- Identify helpful tools for overcoming depression.
- Learn how to find the right therapist.
- Determine which affirmations you'd like to incorporate into your daily life.
- Review ways in which others perceive spirituality, and assess how important spirituality is to your well-being.
- Define the difference between healthy and unhealthy coping mechanisms.
- See how healthy coping mechanisms can play a positive role in your life.
- Identify what external resources you can utilize to help you make healthy adaptations to your style of living.

- Discover how change can be part of your affirmative action plan and liberate you from burdensome ideas.
- Review helpful ways of connecting body, mind, and spirit by changing behaviors.

Have patience with all things, but chiefly have patience with yourself. Do not lose courage in considering your own imperfections, but instantly set about remedying them—every day begin the task anew.

SAINT FRANCIS DE SALES

Depression—Overcoming the Doldrums

Comorbidity is a fancy word for "this ailment and that ailment both exist in this individual." The diagnosis might include two "diseases" (FM and depression) or a "disease" and a symptom cluster (migraines and photosensitivity).

This section concerns two very common pairings: depression and FM or CFID, and depression and CMP.

There is a lot of confusion in published research concerning statistical correlation and causation. The most common error is described in Latin as *post hoc ergo propter hoc,* or, "after this, therefore because of this." In other words, because you had one illness or symptom cluster first, another illness or symptom cluster must have been caused by it. This prompts the question, "Are FM, CFID, and CMP causes of depression?" I believe not, at least not in a direct and causal manner. But like all chronic, debilitating diseases, these are often accompanied by a defined state of depression characterized by low mood, pessimistic outlook, suppression of positive spontaneity, and sleep and appetite disturbance.

illness: a condition marked by pronounced deviation from the normal healthy state; sickness.

morbidity: The relevant incidence of disease.

disorder: a derangement or abnormality of function; a morbid physical or mental state.

disease: a morbid process having a characteristic train of symptoms. It may affect the whole body or any of its parts, and its etiology, pathology, and prognosis may be known or unknown.

symptom: any indication of disease perceived by the patient or health care practitioner.

syndrome: a combination of symptoms resulting from a single cause, or so commonly occurring together as to constitute a distinct clinical picture.

The Psychotherapist's Perspective

Psychotherapists and patients don't always talk about concerns in the same way. A psychotherapist is professionally trained and more likely to speak about a disorder in clinical terms.

"The Blues"

This could be a reaction to an event, a death of someone not extremely close, a loss, or bad news, such as an unwelcome diagnosis or test results. If you've ever lost a beloved pet, you understand this completely. The depressive symptoms arise quickly and generally resolve in days or a few weeks.

Adjustment Disorders (Depressive Type)

These are more pervasive and global in effect, and may continue for months. Most comorbid depressions are of this type. Antidepressants, while often unnecessary, are frequently prescribed for this level of depression.

These antidepressants (usually SSRIs, or selective serotonin reuptake inhibitors) do, at times, speed up the healing process. Prior to such chemical intervention, there should be a cost-benefit analysis of effects versus side effects, as well as a very detailed diagnostic formulation. Unfortunately, some doctors, especially those who are pressured by insurance company affiliates to move patients through quickly, get impatient with depressed patients and ones they cannot "cure" in one visit. In exasperation they push SSRI prescriptions at these individuals with the fervor formerly reserved for antibiotics. Pharmaceutical companies have done a very convincing job in assuring Dr. Primary Care that depression can be wiped out with a Prozac derivative. The good news? If you need an SSRI your family doctor can, and probably will, prescribe one and save you a trip to the psychiatrist. The bad news? Somatic medicine doctors, such as gynecologists and internists, are very poorly trained in the differential diagnoses of mental health issues, and would not be doing you a service.

somatic: bodily, physical.

atypical: not the usual; opposite of typical.

SSRI: selective serotonin reuptake inhibitor. This class of drugs stops reabsorption of serotonin, leaving more available in the brain, which enhances mood.

The best-trained professionals in these disorders are psychologists (usually Ph.D., Psy.D., and Ed.D.) and psychiatrists (M.D. or D.O.). Social workers (M.S.W., L.C.S.W., A.C.S.W.) and professional counselors (L.P.C.) are also trained and might be very knowledgeable (see "Alphabet Soup" later in this chapter). While psychiatrists have held a public information catbird seat for fifty years (due to media fascination with psychoanalysis), most are less qualified for differential diagnosis than a Ph.D. psychologist, and most are prejudiced in favor of using drug therapies nearly exclusively. The most effective treatment for adjustment disorder depression is talk psychotherapy, with or without medication. Equally effective in most nonmedical issue depression is a regular exercise program. Again, this is a chicken and egg question: Is exercise an effective treatment, or is it that the few who can maintain an exercise regimen are able to shrug off depression for other reasons?

Dysthymic Disorder

This is a full-blown depression of more than six-months duration or one where there are thoughts of suicide. It is widespread, more intense, with a full symptom presentation treated with medication (usually SSRIs) and talk psychotherapy. Neither alone is sufficient. In older males this often appears to fit the Walter Matthau *Grouchy Old Men* profile. In both men and women it is often comorbid with a partial obsessive-compulsive disorder. Dysthymic disorder has a very high suicide rate. Usage of stimulant drugs (cocaine, speed, crack, methamphetamines) would be a very dangerous factor in this disorder.

Major Depression

Big dog depression, pervasive and enduring. This may or may not have psychotic features like paranoia or catatonia (mannequin behavior). This disorder requires medication (unusual anti-psychotics, such as Respiradal, Remron, or Zyprexa) and psychotherapy. Think of the despairing wife of the character played by Robin Williams in *What Dreams May Come* who commits suicide from grief, or the silent Chief in *One Flew over the Cuckoo's Nest*.

Bipolar Disorder

Bipolar disorder, actually a sub-type of major depression, is characterized by moods that alternate between deep depression and a manic state that is characterized by impulsive and dangerous behavior, lack of sleep, flights of ideas, and euphoria or irritability. Bipolar disorder is also known as manic depression, or mood swings. Bipolar bears are treated with medication, either lithium carbonate or an antiseizure drug like Tegretol, Limactil, or Resperil. Zyprexa is also being used now. The value of talk therapies is vastly outweighed by the necessity of chemical therapies, yet talk therapy is still very important.

Mental, Nervous Breakdown, and Chemical Imbalance

"Nervous breakdown," "chemical imbalance," and "mental" don't really define any turf, but are merely buzzwords. In general, a person cannot "be committed" anymore. More than 90 percent of in-patient admissions are voluntary, and the rest are emergency placements of actively suicidal/homicidal people. Most placements are short term (several days). Most people who have utilized such a setting agree that it was what they needed at that time.

"Nervous breakdown" is a term from the mid-twentieth century that obscures a great deal of diagnostic turf. It created the illusion that Grandma's "nerves were shot" when in fact she may have been caught in an affair or drinking the cooking sherry and was packed off to the psychiatric unit while the family regrouped. Stress overload is a psycho-physical fact, but the term *nervous breakdown* is an inaccurate and misleading lay term without the referents of causation, symptom presentation, or outcome that better defined terms offer. "Mental" implies something that is not an objective physical fact, but mental phenomena affect all of our lives. Ask a nursing mother what happens when a baby cries in a restaurant and her child is at home. Try to remember, men, when you were fifteen and someone talking about underwear put yours in stress-tent mode. What happens when you think about eating a lemon? These are physical responses to mental stimuli.

The concept of "chemical imbalance" is the latest sacred cow of psychotherapy. The simple truth is that psychiatry discovered chemical supportive care for disorders and then tried to justify it with some new discovery or half-baked research. Do SSRIs work on depression? Sure do! But not any better than talk therapies if the patient and therapist "click," or aerobics, if the patient makes it a regular habit. There are depressions that require pharmacotherapy. However, many depressions could be resolved more quickly with a combination of psychotherapy and SSRIs. But to reason backward that adding a chemical alleviates the disorder or balances the brain chemistry, and thus conclude that there was a "chemical imbalance," is absurd. Are headaches caused by an "aspirin imbalance"? What do these "researchers" make of creativity? Is that a chemical imbalance, too?

Treatment Trends

A steady review of the literature and continuing education shows treatment of depression with talk therapy, pharmacotherapy, and a vigorous exercise program are all equally effective. Any combination of the three is somewhat more effective than any one alone. Over the long haul, the exercise group is most effective at combating depressive relapse. This is no surprise from the behavioral analysis point of view. The exercise group is a self-selected subset of the depressed group that is capable of maintaining a difficult commitment to health that trumps convenience or temporary desire. These are the same people who can quit smoking (if they ever did smoke), and lose weight and keep it off.

Behaviorally, depression is just shortcut thinking, denial, and illogic. "If I stay in bed another hour I'll feel better about getting my day going"; "Maybe I'll feel more like tackling that goal tomorrow"; "I can't do it if I don't feel like doing it"; and so on. I (Jeff) often remember a woman I saw in Queenstown, New Zealand, at A. J. Hackett's bungee jumping station. She was queued up to jump ahead of me and had a lot of trouble deciding to go ahead and jump off the 143-foot high bridge (that's half a football field, or a decent high-rise office building in most towns). She approached the edge, peered over, and backed off, over and over. My jumpmaster, KJ, a very cool Californian and fellow Deadhead, summed it up: "She'll go home and tell people she was in Queenstown, they'll ask, 'Did you bungee jump?' and she'll have to say 'No,' like her whole trip to New Zealand was invalidated in one moment." I asked KJ if he thought she was waiting for courage. He agreed that courage is like the water you can hold in your hands. Every second that goes by, you will have less. Do it now if you want courage as your companion. Fear is constant; courage leaks out with time. You will not feel better about this later. If you want to be a person who can do this, you cannot listen to your internal critic or any excuse-granting entity.

TIPS FOR OVERCOMING DEPRESSION

1. Identify limits that promote wellness (for example, if inadequate sleep affects your ability to cope, stick to your sleep hygiene program). Assess and assist your abilities.

2. Keep to the limits you set and avoid unhealthy temptations. Keep to your routine.

3. Give every day all you have to give, but not one more ounce.

4. Appreciate every day; each one is a gift.

5. Participate in talk therapy.

6. Act on your courage.

7. Exercise positive spontaneity.

8. Exercise your body.

9. Do something special for someone else.

10. Dwell on the positives in your life.

Measuring Limits

If you have FM, CFID, or CMP, the picture is not straightforward. Regardless of courage or decisiveness, your first task is to accurately assess your ability today. You need an objective measure for determining if this is a "terrific" or "semi-terrific" day. If semi-terrific, what limits should you place on yourself to not lose ground in your recovery process? Stepping over those limits, regardless of reason or noble intent, is just not smart. Your goal should be clearly in mind: to increase your participation and appreciation every day, anyway. (Bumper sticker I love: "Praise the Lord anyway.")

Every day you should spend all your available energy pennies, but not one more. One extra penny of effort today will cost the FM, CFID, CMP person a dollar tomorrow. Not smart! Make daily deposits in your well-being bank. If you are not consistent at assessing your abilities, you can easily bankrupt your account. You need to keep this limit sacrosanct.

At the same time, you need to do a balancing act with your unconscious process of self-accommodation and deceit, the permission we give ourselves to loaf, stall, or nonperform. This tendency to give up prematurely, surrender to dread, to drop our own ball at the first sign of difficulty is universal. That's right, universal. Everyone knows the decision to let the Frisbee pass without diving to try to catch it, to allow decline and destruction through premeditated or even spontaneous neglect. This omnipresent human fallacy lies at the heart of a major pain dynamic in chronic illness. The individual experiencing the disease sometimes gives less than 100 percent, sometimes lets things slide, exaggerates the inability, or blames the disease for a failure of effort and will. Other people in the individual's life circle do the same, at least as often. This is the seed of projection that the "sick" person is slacking. The one judging is projecting personal failure. The one judged may sometimes be guilty as charged, but usually not. The key point is that the one judging is also guilty at some time. Thus the projection that the other (sick one) is slacking (I did), and umbrage and emotional escalation follow. Correct response to the judgment? "Don't we all, sometimes, give less than 100 percent? I can only assure you that today, now, I am doing my best. You cannot confirm that; there is no gauge on my forehead to record my effort and current potential. You'll have to take my word for it, as I do yours."

Who we are is more than the body or the personality.

RAM DASS

Tips for Selecting a Therapist

In the days before managed care insurance policies, a therapist was chosen by the patient and the patient's primary doctor. Most people now have mental health insurance coverage through a Managed Behavioral Health Care Organization (MBHCO). So although your regular health insurance is with the Blues, Aetna, United Health Care, or Coventry, your mental health coverage has often been farmed out to an MBHCO, like Magellan, United Behavioral Health, or Cigna Behavioral Health. The fine print on the back of your insurance ID card may include some reference to psychiatric, substance abuse, mental health, or psychological treatment authorizations coming from a different toll-free number. When you call that number to get a referral, be sure to listen carefully to the person or (more often) recording to know with whom you are dealing. MBHCOs make strange bedfellows. Sometimes primary insurance companies use each other's mental health networks. Please refer to the following Alphabet Soup section to determine the type of therapist you need before making the call. I strongly recommend using a speakerphone for this task, as it may take thirty minutes of being on hold and punching buttons to navigate the voicemail trees. Write everything down. Use the Interaction Worksheet for Important Calls and Meetings (in the Useful Tools section at the end of chapter 7), and fill in the suggestions before you call. While you are on hold is a good time to trim nails or clean out desk drawers. When you do succeed in connecting with a real person, here are some helpful tips:

- Write down the person's name and extension number.
- Ask if there is a specific panel, or set of providers, you must use. (Some MBHCOs require this, others use any licensed provider, and still others reimburse their panel better than nonpanel providers.) You'll have a lower co-pay if you stay in-network.
- Get as many names as you can in your preferred geographic area. Many providers listed with various MBHCO panels will not have openings or times you can use. Consider whether driving further is a major factor versus skill level, cost, and personal dynamics.

The difference between the best and worst therapist for you spans a mind-boggling gap (no pun intended).

- Ask the MBHCO representative if you need an authorization. If so, get the authorization number, the number of sessions per authorization, the number of sessions allowed per calendar year, co-pay amounts, and any deductibles you will owe (some plans have separate mental health deductibles).
- Next, call your local community mental health association, your best treating physician, your friends in therapy, and your spiritual advisor. Read the provider list to each one, asking if this therapist knows anything about FM, CFID, CMP, chronic pain management, and other issues important to you. (Mental health associations have lists of providers, including some who state a specialization in health-related issues. That statement does not guarantee competence but it narrows your search field. If you have "out of network" benefits, add the health psychology names to your list of panel providers. The co-pay difference might be negligible.)
- Hopefully, you will have several providers with positive ratings from more than one source. If so, call each and schedule a five-minute phone interview.

If you have traditional "third party" insurance and can choose any licensed provider, have no insurance, or choose to pay cash, skip the MBHCO steps and start with your doctor, friends, advisor, and local mental health association, and ask for names of therapists known to work in this field. Call and interview the most recommended.

Remember, you only need a psychiatrist if you have complicated medication issues. Most of the psychiatrists in the United States just do medication management after their initial evaluation and diagnostic sessions. They generally count on psychologists, licensed counselors, and social workers to do the (necessary) talk therapies. You can always get most of the useful psychotropic drugs prescribed by your other doctors.

After your telephone interviews, schedule a session with the most promising therapist. Plan to see this person two or three times before coming to a decision about continuing in therapy. What you want in a therapist is highly personal, a connection both nurturing and challenging. The therapist you seek is highly empathic and not limited by your current perceptions. Other sections of this book will discuss various therapeutic approaches, such as visualization, biofeedback, cognitive behavioral therapy, hypnosis, and affirmations. The best therapist for you might do all, some, or none of these. There are a number of supplementary resources listed in this book that can add modalities your therapist might not utilize. Do not be afraid to discuss these with that therapist, and possibly do some self-healing exercises. The best therapists will be actively engaged with your therapy. You will feel connected to your therapist, as well as challenged. You will be required to work between sessions on issues. You will be required to "reach deep" in recognizing and challenging your assumptions and beliefs. Plan to stay in therapy for at least one year.

Although I would hope this caution is unnecessary, an ethical therapist never takes advantage of a client, financially, emotionally, or sexually.

Colleges offer a wide variety of degrees and certifications. A board assessing minimum requirements regionally certifies the good colleges. Almost all state colleges and established private schools are certified. The rest advertise in the back of magazines and on the Internet. Frequently, these "diploma mills" sell a degree that is not recognized by any licensing body. Each state and province also has licensing boards to grant annual provider licenses for physicians (including psychiatrists), psychologists, social workers, and counselors. Each professional discipline also recognizes the most trained and persistent practitioners with a higher level of certification.

Hopefully, this quickie course in therapy and therapist selection will help guide you to appropriate treatment if you are in deep distress.

Your condition affects mind, body, heart, and soul. Leaving any aspect untreated is a loss for your whole being. If you feel depressed, have difficulty reacting appropriately to others, have difficulty coping well, or feel you can't go it alone, please seek the help you need. It's okay, we all need help from time to time. I did.

Cognitive-Behavioral Therapy (CBT) and the Patient's Perspective

The power of the mind over bodily functions is phenomenal. A friend of mine is a good example. She suffered severe damage to her lower spine in a car accident when she was twenty-five (and mother of a four year old), leaving her paralyzed from the waist down. They told her she would never walk again. She was persistent and not only retrained her bowels and kidneys to function, she walked again with the aid of braces and drove a car. She returned to college and graduated cum laude from a prestigious law school. Students at this university have a tradition of walking across campus to their final graduation ceremony, but this was a bit too strenuous for her and she needed to be in a wheelchair to go that distance. She convinced her school to change the rules and set a precedent by proceeding with her fellow students to the ceremony. Did I say she was persistent?

We may not be able to completely rid ourselves of pain, but by altering our behaviors, we can teach our minds how to respond to it. In a study done in Belgium, acceptance that pain may not change led to a shift away from pain to non-pain aspects of life.[2]

"Cognitive-behavioral treatment programs have demonstrated the ability to reduce pain, emotional distress, and disability for individuals with chronic pain."[3] CBT operates on the principle that thinking negatively promotes destructive behavior patterns. For example, maybe you're having a bad day and you miss an appointment, and you recriminate yourself with, "I'm stupid, I never remember anything." You have now laid the groundwork for self-esteem destruction. Remember our discussion on identifying blocks to growth in the journaling section? Well, this is one of them. A therapist can use CBT to guide and motivate you to use positive, constructive, and realistic response behaviors to the little curves life throws your way. Think of it as positive rationalization. All of us with these disorders forget things, sometimes very significant things, but does that make us bad? Does it mean that if I forget something I'm a bad parent, rotten friend, or uncaring person? I think not. This therapy helped me to accept chronic pain as part of who I am, and taught me how to use my mind to deal with it in a positive way.

Having chronic pain doesn't mean we're crazy or that our physical difficulties are a result of mental instability. We are really quite fortunate to live in a day where cognitive and behavioral therapy and other mental health treatments are so widely accepted. One would have to ask, if people aren't getting relief from these types of therapy, why are there so many therapists and resources?

Alphabet Soup

Choosing a therapist is an important decision, and your choice will depend as much on personal chemistry as on the person's education. However, knowing what a therapist was required to accomplish in order to earn a particular degree may be of some assistance.

- **Psychiatrists:** Two or three degrees, B.A./B.S., some acquire an incidental Ph.D. or an earned M.A./M.S., then the medical doctorate. All allopathic or osteopathic physicians (M.D. or D.O.) prescribe medications, such as antidepressants, anxiolytics (antianxiety), and mood-stabilizers. A (very) few are also psychotherapists; most of these are psychoanalytically trained, and unless you really like the couch trip, Woody Allen angst thing, this is generally not the psychotherapist you seek. The "super" certification is called "board certified." The best psychiatrists often hold this title. The term psychoanalyst is reserved for those taking an additional five to seven years of psychotherapy training in the Freudian tradition.

- **Psychologists:** They may have three college degrees, B.A./B.S. undergraduate, and M.A./M.S., Ph.D./Psy.D./Ed.D. graduate. These are the crack diagnosticians, the psych testing people, the best-trained therapists, with a bachelor's or master's degree in either arts or science (no significant difference here). A Ph.D. is a doctorate of philosophy in clinical or counseling psychology. This is the benchmark degree that usually takes nine to twelve years of post-high school education. The Psy.D. is a doctorate in psychology, a newer degree that is equally well regarded. The Ed.D. is a doctorate in education. These degrees are also well respected and are often awarded by a school of education counseling psychology program. There are other psychologists generally not interested in psychotherapy, such as school psychologists, researchers, and administrators. Other Ph.D.s have nothing to do with psychotherapy. Radio host "Dr." Laura Schlessinger is a good example of professional misdirection. Her master's degree and license are as a Marriage and Family Therapist (in California). Ms. Schlessinger's doctorate is in a completely unrelated science, physiology. Physiology is not psychology. If she wanted to teach anatomy at a college or give advice on workout routines, her doctorate would be pertinent and informative regarding her training and limitations. As it is presented on the radio show and in her books, however, it is supremely misleading. Based on that Ph.D., she has no more right to a psychological opinion than Colonel Sanders would to lead combat troops. Dr. Phil McGraw on the Oprah show is correctly represented as a trained psychologist. Like him or not, his image and training are consistent. Psychologists do not prescribe medicine. The "super" certification is A.A.B.P. from the American Psychological Association (rare) or the National Register of Psychologists. McGraw surrendered his Texas license after a board complaint.

- **Social Workers:** They have two degrees, a B.A./B.S. and an M.S.W. They may also be licensed (L.M.S.W./L.C.M.S.W.) or hold the "accredited" title (A.C.S.W.) awarded nationally. A few hold doctorates (D.S.W. or Ph.D. in social work, but these generally teach, not treat). Social workers are frequently adept at networking services and at assisting and empowering clients to utilize systems, agencies, and services. Most are trained as psychotherapists. Social service agencies hire many social workers. Some are in private practice. A.C.S.W. is their "super" designation.

- **Licensed Professional Counselors:** L.P.C.s have two or three degrees, B.A./B.S., M.A./M.S., and perhaps a Ph.D. in counseling. Most have bachelor's and master's degrees and a state-issued license. Counselors are trained to provide therapy services and do not have the rigorous research and diagnosis training of psychologists, or the agency networking abilities of social workers. Because their focus is exclusively on therapy skills, they are often well perceived as healers and helpers. There is no recognized certification beyond L.P.C.

Other Designations: These range from very legit and informative to completely bogus designations, depending on the legitimacy of the institution granting the degree or certificate. Some include:

- **A.A.B.P.** The "super" certification for psychologists, from the American Psychological Association.
- **A.A.S.E.C.T.** American Association of Sexuality Educators, Counselors, and Therapists, a designation indicating a great deal of specialized training in sexuality.
- **B.S.N.** Bachelor of Science in Nursing, a four-year degree. Up a step from the R.N. associate degree/license.
- **B.S.W.** Bachelor's in Social Work, nice four-year degree but not ready for prime-time therapy without the addition of at least a master's degree.
- **L.P.N.** Licensed Practical Nurse, between the nurse's aide and the R.N. Requires passing L.P.N. state board exams.
- **M.Div.** Master's in Divinity, a theological degree sometimes held by pastoral counselors.
- **M.S.N.** Master of Science in Nursing, above the B.S.N.

- **N.C.C.P.** National certification in addictions, can be acquired with any degree.
- **N.P.** Nurse practitioner. Advanced R.N.
- **P.A.** Physician's Assistant. Certification by a special board. Does not require the education level of the R.N.
- **R.M.L.P.** Registered Master's Level Psychologist. As it sounds, no Ph.D., some independent practice allowed.
- **R.N.** Registered Nurse, a two-year (A.D.N.) or four-year (B.S.N.) nursing degree and has passed the state board exam required to practice in a particular state.
- **L.L.C.** Limited Liability Company, a business framework, not a degree.
- **P.C.** Professional Corporation, a business.

What You Should Expect from Your Therapist

Regardless of the psychotherapy modality your therapist uses to help you, you should expect to:

- Feel you are understood.
- Feel your therapy is focused on solutions for you.
- Feel the level of care is consistent for your needs. In other words, that your visits are spaced and of duration that is sufficient to meet your needs and accomplish your goals.
- Feel you can build trust with your treating psychologist.
- Be able to trust your therapist to understand your needs for therapy, including type, duration, and termination when your goals are met. If that trust is not mutual, the therapy or the therapist may not be what you need.

Spirituality

What is spirituality? For me (Celeste), this is a difficult topic to define. My scientific mind constantly searches for explanations. I struggle with how to describe what seems to be an amorphous term. I am a spiritual person. I accept that. I do not question it, but how do I relate what I feel to someone else? I found it was easier to answer the question, "What behaviors are part of living a spiritual life?" After reading William Elliott's interviews with "wise and spiritual people" in *Tying Rocks to Clouds,* I determined that spirituality means different things to different people. It is not attached to any one particular religion, and although the term is linked with religious beliefs, it is also part of, but not synonymous with, any secular doctrine.

Vipassana: A meditation practice that teaches awareness of oneself and one's surroundings.

Well-known author Jack Kornfield is a practitioner of Vipassana meditation who teaches internationally. He has a Ph.D. in clinical psychology and is a layman and monk in the Theravada Buddhist tradition. Kornfield believes that spiritual truth is an experience, as well as a belief.[4] He bases his life on Buddhist "truths," like the impermanence of all things and conditions. According to Buddhism you are born and you die, and must adhere to your own "dharma," or right path.

What Kornfield describes as the "Second Truth" is what many spiritual leaders believe, that "there's a mixture of pleasure and pain, light and dark, sweet and sour,"[5] and so with happiness there is sorrow. How would it feel if everything were always the same? What would life be without death?

---

dharma: The laws that govern nature, the universal laws.[6]

The Third Truth he describes is that ultimately all is transient and we possess nothing, not even our own bodies; that it isn't what we have that is important, but what we share with others.

Religious beliefs and practices are an important part of our lives and who we are. The influence of our beliefs is so important that cultural diversity and religious rites should be addressed as elements of whole person health care, yet many people feel uncomfortable talking about their spiritual beliefs.

According to a 2002 report on Spirituality and Medicine at Med CEU[7] (a website that offers continuing education credit for health care providers), "Surveys of the U.S. public in the Gallup Report consistently show a high prevalence of belief in God (95 percent), and 84 percent claim that religion is important to their lives. In one Vermont survey of 115 family health care professionals and 135 patients, 91 percent of the patients and 64 percent of the health care professionals reported believing in God.

This is a key point and difficult to discuss. Many mental health professionals either ascribe to no religion or are fanatical. In either case they may not respect the patient's religious beliefs. Surveys consistently show that only 40 percent of Americans attend religious services at least once a week.

Therapists have perceived authority, and mentioning church can easily make clients feel guilty or negligent, defensive either way. This is not in the spirit of therapeutic nonjudgment or neutrality and it can serve to move clients further away from a potentially helpful resource.

Discussing spirituality as part of your medical care is important. Larry Dossey, M.D., is an internationally recognized speaker on spirituality and medicine and author of numerous books, including *Prayer is Good Medicine: How to Reap the Benefits of Prayer*; *Healing Words: The Power of Prayer and the Practice of Medicine*; *Healing Beyond the Body: Medicine and the Infinite Reach of the Mind*; and many more. Dossey says that surveys show up to 75 percent of patients believe their physicians should address spiritual issues as part of their care, and that 50 percent of patients would like their doctors to pray with them. He also maintains that the majority of doctors pray for their patients.[8]

Doctor Dossey has discussed ways to use your mind to affect your health. He has made many presentations of clinical data and cited many studies that support the idea that thoughts can have a positive effect on the body. He believes that the mind-body phenomenon—the idea that one can profoundly affect the other—has great importance for both patients and doctors.

Praise is well, compliment is well, but affection—that is the last and final and most precious reward that any man can win, whether by character or achievement.

AFFECTION SPEECH, 1907, MARK TWAIN

The central questions of all the great religious traditions pertain to human suffering, the meaning of life, and our relationship to the Divine. In supporting a spiritual approach to the management of these disorders, no particular approach is suggested or promoted. Research on the interaction of faith and healing clearly demonstrates that faith combined with action (for example, prayer) can make a positive change in physical conditions. There is no one religious or spiritual practice that is more important or effective than another for arriving at emotional acceptance and attitude improvement.

Roger Walsh, M.D., Ph.D., has studied religion for more than two decades. He had been an agnostic scientist before his spirituality was awakened. He believes that the great religions offer a great gift. Judaism, Islam, Christianity, the yogis of Hinduism, and the disciplines of Taoism all offer consistent spiritual practices that awaken us and help us reach the goal of self-discovery. There are common teachings among the great religions that he calls the "Seven Perennial Practices."[9]

Bill Withers sang, "We all need somebody to lean on," in his song, "Lean on Me." Sometimes that "somebody" might be a divine aspect or understanding. Regardless of your religious affiliation or lack of one, there are questions you have probably asked at some point: "Why me?" "What now?" and "Which way?" Wayne Dyer pointed out in a lecture that almost all of the names for the Divine contain the key syllable "ah," as in Allah, Jehovah, Buddha, Yahweh, Shiva, Rama, Mazda, God, Krishna, Bahai'ullah. So whatever your "ah" understanding or belief ("ah"gnostics, too!), you will benefit from deepening your connection and clarifying your relationship to your spiritual path.

─────────────   *Personal Testimony*   ─────────────

I (Jeff) was raised in the Lutheran Church and my Christian perspective on disease and suffering was informed by the book of Job and the Passion of Christ. I was taught that here, east of Eden where we reside since "the fall," there will always be death, disease, and suffering. Our faith was to point our attention to the greater reality of God's kingdom, which will free us from these mortal shackles. Our difficulties on Earth are to remind us of our true nature and future. In my current path, Buddhism, the first two tenets, or Noble Truths, hold that "in life there is always suffering" and "suffering is caused by attachment." Accepting the true nature of our current existence is crucial to freedom in either tradition.

Step one: We are in pain; you cannot deny that, personalize it, or wish it away. It is universal.

Step two: Now what? Here the different traditions diverge in practice and emphasis, but each presents a path, practice, or conceptual framework to mitigate suffering and improve our collective lives.

I was comparing scars with a fellow fifty-something friend a while back and noted a big shift in our thinking about them. The scars I chose to share (of many) were from a toxic spider bite and a chest tube insertion after a head-on collision. I suppose when I was younger they were seen as "disfiguring." Now I see them as souvenirs from two times my life was saved through medical interventions. They are "chump change" in the big game of life and death.

I think that from the spiritual perspective, all the suffering of life looks a little like an old scar, a relic of an encounter with our imperfect world and mortal shell. Dr. Dyer also pointed out that while the name of God contains the sound "ah," the

word of God contains "om," and the two sounds join in the prayer Shalom. That
prayer for peace is not the "copasetic" or "A-okay" version of peace, but the peace
of radical acceptance of this truth we live.

SHALOM

Regardless of your belief, spirituality is paramount to being "well-balanced." It is equal in importance to all else, and a source of comfort and support. It has a positive effect on people with chronic pain disorders, such as FM, CFID, and CMP.[10]

The power of empowerment is in the ability to not give up.

Spiritual realities are the underpinnings, the very template of existence.

JEAN HOUSTON

As William Elliot describes her in *Tying Rocks to Clouds,* Jean Houston is "a modern alchemist extracting a new truth from various traditions and sciences." She once worked closely with Margaret Mead. She combines her scientific background in psychology and anthropology with her vast knowledge of myth, religious tradition, and spiritual techniques. She is a leader in human potential through empowerment, an internationally renowned scientist and philosopher, and the author of more than ten books.[11]

Houston reiterates the human need to feel affiliation with, and receive affirmation from, others. We empower each other by what we do. Houston believes we make a spiritual contribution by sharing pain, sparking each other, and being partners with the earth. Our obstacles to empowerment, she believes, are selfishness, unkindness, laziness, and any kind of closing down.[12]

Houston values the powerful shamanic and Native American traditions for their *via positiva.* She honors the "Native American concepts [that] are still reflective of the sensibility and spirit of this place." Each of us must feel some ownership in what is being told or taught. In order to reach our spiritual goals, those goals must be born of something of which we feel a part.

---

skandhas: components of individual consciousness.

via negativa: deep awareness through separation from distraction.

via positiva: laughing, singing, identification with the whole.

Houston says that wounds allow for the opening of ourselves.[13] I agree, when taken in this context. Without FM, CFID, and CMP, I would not have learned to depend upon my self spiritually, nor would I have understood the importance of spirituality—not just religion—in bringing one's whole self into balance. Because of my suffering, I have learned that I am more than a body; I am a spirit. I can do only so much to heal the body, but there is much I can do to heal the heart.

We may choose to acknowledge or accept what is happening to us, or not. I read a story about two families with an almost identical set of circumstances. Each had a handicapped child with similar disabilities. One family refused to accept the little bundle of love as a member of their family, which led to family turmoil; ultimately the family unit splintered, affecting not only the parents and that child, but the other children as well. The second family accepted their disabled child with open arms and thanked God every day for the blessing bestowed upon them. The love they give to that child is returned ten-fold, and their family has grown into an accepting, nurturing, loving family. These two families had similar sets of circumstances, but a difference in perception and a difference in outcome.

I was living a physically, mentally, and spiritually painful life in an incredibly fast-paced world. Everything was urgent, or so it seemed. I was overly driven and based my self-worth on achievements. And yet, my life was not nearly as full then as it is now.

It's true that things were a lot better financially, but I've learned I can survive on much less. What defines a person is not what is received, but what a person contributes, shares, and gives.

Many times I've asked, "Why me? Why do I have to suffer with unrelenting pain every day? Why can't I sleep? Why can't I have the energy others my age have? Why can't I have just one day without pain?" Do these questions sound familiar to you? If so, you need to know that I found the answer to my questions: "God has other plans for me."

I didn't get to this level of awareness, enlightenment, or thinking overnight. It took work and persistence on my part and the part of my Redeemer, but the rewards have been splendid. I am not totally there yet, and probably never will be, but the attempt is what is important. Accepting change can be fulfilling, if you let it.

The destiny of man is in his own soul.

HERODOTUS

Accepting What Is

Acceptance is one of the steps in the grieving process and can have a profound effect on the way we look at our illnesses. Once we are able to admit that chronic pain is part of who we are, we can learn to deal with it. It no longer dominates our personality or what we have to contribute. Acceptance of pain is empowering. When we reach this level of coping with our losses, then we can move on.

In a study reported in the journal *Pain*,[14] researchers found evidence that "acceptance of pain is an independent predictor of mental well-being in patients with chronic pain." Their study concluded that once a chronic pain patient accepts the pain and the fact that it might not change, the patient can and does shift away from "pain to non-pain aspects of life."

From Recognition to Action

- Recognize that until you accept your illness you cannot move forward.
- Accentuate the positives that are a result of your illness. For example, new friends, opportunities for helping others, becoming more spiritual, or any opportunity for personal growth.
- Get a positive role model. This should be someone you see as having more problems than you do, who is exemplary in dealing with them. There is always someone. Mine is the late Christopher Reeve, and now also his late wife, Dana.
- Recognize that your actions do affect others; make them ones that could be a positive role model for someone else.
- Learn something new that can replace something you have lost; for example, a new hobby you can enjoy as much as one that is no longer possible.
- Cut yourself some slack. Don't be overly critical of things you cannot change.
- Find a way to be there for others who have been supportive to you, at least in some capacity.
- Love yourself.
- Learn the importance of self-acceptance as the precursor for accepting others.

Dr. Elisabeth Kübler-Ross was a medical doctor, psychiatrist, and author who was world-renowned for her pioneering work on death, dying, and the grieving process. Through her work she learned that life is like the changing of the seasons from spring to summer, summer to fall, and fall to winter.

It is an ongoing process of adaptation. Like many others in her field, she believed we adjust to change by learning to throw out all the negativity. She believed that we often can be our own worst enemy, and become stagnant if we allow ourselves to be rigid and unchanging. Is religion a blessing or a curse? Through her work with death and dying, Kübler-Ross came into contact with Islam, Buddhism, Judaism, Christianity, and Hinduism. She believed they are all proponents of the same basic truth, and that their differences are in teaching and practice. Her statements regarding religion have left the impression that it is not our affiliation, but in our fervor as participants that we grow spiritually. She once had an incredible vision that she said was like "falling into a waterbed of love." She believed that is what God is like. "It's all love, all wisdom, all understanding, and all compassion for every living thing." She taught patience, tolerance, and love of self.[15]

Nothing is terminal, it is only changing.

ELISABETH KÜBLER-ROSS

According to William Elliott, B. F. Skinner is "possibly the most influential psychologist alive." He authored fourteen books and is considered a leading proponent of behaviorism.

Skinner said, "We don't do anything because of what is going to happen; we do things because of what has happened."[16] We are incapable of knowing what the future holds. We certainly couldn't react to our pain before it happened, and how we react to our environment and those around us is a result of that pain.

Dr. Jon Kabat-Zinn holds several titles, including executive director of the UMMC Center for Mindfulness in Medicine, Health Care, and Society. He is the author of *Full Catastrophe Living* and *Wherever You Go, There You Are*, as well as numerous other books. Kabat-Zinn has used meditation to help people suffering from chronic diseases and stress-related disorders, including abdominal pain, ulcers, and chronic diarrhea. In *Full Catastrophic Living: Using the Wisdom of Your Body and Mind to Face Stress, Pain and Illness,* he writes that a majority of his patients reduced stress-associated pain and improved their health by meditating.[17]

If you know how to worry, you already know how to meditate. Worry is negatively focused meditation.

RICK WARREN, AUTHOR OF *THE PURPOSE DRIVEN LIFE*

Meditation has been shown to have particular usefulness in treating stress and reducing chronic pain.

Baba Ram Dass, formerly known as Richard Alpert, was a Harvard professor who began his search for awareness through psychedelic drugs but ultimately found his path in teaching Eastern spiritual philosophy. Later, after returning to the United States from his travels, he embraced many spiritual beliefs, including the Jewish tradition in which he was raised.

Ram Dass believes that the highest ideal is one of enlightenment, and that this is achieved by three basic practices: quieting the mind, opening the heart, and fulfilling one's karma.

Karma is to become fully alive through honoring the uniqueness of one's incarnation.

RAM DASS

Baba Ram Dass, who has worked extensively with the dying, particularly AIDS patients,[18] has overcome daunting physical challenges brought on by a stroke, and practices Vipassana meditation to quiet his mind. He said, "The biggest obstacle to enlightenment is clinging to one's own mind. It's not the pain of the things the world does to you; it's how you react to the things the world does to you. The way to end suffering is to detach from the desires and clingings of the mind."

He advises patients to lose their personalities and obtain awareness, because once patients get into their awareness, they can heal their spirits and any emotional scarring. A therapist should be only the catalyst for a patient's self-healing.

A NEW SUMMIT OF LIFE—**ALT**ITUDE

Awareness, adaptation, and acceptance.

Lenience with self and others.

Tolerance of change.

His Holiness the Dalai Lama, Tenzin Gyasto, is the fourteenth Dalai Lama of Tibet. He received the Nobel Peace Prize in 1989.

According to the Dalai Lama, if you have compassion for all other beings, you will receive a warmhearted, genuine attitude from others. He believes we see the value of compassion after assessing the value of anger, and says, "By identifying with others, one develops love and compassion."[19] How we respond to others can determine what we get in return. Discontent breeds discontent, birds of a feather flock together, and all that jazz.

And what is the value of anger? Anger is an emotion, and since it is difficult to express more than one emotion at a time, it must take the place of another emotion. Think back to the last time you were angry or felt contempt; what emotion did it replace? Was it peace, happiness, or contentment? We should accept our circumstances, move away from negative emotions, promote positive thoughts, and nurture qualities that create a calm and happy atmosphere for ourselves and those around us.

Laura Huxley was a therapist and author, and widow of the late Aldous Huxley. She believed that things have a certain rhythm and that there are two ideals. One is to encourage life and do no harm, and the other is for a person to "melt into, and participate in, this extraordinary life."[20]

Huxley believed that just because we cannot define the laws of nature doesn't mean they don't exist. We just aren't smart enough to define them. This is much the case with FM and CFID. Just because science cannot explain the cause doesn't mean the cause does not exist. Scientists and researchers just haven't figured it out yet.

Huxley also believed that we are usually our own biggest obstacle to fulfilling our spiritual endeavors.[21]

Pain is the duality of pleasure.

JACK KORNFIELD

Author Stephen Levine, who is a meditation teacher and counselor for the terminally ill, believes that our highest ideal is to reach our own true nature.

His philosophy is to be merciful with himself, try not to judge others, practice Vipassana meditation, practice Vipassana meditation, practice Vipassana meditation, and sing to God.

I love the way he describes what we do when we are in pain. For lack of finding a better way to put it, here is the direct quote from *Tying Rocks to Clouds.* "When we walk across the floor and stub a toe, our conditioning is to send hatred into the pain, to loathe it and really try to put it out of our world, just the opposite of what it is calling out for. It is calling out to be held, to be cradled, to be accepted, to be touched with mercy, and to be explored."[22] To me this was a revelation. It brought about a whole new perspective on learning to deal with pain. I have often said, "The pain is part of who I am now. I accept it so that I can learn. I must deal with it, I can't ignore it, so why let if affect me negatively?" Before learning this, I was the one who hated it and let myself feel victimized. Mind you, I know it will take time, as it did for me, to incorporate this new way of thinking. It is difficult to unlearn certain behaviors and realize that the body is hurt and should be nurtured, to see these disorders as needing to be tended emotionally, spiritually, and physically. Just as one cares for a child's hurt or nurses a wounded animal, learning to treat yourself this way gives the pain a whole new meaning.

Levine believes in being merciful.[23] Being kind to ourselves, understanding there is more than one right way, and being merciful with self and others will allow awareness and freedom. I remember my grandmother saying, "Remember Celeste, there's more than one way to skin a cat." At the time, I was probably ten years old; I thought that was a rather disgusting, perverse thing to say. Perhaps that is why it made such an impression upon me and I am able to remember it. Perhaps that is why my students told me I was a good teacher. There is more than one right way. One small thing can have an immense impact on the way you treat others and the way others treat you.

---

metta: loving-kindness.

Toni Packer is a Zen teacher at the Genesee Valley Zen Center in upstate New York. She maintains that the way we see ourselves is not always the way others see us, because we have control over how we present ourselves.[24] I understand that belief. We are multifaceted individuals. Many of us play different roles—parent, child, sibling, boss, employee, coworker, and friend. We behave differently in each of those roles. As an employee, one certainly wouldn't go to work with the "mother" role in place; that would probably go over like a lead balloon. If you have ever watched the show *Survivor,* you know what I mean. We let others see in us what we want them to see in us. Packer describes this as a sense of self, erected from memory, emotions, and sensations, which, in turn, affects our perception of people and things.

She also says, "Suffering is connected with this sense of self." She believes that suffering is born because we feel victimized. So how does she handle this?

According to an interview with William Elliot,[25] Packer believes that, "The thought of enlightenment can be highly inspirational and can give one rushes or gushes of energy in thinking 'I can get it.' But it is just an idea and thought." She obviously believes in the power of meditation and the effects it can have on one's body, calming and quieting, but only when a person allows the mind to open.

I love the way she describes this opening process. She says, "I don't know how a mind opens up. I couldn't tell you. It is either open or closed. When it is closed, we perform all kinds of practices to get it open. When it is open, we don't know how it happened. We may deduce or think this led to that."[26]

Her advice is to follow Buddha's last words, "Be a lamp unto yourself." She says to learn by yourself what life has to teach you. Don't depend on someone else to do that for you.[27] I agree with that. You must seek your own answers, otherwise there is no ownership in it for you and you will be less likely to stick with it. This applies to any practice, whether it is a new treatment, relationships, spirituality, or even working a crossword puzzle. You will be more likely to retain what you have learned if you don't depend on others to take responsibility for your well-being. Don't expect the doctor or therapist to help you through all the aspects of your health. You must understand that this is your body, most likely (depending upon your beliefs) the only one you will have. Why on earth would we think someone else could possibly be as interested in it as we are? After all, they should be paying most attention to their own.

Swami Satchidananda, born in India, has been a Hindu monk and Eastern spiritual teacher in the United States since 1966. He is the founder of the Integral Yoga Institute and Light of Truth Universal Shrine, which "celebrates the Universal Truth in all religions." He, too, believes that knowing our own true nature is what leads to enlightenment. He calls the highest ideal his famous triad: "Healthy, happy, and useful." If we see the spirit in ourselves, then we can see it in others. He believes that perception begins with God. If we want to see God in other people, then we should look through God's eye.[28]

---

ananda: proper name suffix meaning "supreme happiness," or "bliss."

To have enlightenment without sacrifice is not possible, according to Swami Satchidananda. He says attachment, or the inability to sacrifice or give something up, is the biggest obstacle to becoming enlightened.[29] I totally agree. "It is better to give than to receive." Have you ever watched as someone opens a gift? Many people become embarrassed to receive. The giver is the one who really reaps the reward from the experience.

To attain this bliss we first must know who we are. Swami says, "Then see thyself in your neighbor, love your neighbor as you would love yourself."[30] This is also one of the great commandments in the Judeo-Christian belief system.

Swami Satchidananda equates pain to a process of becoming clean. His master once told him, "Pain is my friend. If the pain is not there, you will not know where the problem is." I can see that this would apply to all aspects of who we are, spiritually, physically, emotionally, and mentally.

As he so eloquently put it, "People come, people go . . . life is like that. Accept it. I am not here to reform the world, but to reform myself. When I have changed myself, then I have changed the world."[31] We have the ability to help ourselves and the example we set can affect others in ways we may never know.

Do everything for God . . . God has given you many gifts—use them for the greater glory of God and the good of the people. Then you will make your life something beautiful for God; for this you have been created. Keep the joy of loving God ever burning in your heart, and share this joy with others. That's all.

MOTHER TERESA

Other Paths

Kathryn E. Ferner, Psy.D.,[32] probably defines the relationship of spirituality best in an article published in the spring 2003 issue of *Paradigm,* titled "Mind-Body-Spirit, Treating the Whole Person." She says, "Treating the mind, body, and spirit together gives us powerful tools for healing, each being irrevocably intertwined."

When we are experiencing times of stress, such as when learning to deal with chronic pain, our spiritual beliefs can give us comfort and guidance on how to go about our lives. Dr. Ferner uses a modified form of the Native American Medicine Wheel to describe what might be called a balanced spiritual life. Those who already have their own spiritual guidelines in place would use those, but Ferner describes most of us as spiritual "nomads."

According to Ferner, Reverend Rosalyn L. Bruyere is a recognized medicine woman of a number of tribes. Bruyere is a minister, healer, and the author

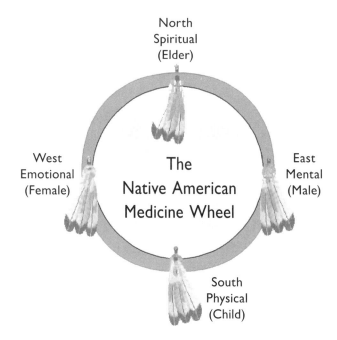

The Medicine Wheel

of *Wheels of Light,* in which she teaches the Sioux version of the wheel. The entire wheel would be too exhausting to teach in the context of one article, but Ferner believes the basic elements are relevant in successful therapy.[33]

The wheel has four directions: north, south, east, and west. The northern point is considered the elder, or the "spiritual" view. Clockwise at 90 degrees is east, considered the male or "mental" direction; south at 180 degrees is the child, or the "physical" aspect of one's life; and at 270 degrees is the west, which represents the female, or "emotional" phase.

Dr. Ferner describes the wheel's use in evaluating progress toward balance. She asks if we have learned something new, taken some fun time to recharge our batteries or get physical exercise, considered our emotional life with journaling or meditation, or maybe spent time in prayer or dream practices to enhance our spiritual life. If there is an over-emphasis in one direction or a deficit in another, then the wheel is out of balance.

William Elliott also talks about balance, and gives a very good example of what it is like to become unbalanced. He discusses his need to be spiritually fulfilled to "save himself," but at one point became so wrapped up in spirituality—what it is and what it means—that he didn't feel whole.[34]

A constipated yogi: one who becomes weighted to the spiritual side.

STEPHEN LEVINE

I like to think of the wheel as though you were sitting on a four-seated teeter-totter. It is important to identify weak areas on that teeter-totter, but it is equally important to identify what Bruyere notes as addictions. Being too weighted in one direction will cause as much of a disruption as neglect. If we are too physical, we may be neglecting our spiritual side. If we are too busy working or being intellectual, we may be neglecting our emotional attributes. Lack of attention to physical or emotional needs may cause overweight to your spiritual side. In other words, if your wheel is out of balance, so are you. Like a teeter-totter, too much or too little will drop at least one seat to the ground.

This is a simplified interpretation of the Medicine Wheel, but understanding the basis for mental, physical, emotional, and spiritual balance will help us learn to heal the various aspects of our lives.

Religion is only one aspect of spirituality, yet for me, without my religion I would have nothing on which to base my spirituality. Religion also offers another powerful avenue for expressing our spirituality—fellowship with others who share our beliefs. Humans have free will, but the choices we make and how we live out these choices are what is really important. In the long run, it is not which religion, but your dedication to your spirituality and how you nurture it, that counts.

You achieve health and wholeness by using your unique beliefs and spirituality to deal with chronic pain. How you choose to grow and change your relationships with others determines what comes back to you.

Life is precious. Who among us hasn't suffered a loss and thought, "If only I had taken the time, if only . . ." Understanding that our time is limited, understanding that we are much more than our illness, is what helps us become better at filling spaces of time. Learning this changes "if only" to "I am so glad that I . . ."

I wanted to change the world. But I have found that the only thing one can be sure of changing is oneself.

ALDOUS HUXLEY

Mindfulness

I try not to waste precious energy on trying to understand that which does not require an explanation. When things seem out of perspective, I try to be mindful of my surroundings or even my pain.

———————————— *Personal Testimony* ————————————

Sometimes when I want to calm myself I think of waking up in the mountains and smelling the aroma of coffee permeating the air around the campsite. I enjoy the solitude within. This is a time to relent, conquer, and transform thoughts of negativity. A once-over body scan finds my muscles relaxing. With each deep inhale, I relax; and with each exhale I release tension and the toxic effects of FM, CFID, and CMP. I put my pain on a shelf for a while and pick it up later when I am better able to cope with it. If you like, come along. We are now walking together through the fragrant pine trees, inhaling their fragrance, to where we hear the gentle sounds of a babbling brook. There is a doe looking at us from across the stream with big, brown, wonder-filled eyes. The birds are chirping to each other; they are aware of our presence, and we of theirs. Perfect harmony. The beautiful butterflies lift their wings in praise of our awe at their beauty; yellow ones, deep blue ones, purple ones. Mountain flowers are gently swaying with the breeze and welcoming us to lie down on their soft fragrant mat. Now, all is at peace. I am leaving you here for a while to bask in your inner tranquility. . . . Evenly breathe in and out deeply, then gradually return to the reality of creation. What a wonderful place to be! Give thanks for the ability to embrace today with continued joyful feelings. Pick up your little packet of pain from the shelf, if you must, but note it is much lighter.

Learning to coexist with nature is a form of mindfulness. There was a time that I would have gone running for a can of insecticide if I had ants at my picnic site. Now I am mindful that they have as much right to be there as I do. Unless they are wreaking havoc, biting, or wanting to share the food, I just ignore them. Although sometimes it is rather fun to watch them going about their day. In and out, up and down, work, work, work. That's when I'm glad I am human. Ants don't have vacation or paid time off. Nature has many things to offer us, if we would just take the time to interact.

Many working in the field of medicine and the mind-body connection have long taught the benefits of remaining positive. The power of positive thinking and optimism is extraordinary. Dr. Bernie Siegel[35] speaks extensively to the subject of changing the body by changing the mind. He cautions, however, not to try to be positive if it is a performance. In other words, don't act happy if you're not happy. Your goal should be peace of mind. As Siegel suggests, treatment modalities such as biofeedback, relaxation training, yoga, visualization, and other consciousness-altering techniques can help us achieve this goal.

Failure is the number one opportunity for achievement.

CELESTE COOPER

Try to find a way to make something positive come from something negative. For instance, my husband and I live in Colorado part of the summer because the constant drastic barometric changes, molds, and so on in the Midwest play a big role in perpetuating coexisting conditions and my other symptoms. We always stop off at the KOA in Limon. One particular year the KOA had acquired new owners. I went in to register, and lo and behold, they didn't have my reservation. I argued, "I made reservations; I would never attempt to make a trip straight through, because of the difficulty of riding for too long." The young girl at the desk was in a quandary until the new owner stepped in and said, "Hmm, Cooper, isn't that the no-show from last night?" They had debited my charge card for not showing up the night before. Well, I put on my defensive hat, which is usually a little lopsided these days because of the brain fog. The new owner was exceptionally nice and said, "Oh that's okay, we have room for you tonight." I thanked her and went on my way. Immediately upon returning to the car, I checked my confirmation; I've learned to question myself more than anyone else does. For goodness sakes, there it was. I had our departure date wrong in my head and we were supposed to be at our next reservation that night. I offered profuse apologies to the new owner, which she kindly accepted. We laughed, and a new friendship began. I had become so frustrated with the brain fog. Honestly, it can be devastating, if you let it. Before I learned acceptance, I used to chastise myself for being so stupid. (Is that negative thinking, or what?) Now I see it as being mindful of brain fog. (Told you cognitive behavioral therapy works.) It is part of who I am, I accept it, I deal with it; and when I do, I open myself up to new possibilities. The owner of that KOA and I have become friends and look forward to seeing one another when we stay there. Had I not made that mistake, I would have missed a wonderful opportunity for a friendship I look so forward to renewing each year.

In a world where there are so many differences of option and media reports of suffering, and so much obsessive dwelling on negativity, it is not easy to maintain a positive outlook. To remain positive may take some extra work. As the age-old adage goes, "Practice makes perfect."

Following are ways to help you get and maintain a positive attitude.

AFFIRMATIONS

I have no duty to be perfect.

I always have options.

I am not my mistakes.

This is a learning experience.

Columbus was looking for India.

Choose once again.

I am learning these lessons faster than I used to learn new things.

I accept that "it's just" or "it's only" means something different to me.

I'm not required to do everything on my "to do" list.

I have the right to expend my energy on the relationships I choose.

I am more than my illness.

Using Affirmations

- Affirmations are positive statements for the here and now.
- Keep them short and easy to remember.
- Write down your favorite affirmations and post them where you can see them frequently.
- Counteract negativity by using one of your affirmations. Practice this until it becomes second nature.
- Commit yourself to one affirmation at a time and repeat it at least every three hours.
- Repeat your affirmation as you look in the mirror every morning and let it set the tone for your day.
- N for "No to negativity" or "Next thought" (from *The A-to-Z Steps to a Richer Life,* by Deepak Chopra).

Guided Imagery

Guided imagery is a form of creative visualization that has been used to help patients suffering from disease, altered body image, or the fear of death. It is a meditation technique in which you visualize your body healing. In order for guided imagery to be effective, you must know how your particular disorder affects your entire body. That is why it is important that you read chapter 1. If you watch the TV show, *Crime Scene Investigation* (CSI), you have an idea of how creative visualization works. Their dynamic filming of blood cells and things like that is actually a form of guided imagery. If you can use this technique to connect the dots between your body and healing energy, you will be able to visualize your body healing. Practitioners of Reiki (ray-kee) incorporate a form of creative visualization in using this Japanese hands-on healing technique.

According to Darlene Cheek at the website Suite101.com, under *Fibromyalgia, Creative Imagery and Healing*, "creative visualization can heighten immune functions, lower blood pressure, speed healing, alleviate depression, reduce perception of pain, lower fatigue, and increase relaxation." She describes it as being like self-hypnosis, except you want to practice until you can actually *see* what you want to happen.[36]

A study at the Norwegian University of Science and Technology (NTNU) in Trondheim, Norway,[37] found that guided imagery was more effective in reducing FM pain than Amitryptyline, which is a commonly prescribed medication.

Meditation—Becoming Full of Yourself

Practicing meditation has been associated with extending life span; heightening awareness; uniting the body, soul, and spirit; and providing a better quality of life. There is no one-size-fits-all meditation, so you may want to explore a few kinds before deciding what is right for you.

Meditation: an active process of focusing the mind into a state of relaxed awareness. To induce a restful trance, which strengthens the mind by freeing it from its accustomed turmoil.

BERNIE S. SIEGEL, M.D., *LOVE, MEDICINE & MIRACLES*

Christian Meditation

I (Celeste) spend time reflecting on what God wants for me. Contemplating this, studying His word, and praying are forms of meditation. This type of prayer or contemplation provides comfort, quiets my soul, and allows me time to focus on the meaning of the trinity—God, Christ, and the Holy Spirit. The power of Christian meditation is awesome for our spirituality.

There are thoughts that are prayers. There are moments when, whatever the posture of the body, the soul is on its knees.

VICTOR HUGO

Prayer

At the conference, "Expanding the Spectrum of Medicine," Dr. Dossey discussed the power of prayer. He said, "Those who fear experiments in prayer might relax and the almighty cannot be harmed by science. Only our prejudices are in danger."[38] Following is part of Dossey's presentation that included a 1988 study by Randolph Byrd.

In a double-blind study done at San Francisco General Hospital on approximately 400 heart patients being treated in the "state of the art" coronary care unit, patients were included in prayer. The patients, randomized and unidentified, were unaware of the study being conducted. Numbers were assigned and a brief description of their health concern was given to various prayer groups. These prayer groups were not given any specific instructions or guidelines, but just told to pray for these people. When the data was analyzed, the prayed-for group had a greater percentage of recovery with no deaths and a shortened recovery period, in comparison to the not-prayed-for group.[39]

Body Scan

The body scan is a type of meditation that uses the mind to induce physical and mental tranquility by methodically bringing attention to each part of the body, from head to toe. Body scanning releases tension and cleanses the mind by allowing you to concentrate on something as simple as breathing.

For your first time using the body scan technique, you may want to use a body scan meditation tape to prompt you. Use whichever relaxation techniques you find helpful. If music therapy aids in your relaxation, there is no reason not to incorporate it, as long as you are in a quiet room, not behind the wheel of a car, and tolerate soothing sounds.

Progressive Muscle Relaxation

Progressive muscle relaxation helps you to release tension and gain serenity by focusing on specific muscles, one at a time, moving methodically from your head to your toes. This is a combination of meditation and gentle active muscle movement. Start by contracting the muscles around your scalp and brow, feel the contraction of the fine muscles, then begin to slowly release. As you are letting go, imagine you are releasing the toxins and the stress, and feel the muscles slowly give way. Stay there until the muscles are completely relaxed. You may feel them start to tighten up again; if they do, start over before moving on. Do this to each and every part of your body as you move from your brow to your eyelids, to your temples, to your mouth. Move on from your mouth to your neck, to your shoulders, and continue on down to the tips of your fingers. Remember to release the tension, breathe calmly, and visualize those toxins and wastes as they leave your body. Continue all the way down to the tips of your toes.

This is a really good exercise to do when you are having a difficult time getting to sleep. You will be amazed at the amount of tension you carry around with you.

I combine body scanning with progressive muscle relaxation for dealing with migraine, chronic pain, and tension.

This is how I practice the body scan and progressive relaxation:

- I lie down on my back in a comfortable, quiet place, usually my bed.
- I allow my eyelids to gently close while feeling the softness of their flowing movement across my eyes.
- I practice diaphragmatic breathing, focusing on the sound of each breath as the air moves in and out of my nose or mouth.
- I begin progressive relaxation by starting at the top of my head and proceeding down my body to the tips of my toes, paying close attention to each individual segment.
- I contract the muscles around the area I am concentrating on, and allow the tension to release as I relax the muscles.
- If I have a hard time releasing the tension, or find my mind keeps drifting back to this area after I have left it, I go back to it.
- For resistant areas, I visualize something comforting as I release the tightened muscles. I might imagine my head full of gelatin that starts to melt as I release the tension in my head. I imagine multiple colors blending into one, full of the strength needed to push out the resistant toxins.
- As I leave each area, I take a deep breath and blow off the cellular waste that had been allowed to accumulate there.
- I allow myself to recognize different sensations, like pain, numbness, tightness, or coldness.
- I move along my body parts, from eyebrows to nose, to mouth, to neck, to shoulders, to arms, to fingers, and so on.
- If the soreness or sensation is deeper, perhaps lodged in my organs where I cannot intentionally contract and release, I visualize something internally

soothing, like warm herbal tea or chicken broth flowing from my mouth down my throat, then coating my stomach and comforting me.

If I'm still awake by the time I get to my toes, I take a deep breath and allow my body to cleanse itself as a whole.

Mindfulness Meditation

Mindfulness meditation is a technique researched and popularized in the United States by Jon Kabat-Zinn, Ph.D. It involves focusing on the present moment, acknowledging thoughts as they come up, and observing them without judgment or interaction. Be aware of the thoughts that are there but don't try to determine whether they are helpful or hurtful thoughts, just that they are there. Pay attention to what is happening in your body and mind at the time it actually is happening.

Kabat-Zinn says that in order to use "mindfulness practice or meditative awareness," you must be open and receptive to learning by doing the following:[40]

- Be nonjudging and patient.
- Nurture the beginners' mind—as though you are seeing everything for the first time.
- Learn to trust yourself and your feelings.
- Let your mind take you where it wants to go.
- Be accepting; he calls this "creating the preconditions for healing." Take each moment as it comes and be open and receptive to whatever happens.
- Let go. Just be and accept things as they are.

Stephen Levine says we should be mindful of our difficulties so that we are aware. Without awareness, we would not be able to correct the problem. He uses anger as an example. "Work with anger is to be as mindful as possible as soon as possible when we notice the first wave, the first ripple of anger."[41] Of course, you must first identify the behavior you would like to change so that you can be aware of making a change.

Mindful Exercise

Mindful exercise is physical exercise plus meditation. While exercising, don't try to solve the problems of the world. If you allow your thoughts to just be, your body will relax and the exercise will be spiritual and relaxing.

Meditation is easy to do. It can be done while sitting, standing, lying down, or even exercising. And it isn't cost prohibitive. There are many good books and tapes available for purchase and at the library. The only investment you have to make is yourself.

As His Holiness the Dalai Lama says, "It takes only one short-tempered person within a family to destroy an otherwise calm and happy atmosphere."[42] This is true, and most difficult to accept when you know that many times *you* are the ill-tempered one. Chronic pain wears on us all. It is not uncommon to have a short fuse when you are in pain. I have learned to identify, or be mindful of, this shameful behavior. When I catch myself being less than cordial, I do a quick mental assessment. Where did that come from? I've noticed that 99.9 percent of the time it is when I am having only a "semi-terrific" day. It is important to make my apologies and go on. I have done a fairly good job at putting my pain in my back pocket, accepting that it is always there with me, but not as the focus of my existence. It is also good to know that when I snap, it is usually because I haven't addressed the pain that is commanding my attention.

People generally have good hearts. When my children are having a difficult time trying to understand the ugliness in the world, I remind them of the heroic contributions of firefighters and others involved in the tragedy of 9-11. Even in the face of vile, foul, and repulsive behaviors from others and ourselves, there is goodness in this world, but sometimes we have to force ourselves to see that goodness within and around us.

Reason is our soul's left hand; faith, her right.

JOHN DONNE

Chapter Conclusion

Developing spiritually allows us to interact harmoniously with the natural way of things. Learning to share your life with supportive loving people, being mindful of your surroundings, living in the now, learning how you can contribute or be of service to others, and bonding with people and nature promotes overall health.

We can overcome obstacles to personal growth through psychotherapy, cognitive/behavioral therapy, hypnotherapy, journal writing, prayer, and meditation.

Discussing and practicing spirituality as part of your medical care is as important as any of your other treatments. As Dr. Dossey emphasized, your mind can have great influence over your body. By nurturing spirituality and mindfulness, we can also intuitively learn about our relationships with others.

Pain is multidimensional. It affects not only our bodies, but also our spiritual practices, relationships with others, and mental well-being. Aristotle called pain "a passion of the soul." It is not an observable event, is purely subjective, and has no objective measurement. It can be treated only through awareness of its presence.

I want to share a story with you regarding the suicide of a young woman who could no longer deal with the intense pain of uncontrolled migraines. I was relating this young woman's story to a friend who responded, "People who commit suicide have a different personality." No, I thought, the mechanism for a person taking his or her own life because of intense physical pain, is not the same as it is for someone with a primary personality disorder. Undoubtedly the mentally ill are in emotional pain, but if treated appropriately, these patients have the opportunity to resolve their emotional pain and thereby, thwart suicidal ideation. In our culture we empathize with people who have a painful terminal illness and contemplate suicide. How is this different from people who endure painful chronic conditions? Why are they treated differently? Why do their complaints fall on deaf ears of people who are supposed to be there to provide assistance? Why should they experience alienation and emotional turmoil in addition to physical pain?

Our pain has often been equated to that of a terminal cancer patient. We feel as though we are in an uphill battle. However, unlike people with a terminal illness, we have the option of climbing that hill. Maybe the affirmation here is . . .

"I have the opportunity to take one more step."

The benefits of meditation come from daily practice that allows us to reap the joys of improved concentration and well-being.

By synchronizing body, mind, and spirit we can learn to minimize the effects of chronic pain on our physical, emotional, spiritual, and mental well-being. By integrating all the aspects of the Native American Medicine Wheel, we can learn to preserve functional capacity, psychological well-being, and overall health.

Jim Donovan, in his *Handbook to a Happier Life,*[43] says you must develop a positive attitude. You are able to achieve that which you affirm because your mind moves in the direction of your dominant thoughts. As an exercise to prove this, he suggests, "Try not to think of the color red. Don't think of red. Think of anything you want but red." I did that exercise and found he was right. I could visualize the color red as sure as anything, and try as I might, I could not get it out of my head. The more I tried not to think about it, the more I did. The point being, if your dominant thoughts are positive thoughts, negative ones can't get in, no matter how hard you try. You have the power to change.

Your life is your message.

RAM DASS

Summary Exercise: Expanding Your Options

1. List two tips for overcoming depression.

_____

_____

2. Explain how spirituality can help you.

_____

_____

_____

3. Define what being mindful means to you.

_____

_____

_____

_____

4. What is your goal for becoming more mindful or spiritual? (Examples: becoming more involved in church, synagogue, or temple; "good deeds" for others; reading self-awareness books; or becoming active in a support group.)

_____

_____

_____

_____

5. Write down three affirmations you wish to practice.

_____

_____

_____

6. What two healthy coping mechanisms do you find play an important part in your life?

_____

_____

_____

7. Describe the four elements to being well-balanced.

_____

_____

_____

_____

Useful Tools
for
Connecting with Your Spiritual Center

On the next pages you will find directions for a three meditations that can help you quiet your mind, relax, and find your center. When you are experiencing chronic pain or having a "semi-terrific" day, there's nothing like meditation for getting through it.

- Breathing Meditation for People with FM, CFID, and CMP
- Guided Meditation for Healing
- New Thoughts on Insomnia

Breathing Meditation for People with FM, CFID, and CMP

1. Sit comfortably.
2. Breathe in slowly and naturally through your nose. Don't try to manipulate your breathing; that is, if your breath is long, let it be long.
3. Feel the strength in your abdomen as you breathe in and out.
4. Let your mind settle by maintaining posture and breathing.
5. Let thoughts and feelings come and go without dwelling on them.
6. Listen and feel your breath as it comes in through your nostrils. Listen to the sounds your breath makes as you exhale through your nose.
7. Practice as time allows and end with one deep diaphragmatic breath releasing all tension and obtaining total relaxation.

Guided Meditation for Healing

Get as comfortable as possible in a place where you can keep distractions at bay for about 20 minutes.

1. Begin by doing a body check for discomfort, numbness, weakness, or pain. Without judgment, color each area with a hue that reflects the dis-ease you feel. I (Jeff) use orange for aches, blue for numbness, grey for weakness, and red for acute pain. If you are aware that a dis-ease will occur if you move, or don't move, add it in as if it were already present. Whatever system of ouchies and colors you pick will work just fine.
2. Begin breathing as deeply as practical and keep the body map in your mind's eye. Accept this map as "where we start".
3. With every breath note the intensity of the colors fading a bit. Note how some colors fade quickly, some more slowly, some completely, others less so. Wonder which might change and in what way. Your focus is on the colors and how they shift. As your mind wanders off task, bring it back gently to breathing and observing.
4. When you sense the fading has reached its peak, begin visualizing warm, gentle rain that blurs the colors beautifully like a soft watercolor painting. Enjoy what you have created; residual pain is always interesting, the tax we pay for aging and changing our health status.
5. Close by affirming your intention to observe and learn from these sensations

New Thoughts on Insomnia

I find that people have more trouble with insomnia than almost any symptom of an illness or syndrome. There is a lot of fear expressed in projecting future impairments from lack of sleep. I tell clients that insomniacs are never original in their complaints. The script for "It's 4 a.m. and I have to get up in 2 hours" was written the day after the clock was invented.

When we sleep we accomplish several things. First, we put our physical body in a fairly stress-free position (relative, of course), which takes postural stress off our muscles, tendons, and bones. This allows our muscles, fascia, tendons, and ligaments to relax. Second, we begin the nightly reconstruction/repair cycle to step up activity as our bodies fix, flush, deconstruct, and replenish all the components battered in our daily grind. Third, we book a mental vacation to Peaceville. Most of our brain goes dormant and hits the reset button. Part, of course, does housekeeping and other functions. Fourth, we cast, direct, and star in our REM Theatre production of dreams *du noir*. Our experience of all this is akin to turning off a switch and entering a different state of consciousness. So my new instructions for insomnia are directed toward experiencing as much of this as possible.

1. Lie down, get comfortable in your bed or chair, and put some soothing instrumental music or environmental sounds on through speakers, earbuds, headphones, or whatever works in your life space.
2. Visualize a peaceful scene, one you remember or construct. Keep adding multisensory details, such as sounds, smells, temperature, and emotional nuances to the visual aspects.
3. Enjoy the peace and refrain from demanding more than this. Rest your body and mind and encourage your imagination. You will probably sleep but even if you don't, you'll still be much better off for relaxing into the peaceful place to which this exercise will take you.

6

Dealing with Circuit Overload

When you have a chronic illness, it's easy to feel overloaded. Energy is a valuable commodity, and lack of it is a perpetuating factor in circuit overload. We, in our unique flock, often seek advice on how to deal with issues that cause us to feel so overwhelmed.

FMily: a loving term created by author Devin Starlanyl for mutually supportive members of the fibromyalgia community.

See my response below to a FMily member who is part of our online FM support group. When I wrote to her, I also copied my response into my journal for future reference.

_____ *Journal Entry* _____

I believe that what you are experiencing is the same thing I call "circuit overload." I have learned that reading and learning about perpetuating factors that can trigger flares is very beneficial. At first, I wanted to do it all. I was so desperate to feel better. Then I recognized it took time to get this bad and it is unreasonable to expect to have immediate knowledge of how to deal with FM, CFID, and CMP.

The objective of this chapter is to help you identify when your circuit is nearing the danger zone. Included within the chapter are thirteen rules for avoiding circuit overload.

On completion, you should be able to do the following:

- List characteristics of brain fog.
- List aggravating factors of brain fog.
- List the two major symptoms of circuit overload.
- Outline time management techniques.
- Identify stress management exercises.
- Review ways to change crisis into opportunity.

People with FM, CFID, and/or CMP are prime candidates for losing their ability to effectively conserve energy and manage their time. We are at higher risk than healthy people for overload and circuit blow out. Pain and fatigue can cause agitation, emotional stress, irritation, restlessness, and the inability to interact with others appropriately. This pool of symptoms is further complicated by disordered thought processes (brain fog), ineffective support structures, and poor time management. This chapter is designed to help you identify what actions and inactions cause overload, so that you can learn to take action before a complete energy loss occurs. You can learn to eradicate, or at least minimize, your episodes of circuit overload.

Brain Fog—Symptoms of Blowout before a Power Failure

The figure below is a visual depiction of the way circuit overload works. Our bodies are conduits for the energy that affects body, mind, and spirit. It is

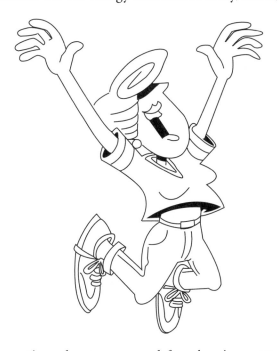

I've only got one nerve left and you're on it!

when we do not take time to recognize overload symptoms that we are at risk for a flare. This power breakdown causes us to physically, mentally, or emotionally retreat to safety—or blow a fuse.

Causes of Brain Fog

According to Ursin and Eriksen, the stress response can be broken down into four areas:

1. Stress stimuli
2. Stress experience
3. The nonspecific
4. General stress response

---

homeostasis: a tendency of biological systems to maintain stability while continually adjusting to conditions that are optimal for survival.

The stress response can upset homeostasis. When the stability of proper body functioning is threatened or impaired, we are in jeopardy. Stress is often blamed for many things, and rightly so. Does this mean that if we control the stress in our lives, we will be rid of the cognitive difficulties some of us suffer? According to what I've read about our conditions, probably not. However, learning to recognize stress stimuli and work through the experience will help us control our reactions.

Know what's weird? Day by day, nothing seems to change. But pretty soon, everything is different.

CALVIN AND HOBBES

People with FM and CFID are at greater likelihood of having cognitive deficit. In other words, we have problems with memory and learning.

Kristina L. Campbell, a student at the University of Missouri, Kansas City, did a dissertation study on the "Neuropsychological Deficits Associated with Chronic Fatigue Syndrome." She was able to conduct her study with Dr. Dennis G. Cowan, Ph.D., consulting neuropsychologist.

The study included 154 physician-diagnosed patients meeting the Centers for Disease Control and Prevention definition for chronic fatigue syndrome. Campbell indicated that, unlike some previous studies, this particular patient population was screened for pre-morbid conditions that can affect cognitive function, such as substance abuse, psychological diagnosis, and neurological deficits related to trauma or disease.

The results of Campbell's study showed that despite some questions regarding the methodology of previous studies, all showed consistent findings of delayed speed of information processing, difficulty with concentration, and attention deficit in these patients. As many as 90 percent of patients with CFID have some degree of cognitive dysfunction, or "brain fog." This is a rather significant percentage.[1]

Fibromyalgia patients have also been studied for cognitive impairment. In a study done by Park, Glass, Minear, and Crofford,[2] Department of Psychology, University of Michigan-Ann Arbor, it was found that FM patients have non-global memory and vocabulary deficits. This confirms why so many of us have trouble recalling events and difficulty finding words, or get them confused. I have found that particularly when I'm writing, I will either use a word totally unrelated to the material or write words, or letters within words, out of sequence. This can be very frustrating. The good news is that although it may be hard to convince some of you, the cognitive deficits associated with these three disorders are "non-global," meaning it is not from Alzheimer's disease.

Devin Starlanyl relates that brain fog, or "fibro fog," is frequently associated with fibromyalgia or fibromyalgia patients with coexisting CMP. It can be aggravated by weather changes, cold, humidity, too much or too little physical exercise, hormonal fluctuations, sleeplessness, anxiety, stress, depression, and mental or physical fatigue. She also believes that reactive hypoglycemia "can be a major contributor," and that the forgetfulness and mental fog associated with it can be significant at the time of a flare.[3] In addition, a diet high in carbohydrates can trigger mental fogginess.[4]

---

fibro fog: brain fog in people with FM.

Chronic pain can cause a myriad of problems. Even though pain and fatigue are obstacles in their own right, they also serve as the foundation for a cascade of other symptoms. All these symptoms, particularly brain fog,[5] detract from the success of coping strategies.

Symptoms of Impending Power Failure

Symptom One—Brain Fog or Cognitive Deficit

Have you noted lapses of short-term memory? Have you lost your sense of direction? Were you formerly the copilot because of your ability to navigate, and now hardly remember the way to the grocery store? Have you noticed that you misplace letters and words when constructing a sentence? Do you lose a word you wanted to use in mid-sentence, or forget names of lifelong friends? If you answered yes to these questions, you suffer from brain fog.

———————————   ***From My Journal***   ———————————

On one particular day I drove to the doctor's office (one I had previously visited twice), only to find myself in an unfamiliar parking lot. I literally sat there and cried with my head in my hands. I was so upset over my inadequacy and the idea that I needed help just to find my way to the doctor.

After a few deep breaths I convinced myself I would get the fog to dissipate, and finally was able to pull enough information from my temporarily absent brain to get to where I needed to go. Thank goodness it was at least in the same town.

Rule Number 1: *Give yourself plenty of time.*

All this and to finally get to the appropriate destination only to have the doctor intimidate me and tell me it was all in my head.

Rule Number 2: *Solicit help from friends and family on "semi-terrific" days.*

All the criteria for circuit overload were definitely in place that day. I now choose to believe that days like that are what make the better days absolutely fantastic!

Brain fog is a semi-humorous term used to describe this collective set of symptoms, but it can be personally devastating. It is easy to become distracted. It makes others feel as though you no longer consider them important enough to remember their names or a date you planned.

Rule Number 3: Write things down in the same place every time, and laugh out loud.

Writing on this topic has been a challenge for me because I suffer some significant symptoms in this area, but the challenge has been good in other ways. I am perpetually learning how to identify overload, which will help me deal with these chronic disorders. It does take effort on my part, and patience with myself.

Rule Number 4: Assess the difference between how much is too much and how much is not enough.

Symptom Two—Lack of Energy

You could blame this "zestlessness" on the nature of the beast or overloaded circuits. It is of the utmost importance that you learn to conserve energy for the times you need it most, and to recognize that you need to recharge before tackling important projects. You wouldn't use a household extension cord to provide electricity to an entire neighborhood. By learning to recognize the energy needed for a task and evaluate the extent of your reserve, you may be able to prevent a circuit breaker fire.

Identifying the underlying cause of your energy depletion, such as too little sleep, too much stress, lack of organization, or too many tasks, will help you figure out how to treat the symptom.

Think of it this way. You are allotted one-hundred joules, or points of energy, for the day; the "otherwise healthy person" probably starts with one hundred and fifty. A hundred-point day is a day when you awaken refreshed and nearly pain-free. If you learn to plan realistically on these days, you can maximize your energy with little threat of running short. It would not be wise to plan a week's worth of chores in that one day, or you will likely bring on exhaustion, brain fog, agitation, restlessness, and irritability. If you drain your car battery completely, you cannot get enough energy to recharge it. The body, mind, and spirit work much the same way.

My second favorite household chore is ironing. My first being hitting my head on the top bunk until I faint.

ERMA BOMBECK

There will also be days when your battery is half-drained before your feet hit the floor. Every morning you should check your voltage. If it is low—say at 50 percent (fifty points for you), plan your activity accordingly. Make sure you leave enough "spark" at the end of the day for overnight "reenergizing." Some days you may have to recharge for the whole day so that you have energy for the next one. This is not a defeat; this is being smart. It is when you allow your energy meter to get too low that you are at the highest risk for a blow out.

Rule Number 5: Avoid the need for a complete overhaul—save at least 1 percent of your energy.

Learn to identify when energy levels are low, and act to prevent a complete drain. This is not the same as wimping out. Only you will know if you are truly pushing the envelope.

Exercising caution does not mean you'll never have another flare, because even with the best of planning, life happens. However, understanding how important energy is and how to optimize it will make coping with symptoms of physical, mental, emotional, and spiritual overload easier to handle.

Making Repairs before a Blowout Occurs

Chronic pain can impair thought processes and interfere with cognitive abilities, especially when you're trying to make emotionally driven decisions.[6] The answer to this dilemma? Do not make emotionally driven decisions. Okay, I can hear you screaming. Me, too. We don't always have this luxury, do we? For example, when we lose someone close to us, it's impossible to make non-emotionally driven decisions. Emotions are not bad. They are part of what makes us who we are, but sometimes we let them, instead of our common sense, drive our decisions. Because of chronic pain and the resulting brain fog, there is an increased risk of making poor decisions. This is a time to solicit support, so there will be no regrets in the future.

Rule Number 6: Get a second opinion.

Be alert to what can happen if you are making life-altering decisions when you are engulfed in pain and/or fatigue.

You should be able to identify some known stressful events by now, ones over which you *do* have some control. Think back to the last time you felt overwhelmed. What was happening at the time? Now write that down. Each time this happens, write it in a diary so you can start to recognize patterns. Avoidance of known stressful events will improve your ability to concentrate. Of course this is not always possible. Life is full of little surprises, some good and some less than good. There are always going to be unavoidable pressures. It is important to learn to minimize stress in between those stressful periods, and make important choices at times that are more acceptable.

Rule Number 7: Avoid known stressors, especially during a critical period.

Clearing Cerebral Dust Bunnies

- Practice deep breathing.
- Challenge your brain on a consistent basis by reading, working crossword puzzles, or playing games that require thought.
- Get organized. Inability to organize can be a symptom of brain fog and a

contributor to impending power failure. (See organizational ideas and how to deal with logjams in the next section.)

- Address the source of anxiety, agitation, fatigue, stress, or depression.
- Identify your symptoms of impending brain fog.
- Avoid distraction.
- Treat your fatigue; use good sleep hygiene.
- Identify medications that might be intensifying brain fog and discuss them with your doctor.
- With your physician's help, identify medications that may be helpful in treating cognitive deficit.
- Discuss biofeedback and neurocognitive feedback with your health care provider.
- Avoid or treat identified aggravating factors of mental confusion. Ask yourself, "Should I be making this decision right now?"
- Say "no" when you feel overwhelmed.
- Accept that you may not remember. Treat yourself and your relationships accordingly.
- Do not drive or make important decisions when you are experiencing brain fog.
- Recharge before a "blowout."
- Access energy needs before tackling a project.
- Minimize multitasking when possible.
- When possible, make life-altering decisions at optimal times.
- Solicit a second opinion when needed.
- Focus on the duty at hand; avoid being sidetracked.
- Remember, if you can, "A flat tire does not create a smooth ride."

Rule Number 8: Exercise your brain to keep it healthy.

I struggled over where to place this topic in the order of the book. Because brain fog is a symptom of trying to do more than your mind is willing to allow, it ended up here. Brain fog can be the source of many symptoms, and it can also be the result of many symptoms, including anxiety. I'm not sure we can make it go away. Like FM, CFID, and CMP, its causes elude us. However, we can do things to help minimize the effects those cerebral dust bunnies have on our self-esteem, mental well-being, and relationships with others. It is an obstacle, but we can mitigate it. It requires constant work, but like anything else, the more we work at it, the better our skills. Share with others what you learn. I've always told my students, "If you really want to learn something, teach it."

Time Management—An Exercise in Energy Conservation

How you act shapes the future. If you behave hatefully or aggressively, it will become automatic, which creates a world around you that is hateful or aggressive.

JACK KORNFIELD, THE OTHER TRUTH

"Wait" Management

In his book *Driving Your Own Karma,* Swami Beyondananda (author Steve Bhaerman) says:

> Do you realize that four out of every five Americans have a serious wait problem? That's right. Studies show that most Americans can't stand waiting. (They can't even sit waiting.) Wait problems are being blamed for everything from heart disease to digestive disorders, high blood pressure, to low income. Think about it: for every minute we spend waiting, most of us lose, on average, a minute off our lives! Ask yourself this question: Am I truly alive while I'm waiting? If the answer is no, then you've shortened your life by that much. Actually, it's not the wait itself that's harmful, but your attitude about your wait. Whenever people say to me, "I hate to wait!" I tell them they have things backward. They should wait to hate instead. And to those people who are always late because they are afraid that if they get there earlier they'll have to sit around doing nothing, I say, "Stop throwing your wait around!"[7]

Unless you are an alien dropped from outer space or have never been to a doctor, you have experienced the waiting game. This can be overwhelming when you are already in pain. In some respects you may feel duped by your medical professional, because to keep a patient waiting beyond the appointment time seems neglectful. However, this is a perfect time to utilize your time management skills.

Rule Number 9: Manage time effectively.

The Swami says times like these are a perfect time to "defile" yourself.

> It's important to defile yourself and defile yourself regularly! Go through some of those files, and for goodness sake throw them out. Donate them to the brainless! Anything! For example, are you still holding on to TV trivia from the early '60s? Are advanced algebra formulas that you will never use occupying valuable cranial real estate?

And you can also forget every negative thing that was ever said to you, not to mention anything negative you might have said. Now go to the photocopy machine in the basement of your mind (the one on the second floor is still not working) and run off copies of every fun, inspiring, happy experience you can remember. Good. Now stick a copy in each of the mental file folders you just cleaned. Just think. In the course of waiting for a bus, you can clear out and replace dozens of stale, spoiled, or downright rotten memories. And if you do your waiting where there isn't even a bus running, you can accomplish much more.[8]

Learn to take along a good book, like *Driving Your Own Karma,* or this one you're reading. Use waiting time to prioritize those items you want to discuss at your meeting with the doctor. Putting yourself in a position where you might be late will only increase your threshold for anxiety, so learn to think of the wait as a long "a-waited" break. You might even find yourself arriving at appointments early just so you can wait. I did.

I (Jeff) distinctly remember meeting some colleagues from another clinic for lunch one day, and waiting forty-five minutes for a sandwich to be served. I was furious and demanded they wrap it to go, as I had an appointment scheduled and no more time for lunch. A week later I received a call from a former patient who was bubbling over with good news on her own spiritual progress and wanted to take me to lunch. When asked if I had a place in mind, I said, "Absolutely, I know the perfect place to talk. They don't even interrupt you to eat." We sat for the two hours it took to cover her exciting changes, drank a lot of tea, and eventually got a meal as well. Getting angry about waiting is one of the pointless misdirections I have endured. The truth is so obvious—use time to clear your emotional vision. As I often tell clients leaving my office, "You are in Missouri, not in Misery; go to the bathroom before you get on the highway. The odds of being stuck on the road by ever-present construction are not in your bladder's favor." Or, "If you get in a line or lane behind an old man wearing a hat (OMWAH, translated, "Oh my, what a hat"), you can only blame yourself for the inevitable wait. Since time began, the OMWAH (and the pipe smoker and the government employee who is on the time clock) has been God's favorite tool for teaching patience. My best friend carries a trove of postcards in his backpack to write whenever the luxury of a delay presents itself.

My other personal revelation on this point was given by a real-life guru, a Tibetan monk who told me the value of my *mala,* or prayer beads. He explained in his halting English that whenever he has to wait for an airplane, a ride, or a meal, he has the opportunity to get caught up on his prayers.

"Mala is your friend when you wait," he said. Believing as many do that a special gift or reward is given on the one millionth recitation of a particular chant, such as *Om mani padhma hum,* he saw every waiting period as a golden opportunity to approach that lofty goal. Once when I stood in line for two hours to see a sand mandala at a Kalachakra initiation, I accomplished four thousand recitations of two different mantras. Regardless of the reward issue, I can vouch for the calming effect and peace of mind this prayer had in what I once would have considered a maddening situation.

Rule Number 10: Activate a self-taught wait exercise class.

The process of respiration is very simple. When you breathe, you inspire. When you don't, you expire.

SWAMI BEYONDANANDA

WAITING STRATEGY

The next time you are near a bookstore or newsstand, invest four dollars in one or two magazines or two that cover your hobbies or interests; not a newsmagazine or work-related publication, just something about an interest or hobby—cooking, surfing, computers, kids, or whatever captures your fancy. Put the magazines under the passenger seat of your car or in a briefcase/purse/backpack. The next time you are pushed into "pause" mode by circumstances, start reading.

Okay, now that we have the waiting issue resolved, we can move on to additional valuable time management techniques.

Prioritizing

Learning what is most important may be difficult in the beginning. Good time management relies on knowing what should or should not be on top of your in-box.

The number one priority for time management is self-management. When you take care of yourself—body, mind, and spirit—you will find you have more energy to tackle the tasks that are high on your priority list. If you have ever been on a commercial aircraft you have heard the words, "If you are traveling with a small child or someone who needs assistance, put your oxygen mask on *first,* then help others." This is prioritizing. By taking care of yourself, you are able to care for others.

Priorities, just like our symptoms, have a way of changing day by day, even minute by minute, or circumstance by circumstance. A priority item at the top of your in box may keep getting shoved down to the bottom by more important matters. Often, seemingly high-priority issues resolve themselves without any intervention.

IT'S YOUR BRAIN, EXERCISE IT

Learn how to identify true priorities such as household chores, duties for work, tasks you do for others, and self-care. Make a list of what you plan to do tomorrow (immediate goals), next week (intermediate goals), or next month (long-term goals). Review your list at the end of the next day and check off tasks accomplished. Now, add and subtract priorities if need be. Keep all your memos and compare them to your first priority list in the following week. Are any of the old priorities still undone? If so, do you need to carry them over to your first priority list the following week? Do this for four weeks and you should be able to identify what your true priorities are and which ones, if left undone, can resolve on their own or in a longer time frame than the one you first imposed.

Organization—Preventing Confusion and Disorder

Chaos breeds discontent in anyone, but for people like us, it is disastrous. The litter around us is more than just clutter; it can also be a safety factor, physically and emotionally. It is extremely important to keep ourselves on track.

The following checklist should be your guide to getting organized. Practicing organization will help you develop coping skills that eventually will save valuable time and precious energy. Once you arrange your life's tools in an orderly fashion, it will be easier for you to set plans and goals in your personal journal, and the planning will help you learn to manage your time.

Rule Number 11: Know your in-box.

Get and Stay Organized

- What is in your in-box? Determine what really needs to be there and get rid of everything else. If you *just can't* rid yourself of all those papers on your desk, items a friend gave you, or Aunt Em's blouse, because you are afraid you might need them one day, throw them in a box and store them in the back of a closet for one year. If you don't need the item in *one year,* get rid of it. Believe me, when you are gone it will mean nothing to your survivors, and if you think it will, give it to them now.

- Practice the in-out rule—when something new comes in, something old goes out. (For example, if you get a new shirt, give an old one you rarely or never wear to someone who can really use it.)

- Put things back in the same place from which they came. When brain fog takes over it is difficult enough to locate things. I once thought I'd found a better place to keep something, and promptly lost it. Oh, I found it all right, long after it had been replaced. Keep things in the *same place!* Don't create disorder where there isn't any.

- If you don't have a place for things, then create one. Make yourself a map or diagram if necessary. My grandmother always said, "There is a place for everything and everything should be in its place."

- Keep frequently used items close by. Don't hide them from yourself. Keep a drawer or box next to your work or leisure area.

- Label things. Don't play a guessing game. Many times I've thought I'd remember what was in a box or a cabinet. Forget it, it doesn't happen. Label, label, and when you run out of labels, buy more. This kind of label is good.

- Once or twice a year take inventory of household goods. The more things you have, the more choices you have. Too many of them are not good for people like us. Keep things simple.

- When in need, ask for help "in deed."

Logjams to Organization

One of the most effective organizational tools is readily available to most of us, but rarely used. Ask someone who has perspective about your stuck point or logjam. Insist on brutal honesty and listen carefully to both the critique and the solution.

Most people approach organization from an ineffective, habitual position. Putting things in piles, waiting for a better time to do something, and postponing a task until all information or parts are present can create personal ineffectiveness.

Rule Number 12: Don't be a clutter bug.

Logjams keep us from moving forward in our lives and our projects. Eric Berne, M.D., psychiatrist and founder of transactional analysis, called this an "until script." Repeatedly in my practice, I see people go stagnant with one of these ineffective strategies. For many people a single unfinished task can block forward momentum in many areas of their lives. Ask yourself, "Am I procrastinating? Do I have forward momentum?"

Ask your friend where you need help, and then ask another and another. You might not like the answers, but listen and consider action anyway. Is your habit more important to you than your progress? In some parts of the world, people have devised a clever way to capture monkeys. A banana is slipped into a narrow-necked jar that is fixed to a table. The monkey reaches into the jar for the banana but cannot pull it out, because the diameter of his grasping fist is wider than the opening of the jar. Instead of opening his hand and releasing the banana inside the jar so that he can remove his hand, allowing him to run for freedom as humans approach, the monkey stubbornly tries to extricate the banana and is captured. Moral: Drop the banana!

Lack of organization can be a major drain on your management of time. Take advantage of having the opportunity to wait, utilize time effectively, and save time for yourself.

The amount of time you would have spent looking for something or constantly rechecking yourself can be spent more productively and will allow you the time to recharge when it's needed.

Rule Number 13: Don't pay tomorrow for a hamburger today.

After all, life will not end because of your temporary brainfuzz. Look at it this way—it's part of the learning curve to getting and staying organized.

Crisis Management—Dealing with Major Life Events

A crisis is really just a regular day compressed into a tiny unit of time. When we enter "crisis mode" a number of interesting brain flips occur.

1. We forget we are on a team. Suddenly we feel like the Lone Ranger on Silver, with the music starting in the background. We don't even see Tonto. Something about that black mask keeps us from realizing that a lot of people will help us for friendship, barter, money, or just for the hell of it. Question yourself and others: "Who might help me?"

2. Focus on the doable, not the impossible. Many times we are really containing damage, not winning the day for the team. Even if you "can't win" the situation, "beat the point spread," as they say in Vegas. There is real value in making things less awful.

3. Things Take Time (TTT). Get this engraved on your watch crystal or the back of your cell phone. The Grand Canyon started as a run-off problem. There is more time than you think in almost any crisis. We are conditioned by movies to believe there is always a large red LED countdown timer

attached to the "bomb" of the problem, and the last second is imminent. Good cinema, but just not so in the real world.

4. Some things can't be fixed. Acknowledge that and stop tearing yourself apart with the agony of not "succeeding." One of my favorite old jokes is about a man who interviews for a job at a remote railway switching station.

> INTERVIEWER: What would you do if two trains were headed for a collision on your route?
> MAN: Telegraph both engines to stop where they are.
> INTERVIEWER: Good. Now what if the telegraph is dead?
> MAN: Set off flares on both sides of the highest point between them.
> INTERVIEWER: Excellent. Now if there were no flares?
> MAN: Use signal flags to stop them.
> INTERVIEWER: Wonderful. And if it were pitch black outside?
> MAN: I'd go get my son.
> INTERVIEWER: Your son? What could he do?
> MAN: Well, nothing. But he loves to watch train wrecks.

5. In Chinese, the symbol for "crisis" literally translates as "dangerous opportunity." If you can't see the opportunity in a crisis, ask someone who can. Paper towels were invented when a giant roll of toilet paper was milled incorrectly. Columbus was aiming for India. If you can't see a golden opportunity or serendipity, at least know that you are gaining wisdom and valuable lessons you can keep and share.

6. "Get mean." Understand that light and dark, rain and shine, birth and death are two sides of the same dance. The arithmetic mean is the "average" we learn in school. Every workday for me, Jeff, contains hours and hours of light duty—playing Candyland while talking to kids, writing reports, or talking on the phone. Then there are thirty to sixty minutes a day when the U.S. Mint can't print money fast enough for me to feel adequately remunerated for my efforts.

7. Finally, there is the story of a condemned prisoner who was offered freedom if he could find the key to making the king happy when sad, and sad when happy. His answer was four words: "This, too, shall pass."

My chiropractor thought I was the wisest of sages when I told him that he and I were required to turn only our little wheels and not worry about the big wheels at all, since our contribution was enough to help them along. After basking in that praise for a minute, I confessed it was from a Grateful Dead song lyric:

Small wheel turn by fire and rod,
Big wheel turn by the grace of God,
Every time that wheel turn 'round,
Bound to cover just a little more ground.
ROBERT HUNTER/JERRY GARCIA, "THE WHEEL"

My (Jeff's) teacher, Lama Surya Das, says his mantra is "Breathe. Smile. Relax." Try it.

Chapter Conclusion

You know about the impaired cognitive function that occurs in so many of us, and how to help deal with it using effective time management techniques. You also know how to confront and deal with crisis. This information should help you identify symptoms of excessive brain wave stimulation and help you to better manage time and crises. As a result, you'll learn to deal with cognitive and emotional overload constructively. Use the exercise at the end of this chapter to your advantage.

When you get into a tight place and it seems you can't go on, hold on, for that's just the place and the time that the tide will turn.
HARRIET BEECHER STOWE

Summary Exercise: Unloading the Gray Matter

1. List three of the characteristics of brain fog.

_____

_____

_____

2. List at least three aggravating factors of brain fog.

_____

_____

_____

3. List the two major symptoms of overload.

_____

_____

4. Outline time management techniques.

_____

_____

5. What is the easiest and most accessible stress management exercise?

_____

_____

6. List three things you could pay someone to do (with money, friendship, or barter) and take off your list of to-dos.

_____

_____

_____

7. Explain ways you could change a crisis into an opportunity, using real or imagined examples.

_____

_____

_____

8. What magazine or book would you choose when you have an opportunity to wait?

_____

9. Review the rules for avoiding circuit overload.

Rule 1: Give yourself plenty of time.

Rule 2: Solicit help from friends and family on "semi-terrific" days.

Rule 3: Write things down in the same place every time, and laugh out loud.

Rule 4: Assess the difference between how much is too much and how much is not enough.

Rule 5: Avoid the need for a complete overhaul.

Rule 6: Get a second opinion.

Rule 7: Avoid known stressors, especially during a critical period.

Rule 8: Exercise your brain to keep it healthy.

Rule 9: Manage time effectively. When the opportunity presents itself, take out the mental trash.

Rule 10: Activate a self-taught wait exercise class.

Rule 11: Know your in-box.

Rule 12: Don't be a clutter bug.

Rule 13: Don't pay tomorrow for a hamburger today.

Brain Fog Relief—Answers to Summary Exercises

1. Short-term memory loss, displacing letters in a written word, difficulty finding common words, loss of sense of direction.

2. Weather changes, cold, humidity, too much or too little physical exercise, hormonal fluctuations, sleeplessness, anxiety, stress, depression, mental or physical fatigue, hypoglycemia.

3. Brain fog and loss of energy.

4. Waiting, prioritizing, organizing.

5. Effective breathing and laughter.

7

Approaching the System Systematically

Learning to cope with chronic pain, fatigue, and brain fog is a difficult task. This chapter includes some of the resources you need in order to deal with your disability, including valuable information regarding your individual rights in dealing with FM, CFID, and/or CMP.

You'll find valuable tools for coping with pain and politics, and you'll read important information regarding ADA (American with Disabilities Act), Social Security benefits, vocational rehabilitation, FMLA (Family and Medical Leave Act), and Temporary Assistance programs.

There are databases of state laws, regulations, and other official government policies that may pertain to your needs. You are encouraged to use them to help you advocate for yourself and for others.

You have the right to compassionate medical care, appropriate testing, and management of your pain. When you finish this chapter you will have a better understanding of how to get the help you need, and will possess a working set of political survival tools.

The ADA and the EEOC

Americans with Disabilities Act

Many people with chronic pain disorders, such as FM, CFID, and CMP, attempt to remain in the workforce in spite of their pain. What statistics do not show is how many of us do not utilize available resources, in part because we are unaware of what protections exist. It is important to remain productive, but it is unjust to have to live to work, instead of working to live. Is it any wonder that so many with chronic pain are depressed? It is very easy to get trapped into living a fractional life, limited to one sphere of life or combination thereof: work, children, addictions, or illnesses.

> The Americans with Disabilities Act of 1990 (ADA) is one of the most compassionate and successful civil rights laws in American history. . . . Since President George H. W. Bush signed the ADA into law, more people with disabilities are participating fully in our society than ever before.[1]

The ADA is administered by the Department of Justice, and its function is to provide federal regulations for nondiscrimination based on disability. It sets guidelines to insure the rights of people with disabilities.

FIVE AREAS OF THE ADA

Title I—Employment
Title II—State and local government programs, services, and transportation
Title III—Public accommodations (places of business)
Title IV—Telecommunications
Title V—Miscellaneous
   This information comes from the Job Accommodation Network (JAN) home page—ADA questions and answers.[2]

There are stringent codes that regulate everything from hiring practices to accommodations for people with disabilities. These include both public and workplace facilities. The codes are quite extensive and cover such things as bathrooms, doorways, ground surfaces, drinking fountains, signs, fitting rooms, wheelchair accommodations, and any other technically feasible alterations to help those with handicaps. They also cover telecommunications, state and local programs, services, and transportation. Most significant to this book are the provisions made for protecting the rights of a disabled individual against employment discrimination.

The ADA General Rule—Statute 42 U.S.C. §12112(a)

> No covered entity shall discriminate against a qualified individual with a disability because of the disability of such individual in regard to job

application procedures, the hiring, advancement and discharge of employees, employee compensation, job training and other terms, conditions and privileges of employment.

Under the employment provisions of the ADA you will hear terms such as "qualified individual," "essential function," "reasonable accommodation," and "undue hardship."

For the purpose of this text you might ask, "How does the ADA assist someone with chronic pain conditions, who may or may not have a visible physical handicap?" Employment discrimination is prohibited against "qualified individuals" with disabilities. This includes people with substantial limiting impairment, but the key words here are "qualified individuals." Disability is defined as "a physical or mental impairment that substantially limits major life activities, such as self-care, performing manual tasks, walking, seeing, hearing, speaking, learning, and working, or a record of such impairment."[3] This does not apply to an individual with a minor, non-chronic condition of short duration, such as a sprain, broken limb, or the flu. Therefore, you will need to have a well-documented medical history detailing the ways in which your condition affects you physically, mentally, and emotionally.

Act of Congress: a statute enacted by Congress, a law voted into the legal code by the Congress of the United States. The Americans with Disabilities Act is an example of an Act of Congress.

The Qualified Individual

A qualified individual is one who is able to perform the essential functions of the position description. If you meet the criteria for disability as a "qualified individual," you and your employer must work together to determine if you can perform the job duties with a "reasonable accommodation." Would the changes influence the essential responsibilities of that job? The employer is not required to eliminate essential elements of the job in order for you to be considered a "qualified individual," simply because you have a disability.[4]

Essential Function

The employer can also assess "essential function." In doing so, the employer asks, "Does the job exist to perform a particular function, how many other employees are there to complete the function, and is the function highly specialized?" Additional questions include, "How much time is spent complet-ing the function and how often would the 'qualified individual' be expected to complete the function, if he or she were part of a team expected to share duties."[5] Even though the ADA provides some protection to the disabled, the employer may make certain inquiries during the interview process in order to determine the applicant's abilities to carry out essential tasks of a particular job description. Pre-employment exams can be required in certain industries if the employer can substantiate that the restriction is based on a "bona fide occupational qualifier." Even with ADA an employer can require an appli-cant to perform the essential function of the job. An employer is not required to remove "essential functions" as a disability accommodation.[6]

Reasonable Accommodation

The ADA protects you from "employer discrimination" in regard to your special needs, but employer accommodations must be considered "reason-able." Modifications to attendance policies to oblige your disability are not required. Other than the legal protection you have for attendance as outlined in the Family and Medical Leave Act (FMLA), you can be held to the same attendance policies set for other employees. "Reasonable accommodation" is an ambiguous area, and the employer is not always required to make the accommodations you would need.[7] In other words, you cannot be discrimi-nated against because of your handicap, but your performance must still meet the expectations of the job description.

When considering the following, please keep in mind that you must be able to perform the tasks of the job and produce at the same level as your coworkers. You will be held to the same job standards, even when "reasonable accommodations" are made.

A "reasonable accommodation" might include any of the following:

- Being allowed to take rest breaks.
- Having ergonomically correct devices and equipment.
- Being provided with a standing and a sitting work station.
- Time off for scheduled doctor and therapy appointments.
- Limited work hours.
- Availability of flextime.
- A modified work schedule.
- Work from home.
- Use of personal equipment and devices in your work area. These might include items like a heating pad, massage unit, or pillow.

It is also a reasonable accommodation to modify training materials or to move a "qualified individual" to a vacant lateral or promotional position more suitable for the person's needs.

---

ergonomics: an applied science for designing and arranging common items for optimal efficiency and safety of use. Human engineering.

The *Technical Assistance Manual* was developed by the Equal Employment Opportunity Commission to help employers and people with disabilities understand and comply with the employment provisions of the ADA. It is a resource directory and guide to the employment provisions of the ADA. The *Technical Assistance Manual* defines reasonable accommodations as "a modification or adjustment to a job, the work environment, or the way things are usually done that enables a *qualified individual* with a disability to enjoy equal employment opportunity." It also provides a list of possible accommodations. There was an addendum to the manual in 2002.[8]

Certain tax credits and deductions are available to employers to encourage them to make reasonable accommodations to comply with the ADA.[9]

- Title I of the ADA prohibits employers of fifteen or more workers, employment agencies, and labor organizations of fifteen or more workers from discriminating against qualified individuals with disabilities.
- Title II of the ADA prohibits state and local governments from discriminating against qualified individuals with disabilities in programs, activities, and services.

United States Department of Labor (USDOL)—
Equal Employment Opportunity[10]

Undue Hardship

Employers are not required to make "reasonable accommodations" if it causes them "undue hardship." Unfortunately, the ADA does not define this term. Influencing factors include size of the employing business or organization, available resources, and the type of business. Basically, "undue hardship" is an action or accommodation that requires a significant expense or unfair action by the employer.

If the employer's business policy and procedures require a medical examination of all potential employees, all medical information is treated as confidential. If the medical exam determines that you are not qualified for the position because of your disability, the disqualification will only apply if there is a "high probability of substantial harm to the employee or others," or the disability relates specifically to the job. In other words, if the job required you to stand for a minimum of two to three hours and modifications could not be made to allow periodic sitting, there would be "high probability" that your pain and fatigue would be harmful to you. As far as company liability and applicant disability consideration (as part of the post-offer, pre-hire medical exam), the potential harm to others relates to the employee's ability to safely perform the "essential functions" of the job. If your medical exam determines you cannot perform the job function you said you could perform on the employment application, the ADA may not provide you with protection. You must still be able to perform the job as it is described in the position description, "with or without reasonable accommodation."[11] In the case of brain fog with fatigue, you could potentially be harmful to others in certain circumstances. If you feel a determination of "high probability of substantial harm" is made in error, you should provide evidence to the contrary from your own personal physician, and proceed from there.

The next question you might have is, "When and how should I approach an employer with these needed accommodations?" This is entirely up to you. There is no requirement that you disclose your disability. However, the employer can ask questions regarding employment and/or background check, as part of the employment interview.[12]

Keep in mind that if you meet the criteria for "disabled individual," your employer may be able to qualify for "perks" for accommodating your needs. Tax incentives available to companies that hire people with disabilities include the Work Opportunity Tax Credit, Disabled Access Credit, and the Architectural/Transportation Tax deduction.[13]

The Equal Employment Opportunity Commission

The Equal Employment Opportunity Commission (EEOC) "has five commissioners and a general counsel appointed by the president and confirmed by the Senate. Commissioners are appointed for five-year, staggered terms. The term of the general counsel is four years. The president designates a chair and a vice chair. The chair is the chief executive officer of the Commission. The five-member Commission makes equal employment opportunity policy and approves most litigation. The general counsel is responsible for conducting EEOC enforcement litigation under Title VII of the Civil Rights Act of 1964 (Title VII), the Equal Pay Act (EPA), the Age Discrimination in Employment Act (ADEA), and the Americans with Disabilities Act (ADA)."[14]

The EEOC enforces the provisions of regulatory statutes regarding discrimination. It is an independent agency under the administrative branch of the federal government, with many field offices that enforce the statutes and process charges filed with the EEOC. If you feel you have been discriminated against because of your disability, you may contact the EEOC for information regarding the ADA and instructions on how to file a written charge. They will initiate an investigation if the initial facts appear to support a violation of law.[15]

An individual is not allowed to go directly to court without first exhausting all administrative resources. After you file the charge, an investigation is initiated by the EEOC. The investigation follows a sequential order as noted below. This information comes from the EEOC website.[16]

- If the evidence establishes that discrimination has occurred, the employer and the charging party will be informed of this in a letter of determination that explains the finding. The EEOC will then attempt conciliation with the employer to develop a remedy for the discrimination.
- If the case is successfully conciliated, or if a case was earlier mediated or settled, neither EEOC nor the charging party may go to court unless the conciliation, mediation, or settlement agreement is not honored.
- If the EEOC is unable to successfully conciliate the case, the agency will decide whether to bring suit in federal court. If the EEOC decides not to sue, it will issue a notice closing the case and giving the charging party ninety days in which to file a lawsuit on his or her own behalf. In Title VII and ADA cases against state or local governments, the Department of Justice takes action.

Title V (the miscellaneous section) of the ADA prohibits any "coercing or threatening" or "retaliation against" a disabled person, or against anyone attempting to help a disabled person.[17]

An employer found guilty of violating the ADA can be fined a substantial amount of money.[18]

Social Security Disability Determination

Chronic Pain and Navigating the System

Of course being able to remain productively employed should be your primary goal, not only for financial independence, but also for the benefits of personal growth and emotional health. However, for some with FM, CFID, or CMP, remaining in the working environment may no longer be an option.

Whether or not you can remain in the workforce depends upon the extent of your disability, your work experience, your past education, and your age. It is unlikely you will find an employer willing to jump through hoops to give you what you need. These needs might include numerous sick days, time off for therapy during normal operation hours, a twenty-hour workweek with full-time benefits, special equipment, ability to move every twenty minutes, or a place to lie down and rest periodically. When your needs become this great, it may become impossible to find an employer willing to make the changes necessary to accommodate your physical requirements. If this is true in your case, it may be time to explore your other options.

Navigating the Social Security system can be an arduous task. If your disability is from chronic pain and brain fog, the application process alone may seem insurmountable. You may require help from a friend or family member in order to complete this process.

Chronic pain can be so severe that it is disabling. If you have reached this point, don't let anyone tell you that you don't have the right to ask for your benefits. Be prepared to carefully document every aspect of your life. This includes the effect of pain and fatigue on your activities of daily living, your relationships, and your ability to remain in the workforce.

This section is intended to give you a better understanding of the way the Social Security application process works, what information you should have readily available, and the steps of the appeals process.

If you have been using the assessment tools and interaction guides throughout this book, then you are off to a good start. It helps others help you if they can obtain an accurate impression of your disability.

I know it is difficult to dwell on your pain. You have heard all about how to do things to take your mind off it, but now you must focus on the pain and fatigue in order to achieve a favorable outcome. Because FM, CFID, and CMP mostly deal with the collection of subjective input, it is often difficult for others to understand how chronic pain and fatigue affect your life. It is important, therefore, to make every effort to help others understand how chronic pain and fatigue affect your ability to function on a daily basis and do tasks that others take in stride. What daily activities should we let others know are causing us difficulty? They include hygiene, dressing, shopping, household chores, work, relationships, leisure, and locomotion.

You have the tools previously provided in this book and the ones in the useful tools section of this chapter to help you document, communicate, and make the application for Social Security less emotionally and physically demanding.

SSDI and SSI—What Is the Difference?

Although SSDI and SSI sound similar, they are very different. SSDI stands for Social Security Disability Insurance and is the benefit you have as a worker. A disability determination will be made for you by the Social Security Administration when it is expected that your disability will continue for at least twelve months or result in death. You and your employers have paid for these Social Security benefits. Generally, you are eligible for benefits before age sixty-five, or the usual retirement date calculated for your present age group. When you apply for SSDI you are asking to receive your benefits early, because your earning capacity has ended due to your disability.

§404.1505 Basic Definition of Disability

(a) The law defines disability as the inability to do any substantial gainful activity by reason of any medically determinable physical or mental impairment which can be expected to result in death, or which has lasted, or can be expected to last, for a continuous period of not less than twelve months. To meet this definition, you must have a severe impairment, which makes you unable to do your previous work or any other substantial gainful activity that exists in the national economy.[19]

SSI, on the other hand, stands for Supplemental Security Income. This is an additional or optional benefit for those who are disabled or blind. To be eligible for SSI you must have been found disabled by the Social Security Administration. However, benefits are based on limited income resources and are not contingent on any contributions to Social Security. You are eligible even if you have never worked, so long as you are a United States citizen. You can get more information regarding SSI from your local Social Security office.[20]

Preparedness Is Next to Godliness

Your first official contact will most likely be the disability interview, which is conducted in the office or by phone. You must be prepared any time you have contact with the Social Security Administration, regardless of how brief you expect your conversation to be. Include the name and title of the person you speak with, date and time, context of your conversation, and outcome of the interaction or meeting. When you have chronic pain, your attention span may not be what it needs to be, so be sure to repeat what you believe you heard back to the representative for clarification. This will help you make sure you understand the information being relayed to you.

When appropriate, provide a written response and keep a copy and any attachments. (See resource section.)

Organizing Your Files

Keep your files organized because the SSA will most likely ask for the following:

- Names of treating doctors
- Doctors' records
- Medical records
- Correspondence
- Medical bills
- Proof of income (employment records)
- Social Security card
- Birth certificate
- Rent/mortgage and utility receipts

Listing Your Doctors

Keep a record of every doctor you see for treatment, including name, address, phone number, specialty, and dates you were treated. Following is an example. (For help with preparing your own records, see the Treating Health Care Provider Log in the useful tools section at the end of this chapter.)

Dr. Family, 1990–present
PRIMARY CARE PHYSICIAN
1800 So. Way To Go Hwy
Blue Horizon, CA 12345
666-777-8888
Fax: 666-777-8889

Dr. Bones, 1989
ORTHOPEDIST—work comp, neck
1600 W. 410 Hwy
Haveacare, CA 12346
222-333-4444
e-mail: DB@soon.com

Dr. Oops, 4/03/09
SOCIAL SECURITY PHYSICIAN
2700 Clay Ground Drive, Suite 40
North Blue Haven, CA 12348
111-222-3334

Dr. Muscle, 5/03/07–present
RHEUMATOLOGIST
1200 E. Way to Go
Blue Horizon, CA 12345
666-777-7888
Fax: 666-777-7889

Documenting for the Medical Record

Give all information to your treating doctor, no matter how insignificant it seems to you. This should include postural difficulties; any nonsymmetrical (abnormally uneven) body areas, with measurements if possible; joint swelling; pictures denoting morning swelling; any numb areas; or any information discussed in the chapter on dealing with your doctor. Be sure to document and take with you to your doctor any lifestyle adaptations made to accommodate your pain and fatigue. This would include such things as hairstyle accommodations, bathing routine alterations, use of ice packs or heating pads, and use of assistive devices. Also include the use of over-the-counter medications and remedies, medical equipment, installation of additional railings, use of jar openers or household assistive devices, or any significant changes in your routine that enable you to cope with your disability.

Try to keep medical records in chronological order. Of course, in order to do this, you must have them. It is a good idea, regardless of whether or not you are filing for Social Security, to always keep your own copies of all your medical records and tests. For very old records you may have to be more general, but try to keep the most recent two years quite specific. Following is an example of how to put your summary in order. (For help with preparing your own summary, see the see the Chronological Health Record form in the Useful Tools section at the end of this chapter.)

HEALTH CHRONOLOGY

1970–8/31/05

Diagnosis of migraine approximately 1960, hysterectomy 1963, gall bladder surgery 1989, irritable bladder 1990, osteoporosis 1998, low back surgery 1999.

12/06/06

Neck pain increasing

• Job change to desk job

4/07

Neck pain

Dr. Electricity (neurologist)

• EMG upper extremities = positive for cervical radiculopathy

• Physical therapy

• Referral to pain management

4/08

Neck pain

Dr. Needles

• Pain injections = helps some

• Plan to follow up again in two weeks

5/09

Overall pain, achy, and extremely fatigued

Dr. Muscle

• MRI head = negative for MS

• Lab work = results pending

• Diagnosis = FM, CMP, and CFID

• Referral back to pain management

• Follow up in one month

Keep copies of all your medical records, including any tests that rule in or out certain disorders. You might be surprised at how little your doctor documents. If this is the case, it is even more important to get your information into your medical record.

The Narrative Report

The Social Security Administration (SSA) will ask your doctor to provide a narrative report of your treatment, tests, and prognosis. They may ask your physician to complete a Residual Functional Capacity Assessment. This questionnaire asks for such information as how much weight you can lift and your ability to stand, bend, sit, climb stairs, grip objects, use assistive devices, and so on. Of course, as previously noted, in order to make statements regarding such issues, your doctor must have made that assessment and documented it. Devin Starlanyl has created a wonderful questionnaire that specifically assesses functional capacity for FM and CMP in her book *The Fibromyalgia Advocate*. (See the Useful Tools section at the end of this chapter to view two SSA Residual Functional Capacity grids.)

Researchers F. Wolfe and J. Potter believe that "if the claimant's physician feels their patient is disabled, he or she writes a strong report in support of the disability. However, if the patient's physician is not certain or does not believe the patient is disabled, the report usually is descriptive, rather than supportive."[21]

Having a physician who is your advocate and willing to assist is not always enough. Following is an excerpt from a mutual agreement between one of my FMily members and me, regarding our physicians and their documentation.

FMily Member

This is a great point about disability application. I found out when I was going through my records, getting ready to file for benefits, my doctor hadn't really documented the severity of my symptoms.

He is an awesome physician, very understanding and supportive of his patients. Nonetheless, maybe because he is so familiar with my symptoms, his notes about my office visits were not very specific. I learned that when I see him I need to make it clear that the severity and debilitating nature of my CFID symptoms should be very clearly documented in his notes.

My Reply

Yes, I totally understand what you are saying. Social Security would not accept my neurologist's records as conclusive because his notes were too vague. I questioned his office manager about this and she told me that often when he has seen a patient for an extended period, and no change is expected because of the patient's condition, he notes little, other than "unchanged."

How Social Security Works

Listing of Impairments

Listing of impairments is a tool that the Social Security Administration uses to see if you meet the criteria for certain medical conditions that would make you disabled.

> The listing of impairments describes, for each major body system, impairments that are considered severe enough to prevent a person from gainful activity. Most are permanent or expected to result in death. For all others, the evidence must show that the impairment has lasted, or is expected to last, for at least twelve months. The presence of an impairment that meets the criteria in the listing of impairments (or that is of equal severity) is usually sufficient to establish disability. Exclusion from the listing of impairments does not mean the individual is not disabled, only that the adjudicator must move to the next step and apply other rules in order to resolve the issue of disability.[22]

The Social Security Administration (SSA) will be looking for medical evidence regarding the nature of your pain, its character, location, onset, duration, frequency, and intensity. Major dysfunction and observable impairments, such as diminished range of motion, atrophy, or other physical inabilities, should be documented and reported. The SSA will also want to know if you (or your physician) have identified precipitating and aggravating factors, such as those discussed previously. Specific treatments and medications and their evaluation will be considered. They will also be looking for documentation of diagnostic criteria regarding your medical diagnosis of FM, CFID, or CMP. Last, but certainly not least, they will be looking for documented functional restrictions and how you go about your daily activities. Your cognitive disabilities may be evaluated by a neurocognitive exam, which presents the type of objective measurements sought by the SSA.

Don't be timid about discussing such issues with your physician. Physicians worth seeing are very busy. When they aren't seeing any significant medical tragedies or miraculous improvements in your condition, they may just acknowledge your complaints as status quo, and therefore, not document them. Offer your assistance as a way of easing the physician's load by documenting using the visual resources provided in this book. Less time will be spent in question-and-answer periods, and you will be less likely to forget something very important to you and your care. If your rapport is as it should be, your physician should welcome the help.

---

functional disability: inability of a person to perform certain activities, such as activities of daily living (housework, laundry, preparing meals, shopping, managing money).

work disability: the inability to perform all or some of an individual's job.

World Health Organization definition of disability: an umbrella term, covering impairments, activity limitations, and participation restrictions. An impairment is a problem in body function or structure; an activity limitation is a difficulty encountered in executing a task or action; a participation restriction is a problem experienced while participating in life situations.[23]

Social Security Benefits

Work Credits

The number of work credits needed for disability benefits depend on your age when you become disabled. Generally you need forty credits, twenty of which were earned in the prior ten years, ending with the year you become disabled. However, younger workers may qualify with fewer credits. The number of work credits you earn will vary according to your income for a particular year, with a maximum of four in one year. The amount of income needed to earn credits changes from year to year.

The rules are as follows:[24]

- Before age twenty-four—You may qualify if you have six credits earned in the three-year period ending when your disability starts.
- Ages twenty-four to thirty-one—You may qualify if you have credit for working half the time between age twenty-one and the time you become disabled. For example, if you become disabled at age twenty-seven, you would need credit for three years of work (twelve credits, assuming you had sufficient income) out of the prior six years (between ages twenty-one and twenty-seven).
- Age thirty-one or older—In general, if you were born after 1929 and become disabled at age thirty-one through forty-two, you'll need twenty-

two credits. The number of needed credits goes up by two for every two years older that you are. As an example, if you are fifty when you become disabled, you'll need twenty-eight credits. If you were born after 1929 and become disabled at age sixty-two or older, you'll need forty work credits. Unless you are blind, you must have earned at least twenty of the credits in the ten years immediately before you became disabled.

Amount

"The amount of your SSDI benefit is calculated by the Social Security Administration based on your average monthly earning (AME)."[25] You can find this information in the Social Security Handbook or at www.ssa.gov/planners/calculators.htm.

Qualifying

As noted in 20 CFR §404.1520, the SSA uses a step-by-step process involving five questions to determine if you are disabled.[26]

1. Are you working? If you are working and your earnings average more than the monthly allowance for that year, you generally cannot be considered disabled.
2. Is your condition "severe"? Your condition must interfere with basic work-related activities for your claim to be considered.
3. Is your condition found in the list of disabling conditions? For each of the major body systems, SSA maintains a list of medical conditions, a "listing of impairments" that are so severe they automatically mean that you are disabled. If your condition is not on the list, the SSA determines if it is of equal severity to a medical condition that is on the list. If it is, you will be considered disabled.
4. Can you do the work you did previously? If your condition is severe but not at the same or equal level of severity as a medical condition on the list, then it must be determined if your condition interferes with your ability to do the work you did previously. If it does not, your claim will be denied.
5. Can you do any other type of work? If you cannot do the work you did in the past, the SSA will want to see if you are able to adjust to other work. They consider your medical conditions, age, education, past work experience, and any transferable skills you may have. If you are deemed able to adjust to other work, your claim will be denied.

Age

According to 20 CFR §404.1563, SSDI applicant ages are categorized as follows:

Younger individual: less than 50 years old
Person closely approaching advanced age: 50–54 years old
Person of advanced age: 55–59 years old
Person close to retirement age: 60–64 years old[27]

Education

According to 20 CFR §404.1564 your educational level will be assessed based on the following criteria:[28]

- Illiterate: No ability to read or write. Someone who cannot read or write a simple message, such as instructions or inventory lists, is considered illiterate, even if the person can sign his or her name. Generally, an illiterate person has had little or no formal schooling.
- Marginal education: Ability in reasoning, arithmetic, and language skills that are needed to perform simple, unskilled jobs. Generally, this is someone who had formal schooling up to sixth-grade level.
- Limited education: Ability in reasoning, arithmetic, and language skills, but not enough to perform most of the more complex job duties required in semiskilled or skilled jobs. Generally, this is someone with a seventh through eleventh grade level of formal education.
- High school education and above: Implies abilities in reasoning, arithmetic, and language skills acquired in formal schooling through at least twelfth grade. Generally, someone with these educational abilities can do semiskilled through skilled work.
- Inability to communicate in English: Since the dominant language of the country is English, it may be difficult for someone who doesn't read, speak, or understand English to work, regardless of the amount of education the person has in another language. Therefore, the ability to communicate in English is considered when evaluating what work the person can do.
- Information about your education: You will be asked how long you attended school and whether you are able to speak, understand, read, and write in English, and do at least simple calculations in arithmetic. Other information will be considered regarding formal or informal education you may have had through your previous work, community projects, hobbies, and any other activities that might help you work.

Residual Functional Capacity

The residual functional capacity assessment—20 CFR §404.1545—accounts for your impairment(s) and any related symptoms, such as pain, that may cause physical and mental limitations and affect what you can do in a work setting.[29] Your residual functional capacity is a composite of the abilities that remain after considering your specific disabilities. For instance, you may have pain that prevents performance of physical tasks, but are still able to reason at your pre-pain state. This is rare, but possible. Residual functional capacity is based on all of the relevant evidence in your case record. Residual functional capacity is what you can still do despite your limitations.

Physical Abilities

When your physical abilities are first assessed, the nature and extent of your physical limitations will be considered. Next the SSA will determine your residual functional capacity for work activity on a regular and continuing basis. A limited ability to perform certain physical demands of work activity, such as sitting, standing, walking, lifting, carrying, pushing, pulling, or other physical functions (including manipulative or postural functions, such as reaching, handling, stooping, or crouching), may reduce your ability to continue past work or do other work.

Mental Abilities

When mental abilities are assessed, the nature and extent of your mental limitations and restrictions are considered first, followed by an evaluation of your residual functional capacity for work activity on a regular and continuing basis. A limited ability to carry out certain mental activities, such as understanding, remembering, and carrying out instructions; and responding appropriately to supervisors, coworkers, and work pressures in a work setting may reduce your ability to work.

Other Abilities Affected by Impairment(s)

Some medically determinable impairment(s), such as skin impairment(s); epilepsy; impairment(s) of vision, hearing, or other senses; and impairments that impose environmental restrictions, may cause limitations and restrictions that affect other work-related abilities. If you have this type of impairment(s), consideration is given to resulting limitations and restrictions that may reduce your ability to do previous work and other work in determining your residual functional capacity.

Total Limiting Effects

When you have a severe impairment(s), but your symptoms, signs, and laboratory findings do not meet or equal those in the "listing of impairments," consideration is given to the limiting effects of all impairment(s), even those that are not severe, in determining residual functional capacity. Pain or other symptoms may cause a limitation of function beyond that which can be determined by anatomical, physiological, or psychological abnormalities alone. As an example, someone with a low back disorder may be fully capable of the physical demands consistent with those of sustained medium work activity, but another person with the same disorder, because of pain, may not be capable on a sustained basis of more than the physical demands consistent with light work activity. In assessing the total limiting effects of your impairment(s) and any related symptoms, all of the medical and non-medical evidence will be considered.

Work Experience (Vocation) and Residual Functional Capacity

Administrative law for Social Security has what is called "the grids." These grids are categorized as sedentary, light, medium, and heavy. The grids are used to guide the decision about whether a claimant is disabled or not disabled, according to the specific rule (law) for the age, education, and previous work experience of the individual claimant.[30]

People with FM, CFID, or CMP may have a sedentary residual functional capacity. Remember, you must meet all the rules before you get to this step in the evaluation process.

If the SSA determines that your maximum sustained work capability is limited to sedentary work because of a severe medically determinable impairment(s), then the sedentary grid for residual functional capacity is used.

The grid includes the rule, the claimant's age, educational background, and previous work experience. (See the sedentary grids and light work grids in the Useful Tools section at the end of this chapter.)

To a great extent our culture defines people by occupation, so when you are no longer able to work, it can be financially and emotionally devastating. It is important to remember that you are not your job. Take this time to learn who you are. Redefine what you have to contribute to society, and above all, don't give up your self-esteem or integrity.

Rule 20 CFR §404.1572: Substantial Gainful Activity, defines gainful employment according to the following categories:[31]

(a) Substantial gainful employment is work activity that is both substantial and gainful.

(b) Substantial work activity is activity that involves implementing significant physical or mental tasks. Your work may be substantial even if it is done on a part-time basis or if you do less, are paid less, or have less responsibility than when you worked in the past.

(c) Gainful work activity is any work activity done for pay or profit. Work activity is considered gainful if it is the kind of work usually done for pay or profit, whether or not it is remunerative.

(d) Other activities. Generally, we do not consider activities like taking care of yourself, household tasks, hobbies, therapy, school attendance, club activities, or social programs to be substantial gainful activity.

Initial Application

Remember the five tips below when navigating the application process:

1. Be honest, but don't elaborate.

2. Don't minimize your symptoms just because you're having a better day than usual. If you have followed the advice in this book, you shouldn't even be thinking about completing the application unless it is a "better day." However, to give a more accurate picture of your condition, you need to consider both good and bad days. Visualize what your day would be like, for instance, if you were trying to juggle work and family responsibilities while experiencing untreated symptoms of FM, CFID, or CMP.

3. Describe your symptoms as you learned in chapter 2: frequency, severity, and duration. Use those handouts!

4. Don't try to be perfect. (This was a difficult task for me. I strive for perfection. It took days and days to fill out those forms, just as it has taken many years to complete this book.)

5. Don't downplay the effects FM, CFID, and CMP have had on all the aspects of your being. Give a comprehensive description of how chronic pain and fatigue have affected you physically, mentally, emotionally, and spiritually.

6. The rate of rejection varies from state to state, but the average seems to be somewhere in the range of two out of every three applicants. Social Security Administration statistics for the year 2007 show 34.1 percent of claims were awarded.[32]

Getting Turned Down—What Next?

Your denial letter will most likely suggest you do some specific type of simple, sedentary work. The SSA gets their suggestions from the Dictionary of Occupational Titles and their suggestion may have little or no relevance to your claim. In my case, their own doctor told them I shouldn't do any type of work that required repetitive hand motion. When they then suggested I get a part-time job as a doll-maker, I was quite sure they hadn't really looked at my case with genuine concern. (By the way, I use a voice-activated program to prepare most of my writing, which takes a great deal of time, compared to direct transcription. It's not conducive to steady employment, but the finished product, regardless of the overwhelming amount of time it takes to prepare, is rewarding in other ways.)

If you disagree with the decision, you can request a review, called an "appeal." There are certain guidelines for filing the appeal, so be sure to verify information with the Social Security Administration.

You do not have to hire an attorney for the appeals action; however, I would strongly suggest it. It can be overwhelming trying to deal with the application process, let alone dealing with an appeal, keeping up with necessary medical record requests and dates for filing, all the while coping with the many associated symptoms of FM, CFID, and CMP.

The Appeals Process

There are four levels of the appeals process:

1. Reconsideration. This is a complete review of the claim by someone other than the individual who made the original decision. All evidence, plus any additional evidence since the initial application, should be submitted. This might include not only medical evidence, but nonmedical sources, such as friends, coworkers, and neighbors who are willing to attest to your normal home, recreational, or work abilities. It will be reevaluated and a new decision will be rendered. Most reconsiderations involve a review of your files without your needing to be present. But when you appeal a decision that you are no longer eligible for disability benefits because your medical condition has improved, you can meet with a Social Security representative and explain why you believe you still have a disability.[33]

It is during this period that the SSA may request that the claimant be examined by one of their doctors. Of course, this doctor is hired by the SSA. Enough said.

If you disagree with the reconsidered decision, they can choose to go to the next level of the appeals process—a hearing.

2. Hearing. A hearing is conducted by an administrative law judge (ALJ) who had no part in either the original decision or the reconsideration of your case. The ALJ will notify you of the hearing.

Before the hearing you may be asked to give the SSA more evidence and to clarify information about your claim. You may look at the information in your file and give new information.

At the hearing the ALJ will question you and any witnesses you bring. Other witnesses, such as medical or vocational experts, may also give the SSA information at the hearing. You or your representative may question the witnesses.

The ALJ will evaluate all the evidence on record, plus any additional evidence brought to the hearing, and will render a decision. A Notice of Decision will be issued to the individual and his or her representative.[34]

At this step of the process it is highly recommended that you have legal counsel familiar with the laws that affect the ALJ's decision.

The ALJ may request expert testimony from medical and vocational experts. These "experts" may or may not have firsthand knowledge of FM, CFID, or CMP. In my experience, finding a doctor who is aware of these conditions was difficult, so you can well imagine the knowledge base of the ALJ's "expert witness." The laws protect the claimant to some extent in that the ALJ must give more weight to the opinion of the claimant's treating doctor than to the opinion resulting from a one-time medical exam requested by SSA or their team. However, the judge's expert witnesses have more impact on the ALJ's decision when the claimant's physician has not adequately addressed and documented key issues in the claimant's medical record. This is why it is so important to make sure your medical records reflect the continuing disabling effect of chronic pain.

During your testimony it may be best to take a multisystem, head-to-toe approach. Leave out absolutely nothing! Most important of all, tell only the truth. An attorney experienced in Social Security disability issues can prepare you for what to expect at the ALJ hearing.

An attorney who specializes in Social Security law will represent your best interest. Federal law sets the maximum attorney fee, and nearly all disability attorneys work on a contingency fee schedule, meaning if you don't win, they don't get paid. The maximum fee allowable by law may change over time. According to others who have been through this process, it is anecdotally noted that it has taken up to three years for a final decision in some parts of the country. Your attorney is obligated to the fee that was allowable at the time you contracted with him or her. So you can see that it is not in your attorney's best interest to delay the process.

Your security and safety feels threatened when the process drags on and on, seemingly forever. When dealing with loss of income and in some cases loss of medical insurance, it is easy to want to blame someone. This is the time to use your fury constructively. Write to your congressional representative! Not only will it make you feel useful, eventually it will also help others. Be the voice.

3. Appeals Council. If you disagree with the hearing decision, you may ask for a review by Social Security's Appeals Council. The Appeals Council may decide to issue its own decision, remand the case to the ALJ to issue another decision, or allow the ALJ's decision to stand.

If the Appeals Council denies your request for review, they will send you a letter explaining the denial. If the Appeals Council reviews your case and makes its own decision, they will send you a copy of the decision. If the Appeals Council returns your case to an administrative law judge, they will send you a letter and a copy of the order.[35]

If you disagree with the Appeals Council's action, the final step is the Federal Court Review.

4. Federal Court Review. A claimant who disagrees with the Appeals Council's action has the right to file a civil suit in Federal District Court. This is the last level of the appeals process. If you bring civil action against the commissioner seeking judicial review of the SSA's final decision, their staff will prepare the record of the claim for filing with the court. There is a related fee for filing a civil action in federal court.[36]

It is a capital mistake to theorize before one has data. Insensibly one begins to twist facts to suit theories instead of theories to suit facts.

SHERLOCK HOLMES

The more extreme measures you have to take, the more likely it is that your case will be tied up for years in the system and you probably won't win. It is imperative that you have your information well organized and are physically, mentally, and emotionally prepared for the stressful and time-consuming process.

An individual shall not be considered to be under a disability unless he furnishes such medical or other evidence of existence thereof as the Secretary may require. An individual's symptoms as to pain or other symptoms shall not alone be conclusive evidence of disability as defined in this section. There must be medical signs and findings, established by medically acceptable clinical and laboratory diagnostic techniques, which show the existence of a medical impairment that results from anatomical, physiological, or psychological abnormalities which could reasonably be expected to produce the pain or other symptoms alleged and which, when considered with all evidence required to be furnished under this paragraph (including statements of the individual or his physician as to the intensity or persistence of such pain or other symptoms which may reasonably be accepted as consistent with the medical signs and findings), would lead to a conclusion that the individual is under disability.*

A Favorable Ruling

Once there is a ruling in a claimant's favor, Social Security benefits begin at the sixth month following the date you last worked (but not more than seventeen months before the month you filed the application). The first five months are considered a waiting period.[37] Disability benefits are payable as of one year before application. In other words, if you quit working due to disability but waited one year before filing for benefits, possibly because you were hoping to get back to work (not uncommon), then you would be eligible as of the day you quit working, back to one year previous. You are eligible for Medicare after two years of your disability determination date.[38] Your case may be set for periodic review by SSA based on the expectation of recovery.

Conclusion

Sure enough, our wish is that we did not have chronic, unending pain; the fact of the matter is . . . we do. Make sure your medical records show an accurate picture of your functional capacity. Apply for benefits in a timely manner; don't give up, even if you are turned down at the initial application, the request for reconsideration, the ALJ hearing, or the appeal. Many times it may seem that you have been treated unfairly, but remember, you must make them understand your disability by using measurable criteria. Let everyone you talk to know how FM, CFID, or CMP has affected and continues to affect your life. It is your lawful right to ask for your benefits.

---

*42 USC §423 [S][A]—Result of the 1984 congressional enactment of the Social Security Disability Benefits Reform Act (Pub L No. 98-406, 98 Stat 1794). Following the outline of Bunnell v Sullivan 947 F 2d 341 (9th Cir 1991).

Patient Rights

As a patient with the chronic, intractable pain of FM, CFID, or CMP, you have the right to appropriate treatment and pain management. Legislation is being passed at both federal and state levels to protect you. This section will provide you with some examples of your rights.

Suffering is the tuition one pays for a character degree.

RICHARD M. RAYNER, M.D.

Patient Bill of Rights Regarding Pain

The American Academy of Pain Management has adopted the following modification of the American Hospital Association's Patient Bill of Rights as part of their framework.[39]

1. The patient has the right to considerate and respectful care.
2. The patient has the right to obtain from his or her credentialed practitioner complete and current information concerning the diagnosis, proposed treatment, and expected prognosis in terms that the patient may reasonably be expected to understand. When it is not advisable to give such information to the patient, the information should be made available to an appropriate person (medical proxy) on the patient's behalf.
3. The patient has the right to receive the necessary information for medical decision-making and the granting of informed consent from the treating credentialed practitioner prior to the start of any procedure or treatment. This information shall include at the minimum: the expected procedure or treatment to be used, who will perform the procedure or treatment, what alternatives exist (if any), what are the likely risks from the procedure or treatment, what may occur if no treatment is undertaken, and the probable duration of incapacitation if any is expected.
4. The patient has the right to refuse any and all treatment to the extent permitted by law, and to be informed of this action.
5. The patient has the right to every consideration of privacy concerning the medical care provided, except when there is imminent risk to the individual or others, or when the practitioner is ordered by a court to breach confidentiality.
6. The patient has the right to be advised if the practitioner, agency, or facility proposes to engage in any form of human experimentation affecting

the care or treatment provided. The patient has the right to refuse to participate in research projects or to withdraw continued consent to participate, without repercussions.

7. The patient has the right to examine and receive an explanation of the bill for professional services rendered.

All pain management activities are to be provided with an overriding concern for the patient, and above all, with recognition of the patent's dignity as a human being.

The National Pain Care Policy Act of 2007 and 2008

On July 11, 2007 at the 110th Congress, House of Representatives first session, Bill HR2994 was introduced by Congresswoman Lois Capps (D-CA) and Congressman Mike Rogers (R-MI). This is a bill to amend the Public Health Service Act with respect to pain care.[40]

The intention of the bill is to improve pain management and quality of life by providing adequate treatment. The bill is initiated to bring about public awareness of pain, and is intended to improve professional training in assessing and treating pain. It promotes funding for research, education, training, improvement of access, and outreach in pain management in the United States.

According to section 3 of the bill, the Institute of Medicine Conference on Pain is to evaluate the adequacy of assessment, diagnosis, treatment, and management of acute and chronic pain. Among other things, the conference is to identify barriers to appropriate pain management and increase education for employers, patients, health care providers, regulators, and third-party payors. The bill also relates to physician concerns over regulatory and law enforcement policies applicable to some pain therapies. This will make physicians less fearful about prescribing appropriate pain medications.

Section 4 of Bill HR2994 calls for a consortium at the National Institutes of Health to establish and maintain a national agenda for basic and clinical research.

Bill HR2994 is comprehensive. In addition to research, training, treatment, and funding, the bill also addresses public awareness and outlines a National Education Outreach and Awareness Campaign. The entire bill is phenomenal and shows forward momentum in recognition of the effects of pain on the individual in the workplace, in relationships, and in our country. We should no longer feel we are responsible for our pain; it does exist, and this is what people who have some power are doing about it. They do care.

We should let them know how much we appreciate their kind consideration for the welfare of the pain patient.

Update: HR2994 did pass the House of Representatives in September of 2008. As of this writing, the bill is yet to receive a Senate vote.

---

act: a statute or bill that has been enacted by a body of people with the power of making laws (legislature).

bill: a proposed law presented for approval to the legislature.

State Laws

Your state has legislation governing issues that affect you as a resident. State laws may vary somewhat from state to state, but most likely, the state you live in will have passed some legislation that addresses pain assessment and management.

The following are examples of legislation at the state level in Missouri and California. You will see that although one is considered more liberal than the other in regard to pain control, both states have adopted similar laws regarding your rights. If you would like to see your state's policies, you can access the information on the Internet by typing in your state's name, followed by the word "statutes."

Missouri Revised Statutes—August 28, 2007
Title XXII: Occupations and Progress
Chapter 334: Physicians and Surgeons-Therapists-Athletic Trainers[41]

Section 334.105—Intractable Pain Treatment Act—definitions:

1. Sections 334.105 to 334.107 shall be known and may be cited as the "Intractable Pain Treatment Act."
2. For purposes of sections 334.105 to 334.107, the following terms have been defined as below.
   - *Board,* the state board of registration for the healing arts;
   - *Intractable pain,* a pain state in which the cause of pain cannot be removed or otherwise treated and for which, in the generally accepted course of medical practice, no relief or cure of the cause of the pain is possible or none has been found after reasonable efforts that have been documented in the physician's medical records;

- *Physician,* physicians and surgeons licensed pursuant to this chapter by the board;
- *Therapeutic purpose,* the use of controlled substances in acceptable doses with appropriate indication for the treatment of pain. Any other use is nontherapeutic.

L. 1995 S.B. 125

Section 334.106—Intractable pain treatment physician may prescribe controlled substances for therapeutic purposes; requirements and exceptions.

1. Notwithstanding any other provision of law to the contrary, a physician may prescribe, administer, or dispense controlled substances for a therapeutic purpose to a person diagnosed and treated by a physician for a condition resulting in intractable pain, if such diagnosis and treatment has been documented in the physician's medical records. No physician shall be subject to disciplinary action by the board solely for prescribing, administering, or dispensing controlled substances when prescribed, administered, or dispensed for a therapeutic purpose for a person diagnosed and treated by a physician for a condition resulting in intractable pain, if such diagnosis and treatment has been documented in the physician's medical records.

2. The provisions of subsection 1 of this section shall not apply to those persons being treated by a physician for chemical dependency because of their use of controlled substances not related to the therapeutic purposes of treatment of intractable pain.

3. The provisions of subsection 1 of this section provide no authority to a physician to prescribe, administer, or dispense controlled substances to a person the physician knows or should know to be using controlled substances, which use is not related to the therapeutic purpose.

4. Drug dependency or the possibility of drug dependency in and of itself is not a reason to withhold or prohibit the prescribing, administering, or dispensing of controlled substances for the therapeutic purpose of treatment of a person for intractable pain, nor shall dependency relating solely to such prescribing, administering, or dispensing subject a physician to disciplinary action by the board.

L. 1995 S.B. 125 § 334.106 subsecs. 1 to 4

Section 334.107—Improperly prescribing controlled substances and failure to keep required records are grounds for license denial, suspension, or revocation.

Nothing in section 334.106 and this section shall deny the right of the board to deny, revoke, or suspend the license of any physician, or otherwise discipline any physician who:

1. Prescribes, administers, or dispenses a controlled substance that is nontherapeutic in nature or nontherapeutic in the manner in which it is prescribed, administered, or dispensed, or fails to keep complete and accurate ongoing records of the diagnosis and treatment plan;

2. Fails to keep complete and accurate records of controlled substances received, prescribed, dispensed, and administered, and disposal of drugs listed in the Missouri comprehensive drug control act contained in chapter 195, RSMo, or of controlled substances scheduled in the Federal Comprehensive Drug Abuse Prevention and Control Act of 1970, 21 U.S.C. 801, et seq. A physician shall keep records of controlled substances received, prescribed, dispensed, and administered, and disposal of these drugs shall include the date of receipt of the drugs, the sale or disposal of the drugs by the physician, the name and address of the person receiving the drugs, and the reason for the disposal or the dispensing of the drugs to the person;

3. Writes false or fictitious prescriptions for controlled substances as defined in the Missouri comprehensive drug control act, chapter 195, RSMo, or for controlled substances scheduled in the Federal Comprehensive Drug Abuse Prevention and Control Act of 1970, 21 U.S.C. 801, et seq.; or

4. Prescribes or administers, or dispenses in a manner which is inconsistent with provisions of the Missouri drug control act contained in chapter 195, RSMo, or the Federal Comprehensive Drug Abuse Prevention and Control Act of 1970, 21 U.S.C. 801, et seq.

L. 1995 S.B. 125 § 334.106 subsec. 5

California Pain Patient's Bill of Rights[42]
Health and Safety Code—Effective October 10, 1997

Existing law, the Intractable Pain Treatment Act, authorizes a physician and surgeon to prescribe or administer controlled substances to a person in the course of treating that person for a diagnosed condition called intractable pain, and prohibits the Medical Board of California from disciplining a physician and surgeon for this action. This bill would establish the Pain Patient's Bill of Rights and would state legislative findings and declarations regarding the value of opiate drugs to persons suffering from severe chronic intractable pain. It would, among other things, authorize a physician to refuse to prescribe opiate medication for a patient who requests the treatment for severe chronic intractable pain, require the physician to inform the patient that there are physicians who specialize in the treatment of severe chronic intractable pain with methods that include the use of opiates, and authorize a physician who prescribes opiates to prescribe a dosage deemed medically necessary.

TEXT: The People of the state of California do enact as follows:
SECTION 1. Part 4.5 (commencing with Section 124960) is added to Division 106 of the Health and Safety Code, to read: Part 4.5

PAIN PATIENT'S BILL OF RIGHTS

Section 124960. The legislature finds and declares all of the following:

(a) The state has a right and duty to control the illegal use of opiate drugs.

(b) Inadequate treatment of acute and chronic pain originating from cancer or non-cancerous conditions is a significant health problem.

(c) For some patients, pain management is the single most important treatment a physician can provide.

(d) A patient suffering from severe chronic intractable pain should have access to proper treatment of his or her pain.

(e) Due to the complexity of their problems, many patients suffering from severe chronic intractable pain may require referral to a physician with expertise in the treatment of severe chronic intractable pain. In some cases, severe chronic intractable pain is best treated by a team of clinicians in order to address the associated physical, psychological, social, and vocational issues.

(f) In the hands of knowledgeable, ethical, and experienced pain management practitioners, opiates administered for severe acute and severe chronic intractable pain can be safe.

(g) Opiates can be an accepted treatment for patients in severe chronic intractable pain who have not obtained relief from any other means of treatment.

(h) A patient suffering from severe chronic intractable pain has the option to request or reject the use of any or all modalities to relieve his or her severe chronic intractable pain.

(i) A physician treating a patient who suffers from severe chronic intractable pain may prescribe a dosage deemed medically necessary to relieve severe chronic intractable pain as long as the prescribing is in conformance with the provisions of the California Intractable Pain Treatment Act, Section 2241.5 of the Business and Professions Code.

(j) A patient who suffers from severe chronic intractable pain has the option to choose opiate medication for the treatment of severe chronic intractable pain as long as the prescribing is in conformance with the provisions of the

California Intractable Pain Treatment Act, Section 2241.5 of the Business and Professions Code.

(k) The patient's physician may refuse to prescribe opiate medication for a patient who requests the treatment for severe chronic intractable pain. However, that physician shall inform the patient that there are physicians who specialize in the treatment of severe chronic intractable pain with methods that include the use of opiates.

Section 124961. Nothing in this section shall be construed to alter any of the provisions set forth in the California Intractable Pain Treatment Act, Section 2241.5 of the Business and Professions Code. This section shall be known as the Pain Patient's Bill of Rights.

(a) A patient suffering from severe chronic intractable pain has the option to request or reject the use of any or all modalities in order to relieve his or her severe chronic intractable pain.

(b) A patient who suffers from severe chronic intractable pain has the option to choose opiate medications to relieve severe chronic intractable pain without first having to submit to an invasive medical procedure, which is defined as surgery, destruction of a nerve or other body tissue by manipulation, or the implantation of a drug delivery system or device, as long as the prescribing physician acts in conformance with the provisions of the California Intractable Pain Treatment Act, Section 2241.5 of the Business and Professions Code.

(c) The patient's physician may refuse to prescribe opiate medication for the patient who requests treatment for severe chronic intractable pain. However, that physician shall inform the patient that there are physicians who specialize in the treatment of severe chronic intractable pain with methods that include the use of opiates.

(d) A physician who uses opiate therapy to relieve severe chronic intractable pain may prescribe a dosage deemed medically necessary to relieve severe chronic intractable pain, as long as that prescribing is in conformance with the California Intractable Pain Treatment Act, Section 2241.5 of the Business and Professions Code.

(e) A patient may voluntarily request that his or her physician provide an identifying notice of the prescription for purposes of emergency treatment or law enforcement identification.

(f) Nothing in this section shall do either of the following:
    1) Limit any reporting or disciplinary provisions applicable to licensed physicians and surgeons who violate prescribing practices or other provisions

set forth in the Medical Practices Act, Chapter 5, (commencing with Section 2000) of Division 2 of the Business and Professions Code, or the regulations adopted there-under.

2) Limit the applicability of any federal statute or federal regulation or any of the other statutes or regulations of this state that regulate dangerous drugs or controlled substances.

Most states have Chronic Intractable Pain Treatment Acts that give guidelines and requirements on treating chronic pain. You may be able to find information about your rights in your state's judicial database. If you feel you have been treated unfairly or inappropriately, you most likely will be able to access this information at your community library or on the Internet.

In response to the development of model guidelines, federal and state statutes, and acts for treatment of intractable pain, the medical community and the legislative branch of government are moving forward. People are speaking out. However, much work still needs to be done to help physicians overcome their fear of treating patients with controlled substances, and to help them understand the laws that protect them and their patients. Many dedicated people are working to help physicians and other health care providers overcome preconceived notions about the treatment of pain. My hopes are that the available guidelines will help physicians utilize acceptable pain management standards and help regulatory agencies, such as the DEA, define appropriate treatment.

It is your most basic human right to have your pain minimized as much as possible. Speak out; learn what your rights are. Share them with your doctor and health care team, and share your opinions with those who can make a difference.

—————————— *Personal Letter* ——————————

Dear Congressmen,

I am contacting you regarding the matter of Canadian prescription drugs for U.S. citizens.

I am a registered nurse who was forced into early retirement because of fibromyalgia and chronic myofascial pain, most likely resulting from hard physical labor over twenty years of caring for others.

Most of the medications required to provide me with some quality of life are new and very expensive.

Our pharmaceutical companies and distributors rape the American public with exorbitant drug costs. Their earnings are quite significant at our expense. For these corporate tycoons to lobby against us, when all we are doing is trying to find affordable health care, is an absolute atrocity. And for our government to allow this is even worse.

The quality of medical care has suffered greatly in the past decade or two. Patients have had to take an active role in their care because of big business, insurance companies, and managed care. We have been forced into becoming advocates for our own care or, it is sad to say, die for the lack of it. This has not always been the case.

We citizens of the "free world" have been told we must go here or go there for our medical care, we can be seen for this but not for that. All for one reason— what insurance policies, including Medicare, dictate. And now our government is attempting to tie our hands even more tightly, putting us between the proverbial rock and hard place by trying to force us to pay higher dollars because a certain drug is manufactured or distributed in the United States. If a physician wants us to take a certain medication, why would these United States be able to say where we purchase that drug, just so we can pad someone else's pocket?

I am well aware that medications and research are necessary and am very grateful for both; however, it is not the scientists making these discoveries who are making all the money.

Please share my concerns with your colleagues and friends.

Sincerely,
Celeste Cooper

Miscellaneous Programs and Help

Workers' Compensation

Workers' Compensation is a form of insurance your employer must provide in the event your disability stems from your work environment. This type of compensation requires that the disability or injury must have occurred during the course of employment. Laws regulating work-comp insurance vary, but they exist in all state and federal governments. The concept behind workers' compensation is to provide the affected employee, regardless of fault, with enough support to avoid requiring public assistance because of an injury or illness that occurred while on the job. Seldom is the compensation the same as the employee's wages.

Generally, this is what happens in a workers' compensation case: A claim is made by the employee with the employer, who is then required to file the claim with the workers' compensation insurance provider within the employee's resident state. The claims representative then decides if the claim is compensable according to the workers' compensation statute of that particular state. If it is found to be compensable, then the provider sets aside a reserve for estimated costs. At this time, the incurred losses are reported to the state workers' compensation bureau. The claim is monitored and bills incurred under the compensation plan are paid. The bureau then makes calculations regarding the amounts and frequency of loss for that particular employer.[43] Hence, if there are too many claims against the employer, their workers' compensation insurance rates go up.[44] You can see why many employers are not happy when you file a claim, and why they would fight to keep compensation down.

Proving the relationship of an illness to job-related activities is a difficult task at best, even though there is much literature regarding the onset of FM after an injury event, CFID after exposures, and CMP from repetitive motion. You will most likely need to engage the services of an attorney who specializes in this area of the law. Finding one who is familiar with these disorders is imperative for success.

Information regarding the Workers' Compensation Act is available from the Workers' Compensation Commission in your state capital, or the federal government agency, should you fall into the category of federally insured workers' compensation.

COBRA

The Consolidated Omnibus Budget Reconciliation Act of 1985 (COBRA) covers many aspects of health care. The discussion here will be limited to the continuation of health benefits after you leave employment as a result of a "qualifying event." A qualifying event can be voluntary or involuntary termination of employment as long as the termination is not related to gross misconduct; or because of a job transition, reduced work hours, entitlement to Medicare, death, or divorce.

COBRA protects you from an interruption in health insurance coverage for you and your dependents. If you are a "qualified individual" you may, however, be responsible for the entire amount, up to 102 percent, of the cost of your health plan.[45]

Generally, if your employer had fewer than twenty employees on more than 50 percent of its business days for the previous year, your employer would not be subject to COBRA. To be a qualified individual[46] you must be a person or beneficiary covered by a group health plan on the day before the qualifying event.

If you qualify for COBRA insurance you should be notified within fourteen days after the plan administrator receives notice of your eligibility. Your employer has thirty days to notify the plan administrator. You or your beneficiaries must make the election within sixty days from the date of loss of health coverage, and you will be responsible for all premiums back to the date of eligibility, regardless of when you make the election within that sixty-day period. You can continue coverage for twelve to eighteen months, depending on the state in which you live and the state of your employer of record. You should contact the plan administrator regarding specific questions. Under COBRA, however, if the Social Security Administration determines you are disabled while the plan is in effect, you may elect to continue the plan for eighteen months, eleven months for dependents. You will need to send the plan administrator an explanation and a copy of the Social Security determination. In this event, the plan may charge you up to 150 percent of the premium cost for the extended period.[47] You will pay dearly for that additional coverage.

If you exhaust your COBRA or other continuation coverage, you may purchase individual coverage. In this instance, under the Health Insurance Portability and Accountability Act (HIPAA) you cannot be turned down on the basis of preexisting conditions.[48] You may find this option financially impossible, however.

Private Disability Insurance

Private disability insurance may be provided or partially provided by your employer, or you can pay for your own individual policy. Policy coverage varies according to the amount of benefit premium, much like a life insurance policy. As a rule, benefits are paid if you are disabled and your disability prevents you from performing your related occupational duties. Each policy will define disability coverage and limits, and can vary based on the type of coverage included.[49] Reports from people in my online support group suggest disability insurance isn't as straightforward as it sounds. People with invisible disabilities, once again, have the arduous task of defending and proving their disabilities. Most insurance companies are reluctant to pay out benefits, but have no hesitation about collecting the premium.

Employee Assistance Programs (EAPs)

Employee Assistance Programs are employer-sponsored programs designed to assist employees with personal needs. They have gained popularity because they seem to work. Employers have found that by providing an EAP, they can actually keep health benefit costs down. If your employer provides an EAP and you are having a difficult time dealing with the side effects of chronic pain, you may want to take advantage of it. It is confidential and you cannot be discriminated against for using it.

ERISA

ERISA stands for Employee Retirement and Income Security Act. According to the U.S. Department of Labor, "ERISA is a federal law that sets minimum standards for most voluntarily established pension and health plans in private industry to provide protection for individuals in these plans."[50]

ERISA was enacted in 1974 and has since been amended because of federal judicial decisions. Two of these amendments are COBRA and HIPAA. Today, ERISA also applies to private employee benefits and employer-sponsored health and disability plans. What does this mean to you? If your health plan is governed by ERISA because it is an employer-sponsored health plan, you will find that the courts remain divided. This is because of the conflicts between ERISA and ADA. If you are treated unfairly or are unable to get necessary treatments because your insurance denies access, or if they refuse to pay a claim, you may have little recourse.[51]

Employers are required to provide you with the same health benefits they offer all their employees. Any employing organization that discriminates against you in this regard is in violation of Title I of the ADA. However, because of health care cost escalation, some employers have opted for self-funded health benefits. These are usually administered by a company experienced in the health insurance industry, but many fall under the jurisdiction of ERISA, as well as of the ADA.

According to the U.S. Department of Labor, ERISA does not cover government group health plans, churches, workers' compensation, unemployment, or disability laws. Therefore, you can see the catch-22 regarding disability.

ERISA does protect you for a full and fair review. However, the review is made by the plan administrator, who is, in the case of employer self-insured plans, the employer. As a result, gaps or overlaps in the act, which was written to protect you, really create a conflict of interest.

If you have been discriminated against by a health insurance provider who falls under the jurisdiction of ERISA, seek legal counsel. Here again, you are best served by employing the assistance of a lawyer who specializes in the ERISA.

FMLA

According to the U.S. Department of Labor, the Family and Medical Leave Act (FMLA) was enacted in 1993 and is enforced by the U. S. Department of Labor's Employment Standards Administration, Wage, and Hours Division. FMLA protects employees who need to take a leave of absence from work for personal or family member–related medical reasons.[52]

FMLA applies to all public agencies, all public and private elementary and secondary schools, and companies with fifty or more employees. These employers must provide an eligible employee with up to twelve weeks of unpaid leave each year for any of the following reasons:

• For the birth and care of the newborn child of an employee.
• For placement with the employee of a child for adoption or foster care.
• To care for an immediate family member (spouse, child, or parent) with a serious health condition.
• To take medical leave when the employee is unable to work because of a serious health condition.

Eligibility

Employees are eligible for leave if they have worked for their employer for at least twelve months, at least 1,250 hours over the past twelve months, and work at a location where the company employs fifty or more employees within seventy-five miles. Whether an employee has worked the minimum 1,250 hours of service is determined according to FMLA principles for determining compensable hours of work. Time taken off work due to pregnancy complications can be counted against the twelve weeks of family and medical leave.[53]

How FMLA Works

The law entitles "eligible employees" to take up to twelve weeks (480 hours) leave either consecutively, in blocks of time, intermittently,[54] or by reducing their normal weekly or daily work schedule when medically necessary.

So how are the twelve weeks in a twelve-month period treated? Although the law provides for unpaid, job-protected leave, the company can require employees to use any paid time off (vacation, and so on) at the time of FMLA leave before taking it as unpaid. This is where your "ownership" in FMLA comes in. Additionally, it can be used by itself or your employer can apply FMLA toward other qualifying leaves of absence. Such absences could be a result of a job-related injury or illness, workers' compensation, or short-term disability. As an example, if you are on workers' compensation leave and you are FMLA eligible, your employer may deduct time from your FMLA time bucket for your absence due to a workers' compensation issue.

How is the FMLA twelve weeks in twelve months determined? The employer determines whether the twelve-month period is for a calendar year or on a rolling twelve-month cycle.[55] Your perception of FMLA protection as a FM, CFID, or CMP patient is important. You do not want to learn about FMLA the hard way, especially when you are trying to juggle family, work, relationships, and your symptoms.

Intermittent absences are granted to eligible employees in certain circumstances. The twelve weeks (480 hours) can be taken in as small of increments as the company's payroll practice allows. As an example, if your employer calculates your time on the job in fifteen-minute increments, then FMLA can be taken in as little as fifteen-minute increments, based on how your physician documents your needs.

As with every aspect of dealing with the system, documentation is *critical* with FMLA. Intermittent time off would likely be the type of FMLA requested by people with FM, CFID, and CMP. Many of the treatments we need must be done consistently, and the unpredictability of a flare can only complicate our ability to cope.

A serious health condition is one that is expected to last more than three consecutive days; requires treatment two or more times by, or under the supervision of, a health care provider; or requires one treatment by a health care provider with a continuing regimen of treatment. Also included are pregnancy or prenatal health care, serious chronic health conditions, permanent or long-term conditions for which treatment may not be effective; and any absences that require multiple treatments.[56] The effects of your FM, CFID, or CMP must be determined on an individual basis. Remember, no two of us are alike. If your symptoms are serious, respond to treatment (for example, rest, sleep, massage, trigger point injections), and are well documented, you may very well be considered eligible for FMLA, *if* your employer's commerce practices comply with FMLA.

It is important for you to use the documentation tools set forth in this book. The documentation help sheets will help your doctor provide the information your employer needs to grant you FMLA. Your physician should document the needs/benefits of your absences. Examples of absences that could be essential to your health might be fifteen to sixty-minute absences from the work area several times a day, an extra fifteen-minute break once a day, or a break of as long as several full days. Regardless of duration your physician should document the medical necessity for these absences. Your employer needs to understand the worst case scenario, so document your health care requirements at their most intense. Of course, you do not want to be off work without pay, but make sure the documentation reflects exactly what you need. I know we have discussed being positive, but in this situation you also need to be realistic. Due to the unpredictably of our symptoms, this should not be difficult to do.

Your employer is required to maintain your current health care coverage; however, you will need to continue your contribution, if applicable, toward premiums. In the event you do not return to work after a FMLA absence, your employer may be able to recoup from you premiums paid in your behalf.[57]

When you return from FMLA leave, your employer must put you back in your previous position or its equivalent with no impact on any of your previously accrued benefits unless you are considered a "key" employee. You are considered a key employee if you work among the highest paid 10 percent of the company's employees living within seventy-five miles of the work site.

If you are considered a key employee and your absence causes "substantial and grievous economic injury to its operations," your employer is not obligated to keep your job open for you. Management does, however, have to let you know you are considered a key employee and that they cannot guarantee your position upon return. They also should offer you the opportunity to return to work at the time they determine your position is essential, and let you know the consequences if you must continue your medical leave.[58]

Your employer may request recertification as often as every thirty days, and some physician's charge each time these forms need to be completed. Once again, it is vitally important to have good rapport with your doctor. Keep those lines of communication open and engage your health care provider as your advocate.

There are specific rules for FMLA benefit application. If you want to maintain your position at work, you should discuss these with your employer. For more information you can contact the Wage and Hour Division listed in most telephone directories in the U.S. Government section under Department of Labor, or visit the website found in the resource section of this book.

FMLA is a very confusing and complicated law. Certain employer commerce practices are required in order for you to be considered an eligible individual. The leave is based on your employer pay practices. As an eligible employee you may be able to request FMLA intermittently, in as little as one-minute increments (depending upon your employer's payroll practices) or for extended periods, totaling up to twelve weeks (480 hours) in a predetermined twelve-month period. The twelve weeks are unpaid, job-protected leave.[59] All this is dependent upon the documentation by your treating physician, who should consider the nature of your illness and medical necessity for utilization of FMLA time. Remember, request more time than you hope you will need.

The way people in democracies think of the government as something different from themselves is a real handicap. And, of course, sometimes the government confirms their opinion.

LEWIS MUMFORD, IN ANNE CHISHOLM, *PHILOSOPHERS OF THE EARTH: CONVERSATIONS WITH ECOLOGISTS*

Vocational Rehabilitation

As a result of illness you may find that you need to change your career focus, either voluntarily or as a result of not being able to keep up with the demands of your current job obligations. The vocational changes you make will depend upon the level of your disability and your treatment needs, experience, education, interests, financial requirements, and age. Only you can determine your energy level and reasons for wanting to work. The important thing to remember is that you should take all of your medical needs under advisement before entering any vocational rehab program.

In some cases, vocational rehabilitation may be offered under workers' compensation or by some type of social service organization. Most likely, if you are able to receive services from a trained vocational counselor, that person can assess your qualifications and help you make informed decisions. The vocational rehabilitation program will probably involve working with you and your attorney to allow you to work part-time, take off work, go back to work, or change your vocation.[60] Just remember that the goal of a successful vocational rehabilitation program should be to maximize your work capacity without draining you.

Because of the provisions of the Rehabilitation Act Amendments of 1998, you may be able to obtain some help from the U.S. Department of Education, Office of Special Education and Rehabilitative Services, or Rehabilitation

Services Administration. In the information memorandum of August 21, 1998, it is suggested that state vocational rehabilitation agencies should provide assistance for counseling and guidance of each individual. Look for such agencies in the state government section of your phonebook.

Before making any decisions about changing your work focus, you might want to take advantage of the numerous resources available on the web. The Social Security Administration has a comprehensive site, called The Work Site, www.ssa.gov/work. You can also check the resource section of this book.

Temporary Assistance Programs

If you require temporary assistance, you may qualify for TANF, Temporary Assistance for Needy Families. This program is backed by federal and state funds, and most states regulate disbursements at the county level through the United States Department of Health and Human Services office. You should be able to find the phone number in your local phone book, in the government section.

Your state probably offers additional assistance for low-income individuals to help with rent or mortgage payments, utilities, and food stamps. Under special provisions, you may also qualify for state Medicaid benefits.

There is a wonderful online site, www.disabilityinfo.gov/, that provides numerous links regarding general income support. Just to name a few, you will find links to Temporary Assistance for Needy Families, food stamps, veterans benefits and welfare, the Red Book on work incentives and employment support, benefits for children with disabilities, computer/electronic accommodations program, rental assistance, HUD counseling, and America's Job Bank.

You may also find emergency assistance through community agencies, homeless shelters, churches and synagogues, community-based meals programs, community health clinics, and domestic violence centers.

Confidentiality and HIPAA

The latest acronym in the alphabet soup of medicine is an odd beast known as HIPAA, or the Health Insurance Portability and Accountability Act. Originally drafted as the Kennedy-Kassebaum Bill to allow individuals to carry over their insurance benefits from job to job, it was intended to plug the gap between termination of one health insurance plan and the start date of a new one, and minimize denial of payments for preexisting conditions. In committee meetings it grew and morphed into an overhaul of the way medical information is managed in the electronic age. HIPAA is neither bad nor good; it is simply the new standard of medical information management. Most of you reading this have encountered the multipage, densely packed HIPAA compliance forms at your doctor's, dentist's, or therapist's offices since April 14, 2003, the deadline for compliance. If you take the time to read these documents you will often be surprised at the exceptions to the doctor-patient confidentiality you thought you enjoyed. Who, might you ask, can see part or all of your records?

- Your insurance companies can request records to determine medical necessity of treatment. They can know your diagnosis, prognosis, treatment dates, and procedures, along with any medical advice given. They may request, through what are called Utilization Review groups, almost anything in your chart.
- Courts and governmental agencies, including Social Security, can request or subpoena records for their purposes. These records can be used to deny benefits under SSI and SSDI. They may surface in divorce or custody hearings.
- Managed care companies with specific "carve out" coverage, "gatekeeper" organizations, and regulatory groups may have access to your records if they are "contracted entities" with your regular insurance provider or treatment providers.
- Phone answering, secretarial, and billing services may also have some access to your records, or at least your identity as a patient.
- Many people sign some very general waivers of confidentiality when interacting with attorneys, insurance companies, and other agencies. Unless these are later limited or defined, your entire record is subject to analysis by any number of groups that might request and receive information. With increased uses of fax machines and e-mail, it makes sense to question what inadvertent leaks might occur because of common-area placement of devices or documents.

The camel is a horse designed by a committee.

ARAB PROVERB

Some True Horror Stories about Breaches of Confidentiality

One woman called my (Jeff's) office incensed by the denial of insurance coverage based on a report of her "alcoholism." I assured her that this was not my opinion or in my records. We later traced it to a reference in the family doctor's notes about responsible alcohol use. Her insurance carrier had paid out a large sum on another policy held by her deceased husband and was trying to avoid covering her. A letter from her doctor and the state insurance commissioner warning set this straight.

A gentleman signed waivers allowing the legal representatives of the company handling his disability benefits to have access to his medical records. The waivers included the words "process notes." This would have given these individuals, the business disability insurance company, and SSI confessions of capital offenses and other extreme behavior that would certainly taint his well-deserved benefit assessment. Quick thinking by his therapist allowed her to call and request he delimit the release to a report and dates of service.

The ex-boyfriend of a receptionist at a clinic hacked into the clinic computers and posted every medical record on the Internet as an act of revenge.

A drug rehabilitation clinic went out of business and all medical charts were found in cardboard boxes on the sidewalks of New York.

HIPAA is designed to minimize these problems, and as such is a welcome overhaul of the legal patchwork covering permission and privilege. It is, however, a cumbersome and unpopular law that requires every medical practitioner to review and rewrite all policies regarding patient records. It increases the size of all files and requires separate folders and cabinets for certain kinds of information. The medical community jokes that it was sponsored by office supply stores for the benefit of paper companies and file drawer manufacturers.

Several advantages to patients are now in play with HIPAA. Clinicians within a practice can consult with one another without the necessity of releases, if the identity of the patient is guarded. This provides an accessible second or third opinion with no red tape. Patients can request a copy of a log of releases presented and honored by the providers. They may request a review of their chart by a designated third party to add, subtract, or correct information they believe is misleading. They may at any time rescind or limit previously signed releases. This does not mean that the groups requesting these limited or denied records will then fulfill their obligations if they are denied access to this information.

Patients with multiple treatment providers, different institutions, laboratories, and specialists might find themselves stymied by these groups, refusing to release information based on pre-HIPAA releases and charts. If you encounter a reply like, "I can't, I don't have a HIPAA-compliant release," by all means, insist that one (or more) be mailed, faxed, or e-mailed to you. Any computer with a scanner and a phone connection can be used to send and receive faxes. It is an excellent idea to keep your own copies of your health information in folders you can physically transport to your doctors' offices.

Psychotherapists have several other wrinkles in their HIPAA compliance requirements. All are allowed to establish a separate chart for "progress notes," one that is extremely difficult to access. This provision was written to allow dynamic therapists to record impressions, analyses, theories, and thoughts of an intensely personal nature. These records could be easily misinterpreted and misused, as they might include speculation on transference and counter-transference issues. Therapists from other theoretical schools use these folders to hold correspondence from other sources and information that could damage the therapeutic relationship if released. Therapists are also bound to contact authorities and break confidentiality in the event of a report of intent to harm self or others, and are mandated to report child or elder abuse. What this means is that if you state that you fully intend to kill yourself, the police will be notified. If you state that you fully intend to harm another person, the police and that person will be notified. If you state that physical, emotional, or sexual abuse of a child or elder has occurred, the therapist will make a mandated call to the social service agency that investigates such situations. Please note that the therapist is not adjudicating the possible abuse. That is for the agency and civil judges to decide. The therapist (and doctor, nurse, teacher, or police officer, who are all mandated reporters) must make the call to report the possibility of abuse.

HIPAA is a first step toward correcting abuses of the insurance industry that were particularly harmful for individuals with chronic conditions. In times past it was not unusual for an insurance company to refuse coverage of an existing illness for five years after an individual changed policies. This led many to stay with jobs they hated or to fear changing positions in a company if their benefits would change, even for a promotion. I remember well the case of a young nurse with Crohn's Disease who had reached her limits working in a practice. The stress of the job kept her condition inflamed and painful, but the expense of medications and treatment kept her stuck in that position. She was lucky to finally find another position with identical health coverage, and that insurer (a local company) allowed the switch without denying her benefits.

Over the last ten years many companies have started to switch health insurers annually or biannually to avoid rate hikes. These switches often overlook necessary treatment continuity and require using different panels of doctors and specialists. This panel is a list of doctors that patients on a particular plan can go to for their mental health treatment. The reason that a managed care company has a panel of providers is to create an artificial shortage of treatment opportunities. This serves to frustrate the consumer and decrease the total number of visits per year. The companies also engage in an insane game of "Mother May I" with their clinical panels, requiring them to submit reams of paperwork on tight schedules in order to get authorizations, and thus payment. They have been known to move their offices without notice, thereby clocking out authorization requests and delaying payment another two months. They seem to deliberately lose authorization requests, and their mazes of branching phone paths and mailboxes virtually guarantee that no problem can be resolved in the patient's favor without several days of unreturned calls. Ask yourself, if these companies pick only the best clinicians for their panels, why do they not take their word that treatment is needed? Why would any of us subject ourselves to unnecessary doctors' office visits and treatments? Unfortunately, HIPAA does not address these system abuses, but it might spark another round of reform.

Chapter Conclusion

Procedural laws may change from time to time as the government attempts to function more effectively and efficiently. Therefore, some of the steps may be slightly different from when this book went to press. Examples of this are a change in the ceiling of attorney fees, additions or deletions of steps in the Social Security appeals process, or new and/or amended standards or statutes set by Congress.

Although there may be procedural changes, the basics of data collection, fact-finding, and documentation will not change. Be persistent in your endeavors to achieve your goals. People have been discriminated against because of disabilities since time began, but this is a new era. Don't allow others to limit your ability to contribute to society, just because your capabilities may be different from theirs. A chronic pain condition is disabling, but with the help of others, you can make a difference.

Useful Tools
for
Navigating the Health Care System

When navigating the health care system, the more organized you can be, the better. Because it is so difficult to arrive at a definitive diagnosis for the conditions covered in this book, you may find that you need to see several health care professionals before you know for sure which conditions you have. Even when you have received a diagnosis, you will still need to navigate the system to receive care that really mitigates your symptoms and disability benefits for which you may qualify.

You will find that health care providers are often on tight schedules with limited time allotted for discussing your needs. The tools included in this chapter will help you handle medical visits efficiently so that your really important questions can be answered; you can remember which providers you've seen for which treatments, and when; and you will be able to accurately summarize your health history. Please feel free to photocopy these worksheets to provide yourself with a lasting supply. The last two tools offered here will give you insight into the criteria used to determine disability benefits.

- Interaction Worksheet for Important Calls and Meetings
- Treating Health Care Provider Log
- Chronological Health Record
- Table for Determining Disability Status for Those Limited to Sedentary Work (Example of a SSA grid)
- Table for Determining Disability Status for Those Capable of Light Physical Work (Example of a SSA grid)

Interaction Worksheet for Important Calls and Meetings

(Keep this worksheet in your diary, next to your telephone, or on your person when going to important meetings.)

Date _____ Time _____ Contact person_____
                                                    (name)   (title)

Conversation key points: (*Outline what you'd like to discuss; or if the contact person contacted you, outline the key points of his or her requests.*)

1. _____

2. _____

3. _____

Try to limit the number of topics in each conversation in order not to become confused. If necessary, ask for another meeting to cover additional topics. It is important that you understand every aspect of this process.

Immediately following the conversation or meeting, summarize what you got out of the interaction. (*If possible, clarify with your contact person before ending the conference.*)

_____

_____

_____

_____

Did you get what you expected from the interaction? If not, be sure to list additional questions and goals here for the next meeting, and keep this record with you.

_____

_____

_____

Next scheduled meeting/interaction:

Date_____Time_____

Treating Health Care Provider Log

Doctor's name _____

Specialty_____

Dates treated _____

Address_____

_____

_____

Phone _____ Fax _____ e-mail _____

Doctor's name _____

Specialty_____

Dates treated _____

Address_____

_____

_____

Phone _____ Fax _____ e-mail _____

Doctor's name _____

Specialty_____

Dates treated _____

Address_____

_____

_____

Phone _____ Fax _____ e-mail _____

Doctor's name _____

Specialty_____

Dates treated _____

Address_____

_____

_____

Phone _____ Fax _____ e-mail _____

Chronological Health Record

Date _____ Doctor _____

Problem/complaint _____

Tests or therapies   Outcomes/results

_____

_____

_____

_____

Follow-up recommendations_____

Date _____ Doctor _____

Problem/complaint _____

Tests or therapies   Outcomes/results

_____

_____

_____

_____

Follow-up recommendations_____

Date _____ Doctor _____

Problem/complaint _____

Tests or therapies   Outcomes/results

_____

_____

_____

_____

Follow-up recommendations_____

| | Table for Determining Disability Status for Those Limited to Sedentary Work Residual Functional Capacity: Maximum Sustained Work Capability Limited to Sedentary Work as a Result of Severe Medically Determinable Impairment(s) | | | |

The Sedentary Grids

Rule	Age	Education	Previous work experience	Decision
201.01	Advanced age	Limited or less	Unskilled or none	Disabled
201.02	. . . . . . do*	. . . . . . do	Skilled or semiskilled—skills not transferable[1]	do
201.03	. . . . . . do	. . . . . . do	Skilled or semiskilled—skills transferable[1]	Not disabled
201.04	. . . . . . do	High school graduate or more—does not provide for direct entry into skilled work[2]	Unskilled or none	Disabled
201.05	. . . . . . do	High school graduate or more—provides for direct entry into skilled work[2]	. . . . . . do	Not disabled
201.06	. . . . . . do	High school graduate or more—does not provide for direct entry into skilled work[2]	Skilled or semiskilled—skills not transferable[1]	Disabled
201.07	. . . . . . do	. . . . . . do	Skilled or semiskilled—skills transferable[1]	Not disabled
201.08	. . . . . . do	High school graduate or more—provides for direct entry into skilled work[2]	Skilled or semiskilled—skills not transferable[1]	do
201.09	Closely approaching advanced age	Limited or less	Unskilled or none	Disabled
201.10	. . . . . . do	. . . . . . do	Skilled or semiskilled—skills not transferable	do

*do = ditto

Rule	Age	Education	Previous work experience	Decision
201.11	. . . . . . do	. . . . . . do	Skilled or semiskilled—skills transferable	Not disabled
201.12	. . . . . . do	High school graduate or more—does not provide for direct entry into skilled work[3]	Unskilled or none	Disabled
201.13	. . . . . . do	High school graduate or more—provides for direct entry into skilled work[3]	. . . . . . do	Not disabled
201.14	. . . . . . do	High school graduate or more—does not provide for direct entry into skilled work[3]	Skilled or semiskilled—skills not transferable	Disabled
201.15	. . . . . . do	. . . . . . do	Skilled or semiskilled—skills transferable	Not disabled
201.16	. . . . . . do	High school graduate or more—provides for direct entry into skilled work[3]	Skilled or semiskilled—skills not transferable	do
201.17	Younger individual age 45–49	Illiterate or unable to communicate in English	Unskilled or none	Disabled
201.18	. . . . . . do	Limited or less—at least literate and able to communicate in English	. . . . . . do	Not disabled
201.19	. . . . . . do	Limited or less	Skilled or semiskilled—skills not transferable	do
201.20	. . . . . . do	. . . . . . do	Skilled or semiskilled—skills transferable	do
201.21	. . . . . . do	High school graduate or more	Skilled or semiskilled—skills not transferable	do
201.22	. . . . . . do	. . . . . . do	Skilled or semiskilled—skills transferable	do

Rule	Age	Education	Previous work experience	Decision
201.23	Younger individual age 18–44	Illiterate or unable to communicate in English	Unskilled or none	do [4]
201.24	. . . . . . do	Limited or less—at least literate and able to communicate in English	. . . . . . do	do [4]
201.25	. . . . . . do	Limited or less	Skilled or semiskilled—skills not transferable	do [4]
201.26	. . . . . . do	. . . . . . do	Skilled or semiskilled—skills transferable	do [4]
201.27	. . . . . . do	High school graduate or more	Unskilled or none	do [4]
201.28	. . . . . . do	. . . . . . do	Skilled or semiskilled—skills not transferable	do [4]
201.29	. . . . . . do	. . . . . . do	Skilled or semiskilled—skills transferable	do [4]

Example 1

The claimant is a younger individual (age 45–49) who has a residual functional capacity for sedentary work. Her education level is illiterate and her previous work experience is unskilled. According to rule 201.17, she would be considered disabled.

Example 2

The claimant is a younger individual (age 45–49) who has a residual functional capacity for sedentary work. Her education level is limited or less and her previous work experience is unskilled or none. According to rule 201.18, she would be considered not disabled.

Table for Determining Disability Status for
Those Capable of Light Physical Work
Residual Functional Capacity: Maximum Sustained Work Capability
Limited to Light Work as a Result of Severe Medically
Determinable Impairment(s)

The Light Work Grids

Rule	Age	Education	Previous work experience	Decision
202.01	Advanced age	Limited or less	Unskilled or none	Disabled
202.02	. . . . . . do*	. . . . . . do	Skilled or semiskilled—skills not transferable	do
202.03	. . . . . . do	. . . . . . do	Skilled or semiskilled—skills transferable[1]	Not disabled
202.04	. . . . . . do	High school graduate or more—does not provide for direct entry into skilled work[2]	Unskilled or none	Disabled
202.05	. . . . . . do	High school graduate or more—provides for direct entry into skilled work[2]	. . . . . . do	Not disabled
202.06	. . . . . . do	High school graduate or more—does not provide for direct entry into skilled work[2]	Skilled or semiskilled—skills not transferable	Disabled
202.07	. . . . . . do	. . . . . . do	Skilled or semiskilled—skills transferable[2]	Not disabled
202.08	. . . . . . do	High school graduate or more—provides for direct entry into skilled work[2]	Skilled or semiskilled—skills not transferable	do
202.09	Closely approaching advanced age	Illiterate or unable to communicate in English	Unskilled or none	Disabled
202.10	. . . . . . do	Limited or less—at least literate and able to communicate in English	. . . . . . do	Not disabled
202.11	. . . . . . do	Limited or less	Skilled or semiskilled—skills not transferable	do

*do = ditto

Rule	Age	Education	Previous work experience	Decision
202.12	. . . . . do	. . . . . do	Skilled or semiskilled—skills transferable	do
202.13	. . . . . do	High school graduate or more	Unskilled or none	do
202.14	. . . . . do	. . . . . do	Skilled or semiskilled—skills not transferable	do
202.15	. . . . . do	. . . . . do	Skilled or semiskilled—skills transferable	do
202.16	Younger individual	Illiterate or unable to communicate in English	Unskilled or none	do
202.17	. . . . . do	Limited or less—at least literate and able to communicate in English	. . . . . do	do
202.18	. . . . . do	Limited or less	Skilled or semiskilled—skills not transferable	do
202.19	. . . . . do	. . . . . do	Skilled or semiskilled—skills transferable	do
202.20	. . . . . do	High school graduate or more	Unskilled or none	do
202.21	. . . . . do	. . . . . do	Skilled or semiskilled—skills not transferable	do
202.22	. . . . . do	. . . . . do	Skilled or semiskilled—skills transferable	do

Example 1

The claimant is advanced age (55–59) and has a residual functional capacity for light work. Her education level of high school graduate or more provides for direct entry into skilled work (meaning her education is related to a particular skill), and her previous work experience is unskilled. According to rule 202.05, she would be considered not disabled.

Example 2

The claimant is closely approaching advanced age (50–54) and has a residual functional capacity for light work. Her education level is illiterate or unable to communicate in English, and she is unskilled. According to rule 202.09, she would be considered disabled.

Epilogue

There are only two ways to live your life.
One is as though nothing is a miracle. The other is as if everything is.

ALBERT EINSTEIN

Twenty years ago, fibromyalgia was virtually unheard of. Today it is one of the most commonly diagnosed musculoskeletal disorders and a hot area of research and debate.

Current research takes many forms. Scientists are closing in on possible causes for FM and CFID, and thanks to the work of Janet Travell and David Simons, there is growing understanding of myofascial disease. Nevertheless, while clinical studies and scientific research have gained headway, further understanding of these elusive disorders is still needed.

Clinicians and researchers are exploring what treatments are most successful, how patients adapt to pain and fatigue, and how pain and fatigue affect quality of life and overall health. Brain scans are now used to document pain sensitivity selective to patients with fibromyalgia. Decreased gastrointestinal (stomach and bowel) protein functioning can be noted in patients with FM, and scientists are studying the association of coexisting conditions, such as irritable bowel syndrome and temporomandibular dysfunction.

Much progress has already been made. Due to the unceasing efforts of concerned scientists, such as Dr. David Simons and Dr. C. Z. Hong and his colleagues, the trigger points of CMP are now better understood, and we've learned that chronic myofascial pain is a disease, not a syndrome. Research into the effects of nerve growth factors indicates that FM may be a neuro-immune-endocrinological disorder, and studies of first-degree relatives point to a possible genetic factor.

Alternative treatment methods to improve quality of life for patients with pain disorders are being studied. New medications and their potentially beneficial interactions are being investigated, along with implantable electronic devices to help control pain. Biochemists are examining the links between immunological responses and CFID, and measuring cognitive impairment in FM and CFID. These are just a few results from dedicated scientists and caring people.

Research and clinical trials are key to uncovering causes and finding successful treatments. Support for research is extremely important for disorders characterized by pain, sleep abnormalities, fatigue, and loss of function. Unfortunately, not all grants are selected for funding. Applications generally go through strenuous review for scientific merit before being selected. Organizations that promote research depend upon funding from many sources, and advocacy does count.

The continued efforts of various organizations support funding for research. The National Fibromyalgia Association not only conducts clinical trials but also recruits participants. The National CFIDS Foundation and the American Fibromyalgia Syndrome Association provide research grants. The CFIDS Association of America has spent millions of dollars on initiatives to bring an end to the pain, disability, and suffering caused by CFID. The American Association for Chronic Fatigue Syndrome reviews clinical trials and research, and advocates for CFID, FM, and associated disorders. Numerous research grants for FM have been funded by the National Institute of Arthritis and Musculoskeletal and Skin Diseases at the National Institutes of Health (NIH). Grant funding continues for research using the fMRI. Thanks to the dedication of these and many other researchers, clinicians, advocates, and funding organizations, there is heightened awareness in the medical and political communities.

We have come a long way since the American College of Rheumatology released classification criteria for FM, and the Centers for Disease Control developed diagnostic guidelines for CFID.

Despite all this progress, the effects of fibromyalgia, chronic fatigue immunodysfunction, and chronic myofascial pain continue to be unpredictable and may intensify at any given moment. You may still encounter obstacles, such as difficulty finding the right physician for you or the ability to participate in a solid treatment plan, but know you are not alone. For every "doubting Thomas" there is a kind, compassionate person who cares. You may have to make some radical decisions regarding your health care in order to get the treatment you deserve, but unless you live in a remote area of the planet, there are resources to help you meet your needs.

These disorders can affect people of all ages, races, and socioeconomic backgrounds. Learning about your disorder is your first line of defense. From there you can learn to identify your symptoms, evaluate what makes them worse or better, and become aware of the effect your coexisting conditions have on your FM, CFID, or CMP. You can relay this information to your physician in a comprehensive manner, providing a basis that will guide your care.

Life is either a daring adventure or nothing. To keep our faces toward change and behave like free spirits in the presence of fate is strength undefeatable.

HELEN KELLER

It is up to you to take control and learn to put your needs into perspective. Seek support. Contact local hospitals or supportive organizations, such as your local Arthritis Foundation, for referrals, resources, and support groups. Get your stress or depression under control through counseling and journal writing. Talk with friends, develop or maintain spiritual fellowship, and advocate for yourself and others with these disorders, or offer your support to someone else in need.

Learn to manage your time so you have time for yourself and for others. In addition, know that if the demands are too great at any particular moment, you can put your crisis management plan into action. If you work and the burden starts to seriously affect your quality of life, know that even if you have to change your lifestyle, living in a prosperous nation makes it possible to get some financial support.

Use the tools in this book to do a self-assessment and set achievable goals for wellness. Embrace the power of a positive attitude. Do things that provide you with a joyful spirit and a richer life.

Many of life's failures are people who did not realize how close they were to success when they gave up.

THOMAS EDISON

It is important to me, for my own mental health, to give something back. This book is that something.

It could not have come to fruition but for the fortitude given me by the grace of God and the support of people who understand my limitations, yet have continued to encourage me, correct my mistakes, fill in the gaps in my work, edit, revise, and write the rest of the book. Many thanks once again to my husband, family, FMily, friends, colleagues, coauthor, and publisher. I hope this project will perpetuate my ability to make contributions to society. I have learned that when one door closes, another opens. I wish the same for you.

Resources for Maximizing Health Care, Relationships, and Emotional Well-Being

We hope you find this resource section useful and helpful. The information is current as this book goes into production, but there are bound to be updates. You'll find many additional web links to help keep you apprised of changes at my website, www.TheseThree.com. It is our intention to provide you with more resources than you may presently have. We wish you good health and good luck.

To help you find what you're looking for more easily, this resource section has been divided into the following categories in the order presented here:

- General Resources
- Fibromyalgia (FM) Resources
- Chronic Fatigue Immunodysfunction Syndrome (CFIDS) Resources
- Chronic Myofascial Pain (CMP) Resources
- Dealing with Coexisting Conditions
- Medications, Herbs, and Supplements
- Assistive Devices and Therapeutic Supplies
- Bodywork, Acupuncture, Massage, and Therapeutic Touch
- Diet
- Exercise
- The Mindfulness Help Section—Managing Emotions, Reducing Stress, Coping, Enriching Spirituality, and Reaching Goals
- Relationships—Resources for Building, Enriching, and Letting Go
- Life's Delights and Clarifications—Journaling
- Legalities and Red Tape—Resources for Overcoming Road Blocks
- Information for Everybody

GENERAL RESOURCES

There are a number of resources that are useful for any of the three major disorders—FM, CFID, and CMP—as well as for coexisting conditions. These would be a logical place to start your investigation.

American Autoimmune Related Diseases Association
22100 Gratiot Avenue, Eastpointe
E. Detroit, MI 48021-2227
586-776-3900
Toll-free: 800-598-4668
Fax: 586-776-3903
aarda@aarda.org
www.aarda.org

American Chronic Pain Association (ACPA)
P.O. Box 850
Rocklin, CA 95677-0850
916-632-0922
Toll-free: 800-533-3231
Fax: 916-632-3208
ACPA@pacbell.net
www.theacpa.org

American College of Rheumatology (ACR)
1800 Century Place, Ste. 250
Atlanta, GA 30345
404-633-3777
Fax: 404-633-1870
acr@rheumatology.org
www.rheumatology.org
At the website click on the patient education tab. The ACR has helpful information not limited to but including all types of arthritis, bursitis, carpal tunnel syndrome, FM, lupus, lyme disease, metabolic myopathies, myopathies, polymyalgia rheumatica and giant cell arteritis, Sjogren's syndrome, spinal stenosis, and tendonitis. They also have a referral network.

American Pain Foundation
201 North Charles Street, Suite 710
Baltimore, Maryland 21201-4111
1-888-615-7246
www.painfoundation.org

National Chronic Pain Outreach Association (NCPOA)
P.O. Box 274
Millboro, VA 24460
540-862-9437
Fax: 540-862-9485
ncpoa@cfw.com
www.chronicpain.org

National Institute of Arthritis and Musculoskeletal and Skin Diseases (NIAMS)
(A division of the National Institutes of Health)
1 AMS Circle
Bethesda, MD 20892-3675
301-495-4484
Toll-free: 877-226-4267
TTY (hearing disabled): 301-565-2966
Fax: 301-718-6366
NIAMSinfo@mail.nih.gov
www.niams.nih.gov

National Organization for Rare Disorders (NORD)
55 Kenosia Avenue
Danbury, CT 06813-1968
203-744-0100
Toll-free voice mail: 800-999-6673
Fax: 203-798-2291
orphan@rarediseases.org
www.rarediseases.org

National Rehabilitation Information Center (NARIC)
8201 Corporate Drive, Ste. 600
Landover, MD 20785
301-459-5900
Toll-free: 800-346-2742
TTY: 301-459-5984
Fax: 301-459-4263
naricinfo@heitechservices.com
www.naric.com
At their website, be sure to click on their nifty search tab to see the latest in research, projects, and other information regarding just about any topic related to a condition that would benefit from rehabilitation. There are many resourceful links.

FIBROMYALGIA (FM) RESOURCES

See American College of Rheumatology in "General Resources"

American Fibromyalgia Syndrome Association
P.O. Box 32698
Tucson, AZ 85751
520-733-1570
Fax: 520-290-5550
www.afsafund.org/default.htm

Fibromyalgia Alliance of America
P.O. Box 21990
Columbus, OH 43221-0990
614-457-4222
Fax: 614-457-2729
masaathoff@aol.com
www.healthywomen.org/resources/healthservices/
nationalorganizations/dbnationalorgs/
fibromyalgiaallianceofamerica

Fibromyalgia International Coalition
6220 Antioch Road, Ste. 212
Merriam, KS 66202
913-384-4673
Fax: 913-384-8998
www.fibrocoalition.org

Fibromyalgia Network
P.O. Box 31750
Tucson, AZ 85751-1750
Toll-free: 800-853-2929
www.fmnetnews.com
The organization publishes a print newsletter, the *Fibromyalgia Network News,* which you can receive in the mail. Use the contact information provided here to subscribe.

The International Association for CFS/ME (IACFS)
This is a nonprofit organization dedicated to chronic fatigue syndrome and fibromyalgia research and patient care (see complete reference in the section on chronic fatigue immunodysfunction syndrome).

National Fibromyalgia Association (NFA)
2121 S. Towne Centre Place, Ste. 300
Anaheim, CA 92806
714-921-0150
Fax: 714-921-6920
www.fmaware.org

National Fibromyalgia Research Association
P.O. Box 500
Salem, OR 97308
503-315-7257
Fax: 503-315-7205
nfra@firstpac.com
www.nfra.net

See National Rehabilitation Information Center (NARIC) in "General Resources."

FM Books and Periodicals

Alternative Treatments for Fibromyalgia and Chronic Fatigue Syndrome: Insights from Practitioners and Patients by Mari Skelly and Andrea Helm. Alameda, Calif.: Hunter House, 1999. Documented experiences by those who work with FM and CFID patients.

The Arthritis Foundation's Guide to Good Living with Fibromyalgia. Atlanta, Ga.: Arthritis Foundation, Longstreet Press, 2001.

The Arthritis Helpbook: A Tested Self-Management Program for Coping with Arthritis and Fibromyalgia by Kate Lorig, James F. Fried, and Maureen R. Gecht, 5th ed. Reading, Mass.: Addison-Wesley Publications, 1986.

The Fibromyalgia Advocate: Getting the Support You Need to Cope with Fibromyalgia and Myofascial Pain Syndrome by Devin J. Starlanyl. Oakland, Calif.: New Harbinger Publications, Inc., 1999.

Fibromyalgia & Chronic Myofascial Pain: A Survival Manual, 2nd ed., by Devin J. Starlanyl, M.D., and Mary Ellen Copeland, M.S., M.A. Oakland, Calif.: New Harbinger Publications, Inc., 2001. Comprehensive review and resources for fibromyalgia and chronic myofascial pain. Author website: www.sover.net/~devstar.

Fibromyalgia and Female Sexuality by Marline Emmal, Ph.D. Victoria, BC, Canada: Trafford Publishing, 2006. About intimacy, menstruation, pregnancy, and menopause.

The Fibromyalgia Help Book: Practical Guide to Living Better with Fibromyalgia by Jenny A. Fransen, R.N., and I. Jon Russell, M.D., Ph.D. St. Paul, Minn.: Smith House Press, 1996.

The Fibromyalgia Survivor by Mark Pellegrino, M.D. Columbus, Ohio: Anadem Press, 2001. Dr. Pellegrino is a physiatrist and FM researcher who has FM. He has also written several other books.

Fibromyalgia Syndrome: Physical Therapy Management by Kathryn Stogner Henderson. New York: The Psychological Corporation, 1999. Includes psychology, physical therapy, medical/nursing, allied health services, and rheumatology.

Finding Our Way: A Guide for Surviving Chronic Pain by Pat Oreilly. Nido, Calif.: Chronic Pain Clearinghouse, 2001. Finding a plan when you have chronic pain.

Making Sense of Fibromyalgia: A Guide for Patients and Their Families by Daniel J. Wallace, M.D., and Janice Brock Wallace. New York: Oxford University Press, 1999.

The National Forum (Newsletter of the National CFIDS Foundation), 103 Aletha Road, Needham, Mass. 02492. www.ncf-net.org/forum.htm. Focus on CFID/ME, FM, GWI, MCS, and related illnesses.

Parting the Fog: The Personal Side of Fibromyalgia/Chronic Fatigue Syndrome by Sue Jones. Reading, Kans.: LaMont Publishing, 2001. Explains symptoms, need for support, and personal reality of FM and CFID.

Winning with Chronic Pain: A Complete Program for Health & Well-Being by H. H. McIlwain, D. F. Bruce, J. C. Silverfield, M. C. Burnette, and B. F. Germain. Amherst, N.Y.: Prometheus Books, 1994.

CHRONIC FATIGUE IMMUNODYSFUNCTION SYNDROME (CFIDS) RESOURCES

American Academy of Environmental Medicine, Referral Network
6505 East Central Avenue, Ste. 296
Wichita, KS 67206
316-684-5500
administrator@aaemonline.org
www.aaemonline.org

The CFIDS Association of America
P.O. Box 220398
Charlotte, NC 28222-0398
704-365-2343
www.cfids.org
Offers information, publications, and brochures.

Good Day-Bad Day Chronic Fatigue Syndrome Research Study
Behavioral Medicine Research Center
Department of Veterans Affairs
University of Miami
200 BMRC, c/o VA Medical Center
1201 NW 16th Street (6th floor)
Miami, FL 33125
Study director: Lina Garcia
305-243-3291
CFSresearch@miami.edu
www.BMRC.Miami.edu
This is an ongoing research study into Chronic Fatigue Syndrome. For more information or to participate in the study go to: www.pandoranet.info/httpwww.pandoranet.inforesearchchronicfatiguesyndromemyalgicencephalomyeliltiscfids.html

Human Ecology Action League (HEAL)
P.O. Box 509
Stockbridge, GA 30281
770-389-4519
Fax: 770-389-4520
HealNatnl@aol.com
www.healnatl.org/
Provides referral and support group information.

The International Association for CFS/ME (IACFS)
27 N. Wacker Drive, Ste. 416
Chicago, IL 60606
847-258-7248
Fax: 847-579-0975
Admin@iacfs.net
www.iacfsme.org
This is a nonprofit organization of research scientists, physicians, licensed medical health care professionals, and others dedicated to chronic fatigue syndrome and fibromyalgia

research and patient care. Website includes periodic reviews of current clinical, research, and treatment ideas on CFS/FM.

The National CFID Foundation
103 Aletha Road
Needham, MA 02492
781-449-3535
www.ncf-net.org

See National Rehabilitation Information Center (NARIC) in "General Resources."

CFIDS Books and Periodicals

The Doctor's Guide to Chronic Fatigue Syndrome: Understanding, Treating and Living with CFID by David S. Bell. Reading, Mass.: Addison-Wesley, 1994.

Enteroviral and Toxin Mediated Myalgic Encephalomyelitis/ Chronic Fatigue Syndrome and Other Organ Pathologies by John Richardson. Binghamton, New York: The Haworth Medical Press, 2001. Covers case studies and theories about viruses and their effects.

Finding Our Way: A Guide for Surviving Chronic Pain by Pat Oreilly. Nido, Calif.: Chronic Pain Clearinghouse, 2001. Finding a plan when you have chronic pain.

Finding Strength in Weakness: Help and Hope for Families Battling Chronic Fatigue Syndrome by Lynn Vanderzalm. Grand Rapids, Mich.: Zondervan Publishing, 1995.

The National Forum (Newsletter of the National CFIDS Foundation), 103 Aletha Road, Needham, Mass. 02492. www.ncf-net.org/forum.htm. Focus on CFID/ME, FM, GWI, MCS, and related illnesses.

Parting the Fog: The Personal Side of Fibromyalgia/Chronic Fatigue Syndrome by Sue Jones. Reading, Kans.: LaMont Publishing, 2001. Explains symptoms, need for support, and personal reality of FM and CFID.

Running on Empty: The Complete Guide to Chronic Fatigue Syndrome (CFID) by Katrina H. Berne, Ph.D. Alameda, Calif.: Hunter House Publishers, 1995. Information on understanding and living with CFID.

Understanding Chronic Fatigue Syndrome: An Empirical Guide to Assessment and Treatment by Fred Friedberg, Ph.D., and Leonard A. Jason, Ph.D. Washington, D.C.: American Psychological Association, 1998.

CHRONIC MYOFASCIAL PAIN (CMP) RESOURCES

Bonnie Prudden Myotherapy
Toll-Free: 800-221-4634
520-529-3979
Fax: 520-529-6679
www.bonnieprudden.com
Provides referrals, educational material, and helpful devices for treating CMP.

Fibromyalgia and Chronic Myofascial Pain with Devin Starlanyl
www.sover.net/~devstar
Provides information for patients, physicians and practitioners, including helpful resources.

MYO
773-583-4145
info@myopain.com
www.myopain.com
Offers teaching on chronic myofascial pain, including trigger point treatment and tools.

Myomed
Inglewood Civic Centre
895A Beaufort Street
Inglewood, WA 6052
Australia
9471-8911
Fax: 9471-8922
www.myomed.com.au
Provides information on chronic myofascial pain and trigger points.

National Association of Myofascial Trigger Point Therapists
Bournemyo@mac.com
www.namtpt.shuttlepod.org
Offers information, education, symptom checker, and therapist referrals.

See National Rehabilitation Information Center (NARIC) in "General Resources." Search keyword "trigger points" at their website.

CMP Books and Periodicals

Acupressure Taping: The Practice of Acutaping for Chronic Pain and Injury by Hans-Ulrich Hecker, M.D., and Kay Liebchen, M.D., translated by Katja Lueders and Rafael Lorenzo. Rochester, Vt.: Healing Arts Press, 2007. This is a self-care manual that shows readers where and how to apply Kinesio tape to relieve muscle spasms and pain in specific muscle groups.

Art of Body Maintenance: Winner's Guide to Pain Relief by Hal Blatman and Brad Ekvall. Cincinnati, Ohio: Danua Press, 2006.

Fibromyalgia & Chronic Myofascial Pain: A Survival Manual, 2nd ed., by Devin J. Starlanyl, M.D., and Mary Ellen Copeland, M.S., M.A. Oakland, Calif.: New Harbinger Publications, Inc., 2001. Comprehensive review and resources for fibromyalgia and chronic myofascial pain: www.sover.net/~devstar.

Myofascial Pain and Dysfunction: The Trigger Point Manual by David Simons, Janet Travell, and Lois Simons, 2nd ed. Philadelphia: Lippincott Williams and Wilkins, 1999.

The National Forum (Newsletter of the National CFIDS Foundation), 103 Aletha Road, Needham, Mass. 02492. Focus on CFID/ME, FM, GWI, MCS, and related illnesses.

Trigger Point Self-Care Manual: For Pain-Free Movement by Donna Finando, L.Ac., L.M.T. Rochester, Vt.: Healing Arts Press, 2005. This book is a self-care manual for lay readers.

Trigger Point Therapy for Myofascial Pain: The Practice of Informed Touch by Donna Finando, L.Ac., L.M.T., and Steven Finando, Ph.D., L.Ac. Rochester, Vt.: Healing Arts Press, 2005. This book is a more technical manual for bodywork professionals.

The Trigger Point Therapy Workbook: Your Self-Treatment Guide for Pain Relief, 2nd ed., by Clair Davies, N.C.M.T. Oakland, Calif.: New Harbinger Publications, 2004. Well-diagrammed self-treatment guide with two new chapters. Chapter 11 shows massage therapists how to effectively treat trigger points and chapter 12 deals with habitual muscle tension. Author website: www.TriggerPointBook.com.

Winning with Chronic Pain: A Complete Program for Health & Well-Being by H. H. McIlwain, D. F. Bruce, J. C. Silverfield, M. C. Burnette, and B. F. Germain. Amherst, N.Y.: Prometheus Books, 1994.

DEALING WITH COEXISTING CONDITIONS

Ankylosing Spondylitis

See National Rehabilitation Information Center (NARIC) in "General Resources."

Spondylitis Association of America
P.O. Box 5872
Sherman Oaks, CA 91413
818-981-1616
Toll-free: 800-777-8189
info@spondylitis.org

Arthritis

See American College of Rheumatology and National Rehabilitation Information Center (NARIC) in "General Resources."

The Arthritis Foundation
P.O. Box 7669
Atlanta, GA 30357
800-283-7800
www.arthritis.org
Provides definition of, and information about, osteoarthritis, and offers free brochures.

Acupuncture and Oriental Medicine Alliance (AOMA)
www.AOMAlliance.org
Provides publications and referrals from The American Association of Oriental Medicine.

Aids for Arthritis
6405 43rd Avenue Ct., NW, Suite B
Gig Harbor, WA 98335
253-851-6896
Toll-free: 800-654-0707
Fax: 253-851-6883

Books and Periodicals

Arthritis Survival: The Holistic Medical Treatment Program for Osteoarthritis by Robert Ivker, D.O., and Todd Nelson, N.D. New York: Penguin Putnam, 2001.

Arthritis Today Supplement Guide from the Arthritis Foundation at www.arthritistoday.org/treatments/supplement-guide/index.php. Offers useful information on numerous supplements from avocado soybean unsaponifiables to valerian, buying tips, safety, and supplements to avoid.

Carpal Tunnel Syndrome

See American College of Rheumatology, and National Rehabilitation Information Center (NARIC) in "General Resources."

Association for Repetitive Motion Syndromes (ARMS)
P.O. Box 471973
Aurora, CO 80047-1973
303-369-0803
www.certifiedpst.com/arms
Offers a quarterly newsletter with current information on such topics as medical research, treatment alternatives, insurance and legal issues, and ergonomic concerns.

Depression

National Foundation for Depressive Illness
P.O. Box 2257
New York, NY 10116
Toll-free: 800-248-4344

Center for Mental Health Services, Substance Abuse, and Mental Health Services Administration
P.O. Box 2345
Rockville, MD 20847-2345
Toll-free: 877-726-4727 (877-SAMHSA-7)
Helpline at **1-800-662-HELP** (1-800-662-4357)
SHIN@samhsa.hhs.gov
www.samhsa.gov

National Institute of Mental Health
6001 Executive Boulevard
Room 8184, MSC 9663
Bethesda, MD 20892-9663
301-443-4513
Toll-free: 866-615-6464
TTY (hearing disabled): 301-443-8431
Fax: 301-443-4279
nimhinfo@nih.gov
www.nimh.nih.gov

Dry Eye Syndrome

National Eye Institute
Information Office
31 Center Drive, MSC 2510
Bethesda, MD 20892-2510
301-496-5248
2020@nei.nih.gov
www.nei.nih.gov

Endometriosis

The Endometriosis Association
8585 76th Place
Milwaukee, WI 53223
414-355-2200
Fax: 414-355-6065
www.endometriosisassn.org

The National Institutes of Health
www.nichd.nih.gov

Books and Periodicals

The Endometriosis Sourcebook: The Definitive Guide to Current Treatment Options, the Latest Research, Common Myths about the Disease and Coping Strategies by Mary Lou Ballweg. Chicago: Contemporary Books, 1995.

Headaches

American Academy of Neurology
1080 Montreal Avenue
St. Paul, MN 55116-2325
651-695-2717
Toll-free: 800-879-1960
memberservices@ann.com
www.aan.com
This is a professional organization that offers no-fee headline news related to neurology, science, and advocacy.

American Headache Society (ACHE)

19 Mantua Road

Mount Royal, NJ 08061

856-423-0043, Option 1

achehq@talley.com

www.achenet.org

ACHE is a professional society of health care providers dedicated to the study and treatment of headache and face pain, offering articles and videos for patients.

National Headache Foundation

820 N. Orleans, Ste. 217

Chicago, IL 60610

Toll-free: 888-643-5552

info@headaches.org

www.headaches.org

Information includes education, publications, clinical trials, and a blog. There is a fee for on-line membership.

Books and Periodicals

Handbook of Headache Management: A Practical Guide to Diagnosis and Treatment of Head, Neck and Facial Pain, 2nd ed., by J. R. Saper, S. D. Silberstein, C. D. Gordon, R. L. Hamel, and S. Swidan. Philadelphia: Lippincott Williams & Wilkins, 1999. Covers epidemiology, classifications, diagnostic evaluation, mechanisms and theories of head pain.

Migraine by Oliver Sacks, M.D. New York: Vintage Books, 1999.

Trigger Point Therapy for Headaches & Migraines: Your Self-Treatment Workbook for Pain Relief by Valerie DeLaune, L.Ac. Oakland, Calif.: New Harbinger Publications, Inc., 2008.

Interstitial Cystitis

Interstitial Cystitis Association

100 Park Avenue, Ste. 108A

Rockville, MD 20850

Toll-free: 800-435-7422

Fax: 301-610-5308

icamail@ichelp.org.

www.ichelp.org

Irritable Bowel Syndrome Self-Help and Support Group

IBS Association

1440 Whalley Ave. #145

New Haven, CT 06515

Phone: 203-404-0660

For Canada:

P.O. Box 94074

Toronto, ON M4N 3R1

Canada

416-932-3311

ibsa@ibsassociation.org

www.ibsassociation.org

Lupus (SLE)

American Lupus Society

3914 Del Amo Boulevard, Ste. 922

Torrance, CA 90503

Toll-free: 800-331-1802

Lupus Foundation of America, Inc.

National Office

2000 L Street, N.W., Suite 710

Washington, DC 20036

202-349-1155 –0121

Toll-free: 800-558-0121

Fax: 202-349-1156

www.lupus.org

Local chapter information available at the website.

Meralgia Paresthetica

See National Organization for Rare Disorders in "General Resources."

Multiple Chemical Sensitivities (MCS)

The Collaborative on Health and the Environment

c/o Commonweal

P.O. Box 316

Bolinas, CA 94924

www.healthandenvironment.org/index.php

What Is Multiple Chemical Sensitivity
Registered Office
Unit 34 Heysham Business Park
Middleton Road
Heysham, Lancs LA3 3PP
www.multiplechemicalsensitivity.org
This website has many useful and informative links related to MCS. Organic products offered. This is a UK-based organization.

Multiple Sclerosis

National Multiple Sclerosis Society
National Chapter
1800 M Street, N.W.
Suite 750 South
Washington, D.C. 20036
Toll-free: 800-344-4867
www.nationalmssociety.org
In addition to providing helpful information and support, this organization can help you find a chapter near you.

International MS Support Foundation
9136 E. Valencia
Suite 110–PMB–83
Tuscon, AZ 85747
jsumpton@imssf.org
www.imssf.org

Osteoporosis

National Osteoporosis Foundation
1232 22nd N.W.
Washington, DC 20037-1292
202-223-2226 • Toll-free: 800-231-4222
www.nof.org

Peripheral Neuropathy

Neuropathy Association
60 E. 42nd, Ste. 942
New York, NY 10165
212-692-0662
Fax: 212-692-0668
info@neuropathy.org
www.neuropathy.org

Books and Periodicals
Numb Toes and Aching Soles: Coping with Peripheral Neuropathy by John A. Senneff. San Antonio, Tex.: Medpress, 1999.

Piriformis Syndrome
See National Rehabilitation Information Center (NARIC) in "General Resources."

Polymyalgia Rheumatica
See National Institute of Arthritis and Musculoskeletal and Skin, and American College of Rheumatology in "General Resources."

Posttraumatic Stress Disorder
See National Institute of Mental Health (NIMH) under Depression in this section on coexisting conditions.

National Center for Posttraumatic Stress Disorder (NCPTSD)
VA Medical Center 116D
White River Junction, VT 05009
802-296-6300
ncptsd@ncptsd.va.gov
www.ncptsd.org

Raynaud's Phenomenon or Disease
See National Institute of Arthritis and Musculoskeletal and Skin Diseases, and American Autoimmune Related Diseases Association in "General Resources."

Reflex Sympathetic Dystrophy Syndrome (RSDS) or Complex Regional Pain Syndrome
Reflex Sympathetic Dystrophy Syndrome Association (RSDSA)
P.O. Box 502
Milford, CT 06460
203-877-3790
Toll-free: 877-662-7737
Fax: 203-882-8362
info@rsds.org
www.rsds.org/index2.html

American RSD Hope Group
P.O. Box 875
Harrison, ME 04040-0875
207-583-4589
rsdhope@mail.org
www.rsdhope.org
This is an organization that is staffed with volunteers. They ask for your patience if they do not respond to you immediately.

Restless Leg Syndrome

Restless Leg Syndrome Foundation, Inc.
1610 14th St NW, Ste. 300
Rochester, MN 55901
507-287-6465
Toll-free: 877-INFO-RLS
Fax: 507-287-6312
rlsfoundation@rls.org
www.rls.org

Worldwide Education & Awareness for Movement Disorders (WE MOVE)
204 West 84th Street
New York, NY 10024
212-875-8312
wemove@wemove.org
www.wemove.org

Sjogren's Syndrome

See American College of Rheumatology in "General Resources."

See American Autoimmune Related Diseases Association in "General Resources."

See National Organization for Rare Disorders (NORD) in "General Resources."

Sleep

National Sleep Foundation
1522 K Street NW, Ste. 500
Washington, DC 20005
202-347-3471
Fax: 202-347-3472
nsf@sleepfoundation.org
www.sleepfoundation.org
You will find discussion of disorders related to sleep not exclusive to but including allergies, bruxism (grinding of teeth), FM, hypersomnia, insomnia, PLM, and RLS.

Temporomandibular Dysfunction (TMD/TMJ)

National Institute of Dental and Craniofacial Research
National Institutes of Health
9000 Rockville Pike
Bethesda, MD 20892
301-496-4261
nidcrinfo@mail.nih.gov
www.nidcr.nih.gov

The TMJ Association
P.O. Box 26770
Milwaukee, WI 53226-0770
262-432-0350
Fax: 262-432-0375
info@tmj.org
www.tmj.org

American Association of Oral and Maxillofacial Surgeons
9700 West Bryn Mawr Avenue
Rosemont, IL 60018-5701
847-678-6200
Toll-free: 800-822-6637
www.aaoms.org

Thoracic Outlet Syndrome (TOS)

American TOS Association
2263 W. New Haven Avenue #454
W. Melbourne, FL 32904
888-300-1954
atosa.org

See National Rehabilitation Information Center (NARIC) in "General Resources."

Books and Periodicals

Thoracic Outlet Syndrome: A Common Sequela of Neck Injuries by Richard J. Sanders, M.D., and Craig Haug, M.D. Philadelphia: Lippincott, 1991.

Trigeminal Neuralgia

Trigeminal Neuralgia Association
925 Northwest 56th Terrace, Ste. C
Gainesville, FL 32605-6402
352-331-7009
Toll-free: 800-923-3608
patientinfo@tna-support.org
www.fpa-support.org

Vulvodynia

National Vulvodynia Association
P.O. Box 4491
Silver Spring, MD 20914-4491
303-299-0775
Fax: 301-299-3999
www.nva.org

Vulvar Pain Foundation
203½ North Main Street, Suite 203
or P.O. Drawer 177
Graham, NC 27253
336-226-0704
Fax: 336-226-8518
www.vulvarpainfoundation.org

MEDICATIONS, HERBS, AND SUPPLEMENTS

American Botanical Council
6200 Manor Rd
Austin, TX 78723
512-926-4900
Toll-free: 800-373-7105
Fax: 512-926-2345
abc@herbalgram.org
www.herbalgram.org
Provides an herbal library, programs, and services.

Herb Research Foundation
4140 15th Street

Boulder, CO 80304
303-449-2265 • Fax: 303-449-7849
www.herbs.org
Provides information and referrals on botanical medicine worldwide.

National Council on Patient Information and Education
4915 Saint Elmo Avenue, Suite 505
Bethesda, Maryland 20814-6082
301-656-8565
www.talkaboutrx.org
Provides education on safe use of medications.

Pharmaceutical Research and Manufacturing of America (PHRMA)
950 F Street, NW, Ste. 300
Washington, DC 20004
202-835-3400
Fax: 202-835-3414
www.phrma.org
Provides a pharmaceutical manufacturing information booklet about assistance with medication costs.

www.wholehealthMD.com
This is an excellent resource for checking doses, interactions, and safety for the use of herbs, vitamins, and other supplements.

Books and Periodicals

Alternative Health & Medicine Encyclopedia, 2nd ed., by James E. Marti. Detroit, Mich.: Visible Ink Press, 1997.

Alternative Treatments for Fibromyalgia and Chronic Fatigue Syndrome: Insights from Practitioners and Patients, 1st ed., by Mari Skelly and Andrea Helm. Alameda, Calif.: Hunter House Publishers, 1999.

The American Pharmaceutical Association Practical Guide to Natural Medicines, 1st ed, by Andrea Peirce. New York: William Morrow, 1999.

The Chopra Center Herbal Handbook: Forty Natural Prescriptions for Perfect Health by Deepak Chopra, M.D., and David Simon, M.D. New York: Three Rivers Press, 2000.

The Doctors Book of Home Remedies for Preventing Disease by *Prevention Magazine* Editors. New York: Bantam Paperback Editions, 2000.

Plants that Heal by Joel L. Swerdlow, Ph.D. Washington, DC: National Geographic Books, 2000.

Your Guide to Alternative Medicine: Understanding, Locating, and Selecting Holistic Treatments and Practitioners by Larry P. Credit, Sharon G. Hartunian, and Margaret J. Nowak. New Hyde Park, New York: Square One Publishers, 2003.

ASSISTIVE DEVICES AND THERAPEUTIC SUPPLIES

Physical Therapy and Medical Equipment Suppliers

Allegro Medical—Online Medical Supply Store
1833 West Main Street, Suite 131
Mesa, AZ 85201
Toll-free: 800-861-3211
www.allagromedical.com
This online medical supply store offers a wide variety of home medical supplies and assistive devices, such as canes, walkers, wheelchairs, and electric scooters. They also offer orthopedic products, such as orthotics and carpal tunnel splints; Kinesio tape, other brands of athletic tape, and taping books; the Theracane for self-treatment of TrPs, and a good selection of electric muscle stimulation units.

The Comfort Store
459 Orange Point Drive, Suite H
Lewis Center, Ohio 43035
740-549-3900
Toll-free: 888-867-2225
Fax: 740-549-4148
sales@sitincomfort-store.com
www.sitincomfort.com
This site is a good source for the Theracane for self-treatment of TrPs (a search for Theracane within the site provides easy access). The site also offers ergonomic chairs, orthopedic back supports, body pillows, memory foam pillows, massagers and massage tools, exercise balls, and more.

OPTP (Orthopedic Physical Therapy Products)
3800 Annapolis Lane, Suite 165
P.O. Box 47009
Minneapolis, MN 55447-0009
763-553-0452
Toll-free: 888-819-0121
Fax: 763-553-9355
customerservice@optp.com
www.OPTP.com
Offers a wide variety of products for self-treatment of TrPs, including the Theracane (a search for Theracane within the site provides easy access). Also offers lumbar supports, cervical rolls, exercise straps, foam rollers, and books and information about back care.

VitalityWeb Backstore
13820 Stowe Drive
San Diego (Poway), CA 92064-8800
858-218-1320
Toll-free: 800-796-9656
Fax: 858-218-1321
sales@vitalityweb.com
www.vitalityweb.com
This online store for back care supplies is an excellent source for a variety of electric muscle stimulation units (TENs and Microstims), electrodes, and related supplies. It also offers a wide selection of ergonomic chairs and recliners, memory foam mattresses and pillows, neck rolls, lumbar supports, massage equipment, and more.

Wisdom King
4015 Avenida de la Plata
Oceanside, CA 92056
Toll-free: 877-931-9693
Fax: 760-450-0675
www.wisdomking.com
This online physical therapy supply store is an excellent source for a wide range of physical therapy supplies, including TENS electric muscle stimulation units, electrodes, and related supplies; Kinesio tape and other brands of athletic tape, including some that are latex free; the Theracane for self-treatment of TrPs; home traction units; exercise balls; therabands; heat and cold treatments; and more.

Yoga Props and Supplies

Drishti—Yoga Clothing & Essentials
130 E. Canyon Perdido Street
Santa Barbara, CA 93101
Toll-free: 877-DRISHTI (374-7484)
Fax: 805-963-0887
ordersupport@drishtiyoga.com
www.drishtiyoga.com
Along with a large selection of yoga clothing, offers yoga mats, blocks, bolsters, blankets, and straps to support your yoga practice despite physical challenges. Also offer meditation cushions and benches and yoga and exercise balls.

Hugger Mugger Yoga Products
1190 S. Pioneer Road
Salt Lake City, UT 84104
Toll-free: 800-473-4888
Fax: 801-268-2629
comments@huggermugger.com
www.huggermugger.com
Offers a wide variety of yoga bolsters, pillows, mats, blocks, straps, and blankets to support your yoga practice despite physical challenges. Also offers yoga clothing, Pilates equipment, and several yoga and Pilates DVDs.

Self-Massage Tool for Spinal Acupressure

The MA Roller
6207 Biltmore Avenue
Baltimore, MD 21215-3603
410-358-1777
Toll-free: 800-830-5949
Fax: 410-358-1778
Made of solid maple, the MA Roller is a self-massage tool that promotes deep relaxation. It is designed to stimulate acupressure points in the muscles that run along either side of the spine, working to open the twelve organ meridians of traditional Chinese medicine for overall improved health. Caution: You could find that the pressure exerted by the MA Roller is too intense if you suffer from the body-wide pain of fibromyalgia.

Voice-Activated Computer Software

Nuance, Inc.
1 Wayside Road
Burlington, MA 01803
781-565-5000
Fax: 781-565-5001
www.nuance.com
For those who experience physical difficulties when working at a keyboard, this company produces a variety of voice-activated computer software products that allow you to produce documents in any Microsoft Office application by speaking into the computer, rather than typing at the keyboard. With some of their products you can even cruise the Web by voice. Most of this book was written using their popular product Dragon Naturally Speaking. Be sure to check with the company to make sure that the product you order will be compatible with your computer's operating system.

BODYWORK, ACUPUNCTURE, MASSAGE, AND THERAPEUTIC TOUCH

American Association of Oriental Medicine
P.O. Box 162340
Sacramento, CA 95816
916-443-4770
Toll-free: 866-455-7999
Fax: 916-443-4766
www.aaaomonline.org
Offers publications and referrals.

American Academy of Medical Acupuncture
1970 E. Grand Avenue
Suite 330
El Segundo, California 90245
310-364-0193
administrator@medicalacupuncture.org
www.medicalacupuncture.org
Provides an M.D. and D.O. membership directory and referrals.

American Chiropractic Association
1701 Clarendon Boulevard
Arlington, VA 22209
703-276-8800
Fax: 703-243-2593
www.amerchiro.org
Offers health tips, information, and referrals

American Holistic Nurses Association
323 N. San Franscisco Street, Suite 201
Flagstaff, AZ 86001
928-526-2196
Toll-free: 800-278-2462
www.ahna.org

American Massage Therapy Association
500 Davis Street, Ste. 900
Evanston, IL 60201
864-0123
Toll-free: 877-905-2700
Fax: 847-864-1178
info@amtamasssage.org
www.amtamassage.org
Provides referrals.

Associated Bodywork & Massage Professionals
25188 Genesee Trail Road
Golden, CO 80401
303-674-8478
Toll-Free: 800-458-2267
Fax: 800-667-8260
expectmore@abmp.com
www.abmp.com
Offers information and referrals.

Cranial Academy
8202 Clearvista Parkway, # 9D
Indianapolis, IN 46256-1496
317-594-0411
Fax: 317-594-9299
info@cranialacademy.org
www.cranialacademy.com

Healing Touch Program: Worldwide Leaders in Energy Medicine
20822 Cactus Loop
San Antonio, Texas 78258
210-497-5529
Fax: 210-497-8532
info@HealingTouchProgram.com
www.healingtouchprogram.com
Offers information and referrals.

International Association of Healthcare Practitioners
11211 Prosperity Farms Road, Suite D-325
Palm Beach Gardens, FL 33410-3487
Toll-free: 800-311-9204
Fax: 561-622-4771
iahp@iahp.com
www.iahp.com
Their list of referrals to practitioners includes, but is not limited to, Aston therapeutics, craniosacral therapy, Feldenkrais method, lymph drainage, process acupressure, qigong, and many other helpful practices.

International Institute of Reflexology
P.O. Box 12462
St. Petersburg, FL 33733
727-343-4811
iir@tampabay.rr.com
www.reflexology-usa.net
Provides information and referrals.

International Rolf Institute
5055 Chaparral Ct. Ste. 103
Boulder, CO 80301
303-449-5903
Toll-free: 800-530-8875
Fax: 303-449-5978
www.rolf.org
Provides information and referrals.

Qigong Institute—East-West Academy of Healing Arts
617 Hawthorne Ave
Los Altos, CA 94024
www.qigonginstitute.org
Provides information and referrals.

National Certification Commission for Acupuncture and Oriental Medicine (NCCAOM)
76 South Laura Street, Ste. 1290
Jacksonville, FL 32202
904-598-1005
Fax: 904-598-5001
www.nccaomwww.org
Offers news, upcoming events, and referrals.

National Certification Board for Therapeutic Massage and Bodywork
1901 South Meyers Road, Ste. 240
Oakbrook Terrace, IL 60181
630-627-8000
www.ncbtmb.com
Provides information and referrals.

Nurse Healers Professional Associates, Inc.
P.O. Box 419
Craryville, NY 12521
518-325-1185
Fax: 509-693-3537
www.therapeutic-touch.org
Provides information and referrals.

Reiki Alliance
413-323-4381
reikihearts@aol.com
www.reikialliance.com
Provides information and referrals.

The Upledger Institute
11211 Prosperity Farms Road
Palm Gardens, FL 33410
561-622-4334
Toll-free: 800-233-5880
www.upledger.com
Offers training, information, and referrals for craniosacral therapy. When you click on the referral tab you will be redirected to International Association of Healthcare Practitioners to search for a practitioner. See International Association of Healthcare Practitioners.

Books and Periodicals

The Acupressure Atlas by Bernard C. Kolster, M.D., and Astrid Waskowiak, M.D., translated by Nikolas Win Myint. Rochester, Vt.: Healing Arts Press, 2007.

CranioSacral Therapy, 1st ed., by John Upledger and Jon Vredevoogd. Vista, Calif.: Eastland Press, 1983.

CranioSacral Therapy II: Beyond the Dura by Dr. John Upledger. Vista, Calif.: Eastland Press, 1987.

The Endless Web: Fascial Anatomy & Physical Reality, 1st ed., by R. Louis Schultz and Rosemary Feitis. Berkeley, Calif.: North Atlantic Books, 1996.

Healthy Pleasures by Robert Ornstein, Ph.D., and David Sobel, M.D. N.Y.: Da Capo Press, 1990. How enjoying such things as a hug, a movie, or a favorite dessert can affect immune responses in a positive way.

Intuitive Reiki for Our Times: Essential Techniques for Enhancing Your Practice by Amy Z. Rowland. Rochester, Vt. : Healing Arts Press, 2006.

Job's Body: A Handbook for Bodywork, 3rd ed., by Deane Juhan. Barrytown, N.Y.: Station Hill Press, 2002.

Mosby's Visual Guide to Massage Essentials by Sandra Fritz. Philadelphia: Mosby Trade Books, a division of Elsevier, 1997.

The Myofascial Release Manual, 4th ed., by Carol J. Manheim. Thorofare, N.J.: Slack, Inc., 2008.

The Reflexology Atlas by Bernard C. Kolster, M.D., and Astrid Waskowiak, M.D. Translated by Nikolas Win Myint. Rochester, Vt.: Healing Arts Press, 2005.

Rolfing: Reestablishing the Natural Alignment and Structural Integration of the Human Body for Vitality and Well-Being, 2nd ed., by Ida P. Rolf, Ph.D. Rochester, Vt.: Healing Arts Press, 1989.

Total Reflexology by Martine Faure-Alderson, D.O., translated by Jon E. Graham. Rochester, Vt.: Healing Arts Press, 2008. Includes a number of very precise reflexology maps of the feet.

Traditional Reiki for Our Times: Practical Methods for Personal and Planetary Healing by Amy Z. Rowland. Rochester, Vt.: Healing Arts Press, 1998.

Trigger Point Self-Care Manual: For Pain-Free Movement by Donna Finando, L.Ac., L.M.T. Rochester, Vt.: Healing Arts Press, 2005. This book is a self-care manual for lay readers.

Trigger Point Therapy for Myofascial Pain: The Practice of Informed Touch by Donna Finando, L.Ac., L.M.T., and Steven Finando, Ph.D., L.Ac. Rochester, Vt.: Healing Arts Press, 2005. This book is a more technical manual for bodywork professionals.

The Trigger Point Therapy Workbook: Your Self-Treatment Guide for Pain Relief, 2nd ed., by Clair Davies, N.C.M.T. Oakland, Calif.: New Harbinger Publications, 2004. Well-diagramed self-treatment guide with two new chapters. Chapter 11 shows massage therapists how to effectively treat trigger points and chapter 12 deals with habitual muscle tension. Author website: www.TriggerPointBook.com.

Anthology of T'ai Chi & Qigong: The Prescription for the Future, DVD featuring Bill Douglas. 2000. www.worldtaichiday.com. Also available through Amazon.com.

DIET

American College for Advancement in Medicine (ACAM)

American College for Advancement in Medicine
8001 Irvine Center Drive
Suite 825
Irvine, CA 92618
949-309-3520
Toll-free: 800-532-3688
Fax: 949-309-3538
www.acamnet.org

ACAM is a nonprofit association dedicated to educating physicians and other health care professionals on the latest findings and emerging procedures in complementary, alternative, and integrative (CAIM) medicine. They have a referral network for finding a health care provider trained in nutritional medicine.

American Dietetic Assocation.

120 South Riverside Plaza, Ste. 2000
Chicago, IL 60606-6995
Toll-free: 800-877-1600
www.eatright.org

Provides food and nutritional information. They suggest that one dietary guideline does not fit all individual nutritional needs. Also see USDA Center for Nutrition Policy and Promotion.

Center for Science in the Public Interest

1875 Connecticut Ave. NW, Ste. 300
Washington, DC 20009
302-332-9110
Fax: 302-265-4954
www.cspinet.org

Directory of mail-order organic and hormone-free beef. General information on diet and nutrition.

USDA Center for Nutrition Policy and Promotion

3101 Park Center Drive
Room 1034
Alexandria, VA 22302-1594
MyPyramid.gov

The USDA provides educational information on basic nutrition and interactive tools to help you. Diet recommendations are not a one size fits all. The USDA and Heath and Human Services will jointly publish and release the seventh edition of their *Dietary Guidelines for Americans* in the fall of 2010.

Books and Periodicals

Eating Well for Optimal Health: The Essential Guide to Food, Diet & Nutrition by Andrew Weil, M.D. New York: Alfred A. Knopf, 2000.

Foods That Fight Pain: Revolutionary New Stategies for Maximum Pain Relief by Neal Barnard, M.D. New York: Harmony Books, 1998.

Sugar Blues: Overcoming the Hidden Dangers of Insulin Resistance by Miryam Ehrlich Williamson. New York: Walker Books, 2001. Author website: www.mwilliamson.com/aboutbsb.htm.

Zone-Perfect Meals in Minutes by Barry Sears. New York: Harper Collins, 1997.

EXERCISE

Books and DVDs

Facilitated Stretching by Robert E. McAtee and Jeff Charland. Champaign, IL: Human Kinetics Publishers, 2007.

Pain Free: A Revolutionary Method for Stopping Chronic Pain by Pete Egoscue with Roger Gittnes. New York: Bantam Books, 1998.

Stretching, 20th Anniversary Revised Edition, by Bob Anderson. Bolinas, Calif.: Shelter Publications, Inc., 2000. This book shows how to stretch and strengthen muscles at every level of physical ability.

The Therapeutic Yoga Kit: Sixteen Postures for Quiet Yin Awareness by Cheri Clampett and Biff Mithoefer. Rochester, Vt.: Healing Arts Press, 2009. Presents adapted postures to promote recovery from injury and illness and relief from stress and fatigue. Includes a deck of sixteen posture cards and a 75-minute audio CD along with a 256-page book.

Yaz Exercise (for those who need therapeutics without inducing symptoms). www.yazinc.com.

Stretch for Health, DVD by fitness expert Dawn Jones, available from Smith House Press. To order call the company's toll-free number: 888-220-5402.

Chronic Fatigue: Your Complete Exercise Guide by Neil F. Gordon. Champaign, IL: Human Kinetics Publishers, 1993. Diagrams and illustrations with explanations.

Pain Erasure The Bonnie Prudden Way. New York: M. Evans and Company, Inc., 2002. www.bonnieprudden.com. CMP stretch & exercise.

Simple Relief through Movement by Stacie L. Bigelow. New York: John Wiley & Sons, 2000. Explains why movement is important and what movements can be performed by FM patients.

THE MINDFULNESS HELP SECTION—MANAGING EMOTIONS, REDUCING STRESS, COPING, ENRICHING SPIRITUALITY, AND REACHING GOALS

Association for Humanistic Psychology
P.O. Box 1190
14B Beach Road
Tiburon, CA 94920
415-435-1604
ahpoffice@aol.com
www.ahpweb.org
Provides publications and referrals.

Massachusetts General Hospital—Benson-Henry Institute for Mind-Body Medicine
151 Merrimac Street
4th Floor
Boston, MA 02114
617-643-6090
Fax: 617-643-6077
massgeneral.org/bhi
Offers stress reduction information and resources.

Books and Periodicals

Anatomy of an Illness as Perceived by the Patient by Norman Cousins. New York: W. W. Norton & Co., Inc., 1979. How to use humor and laughter to overcome an "incurable" disease.

Anger: The Misunderstood Emotion, Rev. ed., by Carol Tavris. New York: Touchstone, 1989.

The Complete Idiot's Guide to T'ai Chi and Qigong by Bill Douglas. New York: Alpha Books, 1999. In additions to being an author, Bill Douglas is the director of the nationally known consulting company, Stress Management and Relaxation. His program is used by the University of Kansas Medical Research Institute, Inc., for measuring the benefits of t'ai chi and qi gong.

Creating Affluence: The A-Z Steps to a Richer Life by Deepak Chopra, M.D. San Rafael, Calif.: New World Library and Novato, Calif.: Amber-Allen Publishing, 1998. Among other books by this author: *Seven Spiritual Laws of Success; Perfect Health: The Complete Mind/Body Guide; Ageless Body, Timeless Mind.*

Creative Visualization: Use the Power of Your Imagination to Create What You Want in Your Life by Shakti Gawain. New York: Bantam, 1997. Also available from this author is the *Creative Visualization Workbook.*

Driving Your Own Karma: Swami Beyondananda's Tour Guide to Enlightenment by Swami Beyondananda, with Steve Bhaerman. Rochester, Vt.: Destiny Books, 1989.

Feeling Good: The New Mood Therapy by David Burns. New York: Quill/Harper Collins, 2000.

Flying Without Wings: Personal Reflections on Loss, Disability, and Healing by Dr. Arnold Beisser, New York: Bantam Books, 1990. How to manage pain and live a rewarding life, written by a disabled psychiatrist.

Full Catastrophe Living: Using the Wisdom of Your Body and Mind to Face Stress, Pain and Illness by Jon Kabat-Zinn. New York: Delta Book by Dell Publishing, a division of Bantam Doubleday Dell Publications Group, 1990. Other books by this author include *Wherever You Go There You Are: Mindfulness Meditation in Everyday Life,* and many more.

Getting Unstuck: Breaking through Your Barriers to Change by Sidney B. Simon. New York: Grand Central Publishing, 1989.

Handbook to a Happier Life: A Simple Guide to Creating the Life You've Always Wanted by Jim Donovan. Novato, Calif: New World Library, 2003.

Healers on Healing by Richard Carlson, Ph.D., and Benjamin Shield. Los Angeles: Jeremy P. Tarcher, 1989. Essays and articles by leaders in healing and alternative approaches, including Bernie Siegel, Gerald Jampolsky, Hugh Prather, and Lynn Andrews.

Health and Healing by Andrew Weil, M.D. Boston: Houghton Mifflin, 1998. History, theory, and treatments in osteopathy, holistic, eastern, and other medical treatments and philosophies.

Healthy Pleasures by Robert Ornstein, Ph.D., and David Sobel, M.D. New York: Da Capo Press, 1990. How enjoying such things as a hug, a movie, or a favorite dessert can affect immune responses in a positive way.

Humor and Healing by Bernie Siegel, M.D. Audiobook. Louisville, Colo.: Sounds True, 1990. Siegel is also author of *Love, Medicine and Miracles*, and many other books.

Living Well with a Hidden Disability: Transcending Doubt and Shame and Reclaiming Your Life by Stacy Taylor, M.S.W., L.C.S.W., with Robert Epstein, Ph.D. Oakland, Calif.: New Harbinger Publications, Inc., 1999.

Love, Medicine and Miracles: Lessons Learned about Self-healing from a Surgeon's Experience with Exceptional Patients by Bernie Siegel. New York: Harper and Row, Publishers, 1988.

MBS-Healing. A discussion on healing from the mind/body/spirit perspective by patients, practitioners, and others interested in exploring those ideas and therapies that view the person as a whole. To subscribe, send an e-mail message to: MBS-Healingrequest@maelstrom.

StJohns.edu and in the body of the message type "subscribe mbs-healing."

Peace, Love and Healing: Body-Mind Communication and the Path to Self-Healing and Exploration by Bernie Siegel. New York: Harper & Row Publishers, 1988.

Perfect Health: The Complete Mind/Body Guide, Revised and Updated Edition, by Deepak Chopra, M.D. New York: Three Rivers Press, 2000.

Prayer Is Good Medicine: How to Reap the Benefits of Prayer, by Larry Dossey, M.D. New York: Harper Collins, 1996. Other books by this author: *Healing Words: The Power of Prayer and the Practice of Medicine; Space, Time & Medicine; Beyond Illness; Recovering the Soul: A Scientific and Spiritual Approach; Healing Beyond the Body: Medicine and the Infinite Reach of the Mind; Meaning & Medicine;* and more.

The Purpose Driven Life: What on Earth Am I Here For? by Rick Warren. Grand Rapids, Mich.: Zondervan, 2002. A Christian-based book and video that helps you understand what your purpose is. www.zondervan.com.

Staying Well with Guided Imagery: How to Harness the Power of Your Imagination for Health and Healing by Belleruth Naparstek. New York: Warner Books, 1994.

Teach Only Love by Gerald G. Jampolsky. Hillsboro, Ore.: Beyond Words Publishing, Inc., 2004.

Simplify Your Life: 100 Ways to Slow Down and Enjoy the Things that Really Matter by Elaine St. James. New York: Hyperion, 1994. Short essays on how to identify priorities and act accordingly.

The 22 (Non-Negotiable) Laws of Wellness by Greg Anderson. New York: HarperCollins, 1996. Personal success stories on beating impossible odds.

Tying Rocks to Clouds: Meetings and Conversations with Wise and Spiritual People by William Elliott. New York: Doubleday, 1995.

When I Say No I Feel Guilty by Manuel J. Smith, Ph.D. New York: Bantam, 1988.

Audio and Video Resources

Mindfulness Meditation: Cultivating the Wisdom of Your Body and Mind by Jon Kabat-Zinn. Audio recordings on cassette tapes. New York: Simon & Schuster Sound Ideas, 1995. A new abridged edition of these recordings was produced in 2002 and is available on CD from Simon and Schuster Audio.

Minding the Body, Mending the Mind by Joan Borysenko, Ph.D. Audio recording on CD. New York: Bantam Books, 1993. Learning to relax and the emotional effects of stress.

RELATIONSHIPS—RESOURCES FOR BUILDING, ENRICHING, AND LETTING GO
Books and Periodicals

The Book of Questions by Gregory Stock, Ph.D., New York: Workman Publishing, 1987. A book on self-discovery and how to talk with family and friends.

The Dance of Anger: A Woman's Guide to Changing the Patterns of Intimate Relationships. By Harriet Lerner, Ph.D. New York: HarperCollins Publishers, Inc., 2005.

The Dance of Intimacy: A Woman's Guide to Courageous Acts of Change in Key Relationships by Harriet Lerner, Ph.D. New York: Harper & Row, 1989. Steps to take to maintain or avoid intimacy.

Helping Yourself Help Others: A Book for Caregivers by Rosalyn Carter, with Susan K. Golant. New York: Three Rivers Press, 1995.

Living, Loving & Laughing with Pain by Jacqueline J. Pliskin. Words and Pictures, 1995. Note: This book is out of print but several used copies are available on the Web.

Love is Never Enough: How Couples Can Overcome Misunderstandings, Resolve Conflicts and Solve Relationship Problems through Cognitive Therapy by Aaron T. Beck. New York: Harper & Row, 1988.

Love & Survival: 8 Pathways to Intimacy and Health by Dean Ornish. New York: HarperCollins, 1998.

Love is the Answer by Gerald Jampolsky and Diane V. Cirincione. New York: Bantam, 1990. Others by Gerald Jampolsky include *Love Is Letting Go of Fear* and *Forgiveness: The Greatest Healer of All.*

Mainstay: For the Well Spouse of the Chronically Ill by Maggie Strong. Cambridge, Mass.: Bradford Books, 1997.

Mayo Clinic on Chronic Pain: Lead a More Active & Productive Life by David Swanson. New York: Kennsington Publishing Coporation, 1999.

Reclaiming Intimacy in Your Marriage: A Plan for Facing Life's Ebb and Flow . . . Together by Robert and Debra Bruce. Minneapolis, Minn.: Bethany House, 1996.

Seniors Guide to Pain-Free Living: All Natural Drug-Free Relief for Everything that Hurts by Doug Dollemore. Emmaus, Pa.: Rodale, 2000.

Silver Linings: Triumphs of the Chronically Ill and Physically Challenged by Shaena Engle (ed.). Amherst, N.Y.: Prometheus Books, 1977.

Sex, Love & Chronic Illness by Lucille Carlton. National Parkinson Foundation, 1994. This book is out of print but used copies are available on Amazon.com.

Shadows of Pain: Intimacy & Sexual Problems in Life by Vimala Pillari. Amsterdam, The Netherlands: Jason Aaronson, 1997.

The Ultimate Guide to Sex and Disability: For All of Us Who Live with Disabilities, Chronic Pain, and Illness by Miriam Kaufman, Cory Silverberg, and Fran Odette. San Francisco: Cleis Press, Inc., 2007.

LIFE'S DELIGHTS AND CLARIFICATIONS—JOURNALING
Books and Periodicals

The New Diary: How to Use a Journal for Self-Guidance and Expanded Creativity by Tristine Rainer. New York: Jeremy P. Tarcher, Inc., 2004. How to clarify goals and tap inner resources.

Recovering: A Journal by May Sarton. New York: W. W. Norton, 1986. A personal testimony.

A Trail Through Leaves: The Journal as a Path to Place by Hannah Hinchman. New York: W.W. Norton, 1997. Self-expression through drawing.

Writing Down the Bones: Freeing the Writer Within, 2nd ed., by Natalie Goldberg, Boston: Shambhala Publications, Inc., 2005. Includes writing exercises for self-expression.

LEGALITIES AND RED TAPE—RESOURCES FOR OVERCOMING ROAD BLOCKS

Americans with Disabilities Act (ADA) website. www .ada.gov.

Disability.gov

Direct questions about specific federal government programs for the disabled to:

800-333-4636 (voice and TTY)

Direct questions regarding the ADA (Americans with Disability Act) to:

Information Hotline: 800-514-0301

www.disability.gov.

Provides information and resources for housing, education, community, and health.

Equal Employment Opportunity Commission (EEOC)

131 M Street, NE

Washington, DC 20507

800-669-4000, TTY: 800-669-6820

202-663-4900, TTY: 202-663-4494

www.eeoc.gov

Find your Senator. www.senate.gov.

Find your representative. www.clerkweb.house.gov.

Job Accommodation Network

P.O. Box 6080

Morgantown, WV 26506-6080

800-526-7234

TTY (hearing impaired): 877-781-9403

www.jan.wvu.edu

National Disability Rights Network

900 2nd St., Ste. 211

Washington, DC 20002

202-408-9514,

TTY (hearing impaired): 202-408-9521

Fax: 202-408-9520

www.napas.org

Social Security Administration (SSA) website

Office of Public Inquiries

Windsor Park Building

6401 Security Blvd.

Baltimore, MD 21235

Toll-free: 800-772-1213

Toll-free TTY (hearing impaired): 800-325-0778

www.ssa.gov

The SSA suggests contacting your local social security office first.

U.S. Department of Education

Office of Vocational and Adult Education

400 Maryland Avenue, SW

Washington, DC 20202

Toll-free: 800-872-5327.

www.ed.gov/about/offices/list/ovae/index.html?src=mr

U.S. Department of Health and Human Services

200 Independence Avenue, S.W.

Washington, D.C. 20201

Telephone: 202-619-0257

Toll Free: 1-877-696-6775

www.hhs.gov

Provides information on financial assistance, health, grants, diet and exercise, environment, and prevention.

U.S. Department of Health and Human Services and Substance Abuse & Mental Health Services Administration (SAMHSA)

National Clearinghouse for Alcohol and Drug Information, Division of Communications and Education

SAMHSA's Health Information Network

P.O. Box 2345

Rockville, MD 20847-2345

877-726-4727

TTY (hearing impaired): 800-487-4889

Fax: 240-221-4292

www.samhsa.gov

The HHS and SAMSHA National Clearinghouse for Alcohol and Drug Information offers quick facts on drugs and alcohol at: http://ncadi.samhsa.gov

U.S. Department of Labor

200 Constitution Ave., NW

Washington, DC 20210

866-4-USA-DOL, TTY: 877-889-5627

www.dol.gov

Provides information on workplace rights and benefits, getting or leaving a job, workplace safety and health, and workplace statistics.

In your local telephone book, check the "Helpful Numbers" and "Government" sections.

Books and Publications

Administrative Law and Procedure by Elizabeth C. Richardson. Albany, N.Y.: J. D. Delmar Publishers, Inc. and Lawyers Cooperative Publishing: A division of Thomson Legal Publishing, 1996.

"The Appeals Process," Social Security Administration. SSA Pub. No. 05-10141, October 1999. Toll-free: 800-772-1213; TTY (hearing disabled) toll-free: 800-325-0778. www.ssa.gov.

Ballentine's Law Dictionary by Jack G. Handler. Albany, N.Y.: J. D. Delmar Publishers, Inc. and Lawyers Cooperative Publishing: A division of Thomson Legal Publishing, 1994.

Legal Nurse Consulting: Principles and Practice by Julie Brewer Bogart, R.N., M.N. Boca Raton, Fla.: CRC Press, 1998.

INFORMATION FOR EVERYBODY

American Association of Naturopathic Physicians
4435 Wisconsin Avenue, NW, Ste. 403
Washington, DC 20016
202-237-8150
Toll-free: 866-538-2267
www.naturopathic.org
Provides referrals.

American Medical Association
515 N. State St.
Chicago, IL 60610
Toll-free: 800-621-8335
www.ama-assn.org

American Nurses Association (ANA)
8515 Georgia Avenue, Suite 400
Silver Spring, MD 20910-3492
301-628-5000
Toll-free: 800-274-4262
Fax: 301-628-5001
www.nursingworld.org

American Osteopathic Association
142 E. Ontario Street
Chicago, IL 60611
Toll-free: 800-621-1773
Fax: 312-202-8200
www.osteopathic.org

The Centers for Disease Control and Prevention (CDC)
1600 Clifton Road
Atlanta, GA 30333
Toll-free: 800-232-4636,
TTY (hearing impaired): 888-232-6348
www.cdc.gov

Healthscout
www.healthscout.com.
Healthscout is a consumer-oriented health website that offers a newsfeed and information on disease, addictions, sex and relationships, and alternative medicine. It also has handy tools, such as a symptoms checker, a drug checker, an ideal body weight calculator, heart healthy diet recommendations, and fitness guides.

Merriam Webster online dictionary. www.m-w.com.

National Center for Homeopathy
101 S Whiting Street
Suite 16
Alexandria VA 22304
703-548-7790
www.nationalcenterforhomeopathy.org
Offers information on homeopathy, resources, and referrals.

National Foundation for the Treatment of Pain
P.O. Box 70045
Houston, Texas 77270-0045
713-862-9332
www.paincare.org
In addition to helpful information, the organization also provides outreach and advocacy for intractable pain.

National Institutes of Health (NIH) Clinical Research Program
10 Center Drive
Bethesda, MD 20892
301-496-2563
Fax: 301-402-2984
To participate in a clinical trial:
10 Cloister Court
Building 61
Bethesda, MD 20892
800-411-1222
Fax: 301-480-9793
prpl@mail.cc.nih.gov
www.clinicalresearch.nih.gov with link to
www.clinicaltrials.gov
Provides information about participating in clinical trials.

Web MD. www.webmd.com

World Book Online. www.worldbook.com

Books and Periodicals

The Anatomy Coloring Book by Wynn Kapit and Lawrence Elson. New York: Harper & Row, 1977.

The Body in Pain: The Making and Unmaking of the World by Elaine Scarry. New York: Oxford University Press, 1985.

Miller-Keane Encyclopedia & Dictionary of Medicine, Nursing, and Allied Health, 6th ed, by Benjamin F. Miller, M.D., and Claire Brackman Keane, R.N.B.S., M.Ed. Philadelphia: W. B. Saunders Company, 1997.

Glossary of Acronyms

AAPM	American Academy of Pain Management
ACPA	American Chronic Pain Association
ACR	American College of Rheumatology
ADA	Americans with Disabilities Act
ADEA	Age Discrimination in Employment Act
ALJ	administrative law judge
AME	average monthly earning
ANA	antinuclear antibody
AS	ankylosing spondylitis
ANS	autonomic nervous system
ATOIMS	automated twitch-obtaining intramuscular stimulation
ATP	adenosine triphospate
CAM	complementary alternative medicine
CBT	cognitive behavioral therapy
CDC	Centers for Disease Control and Prevention
CFID	chronic fatigue immunodysfunction
CMTPT	Certified Myofascial Trigger Point Therapist
CMP	chronic myofascial pain
CNS	central nervous system
COBRA	Consolidated Omnibus Budget Reconciliation Act
CRPS	complex regional pain syndrome
DEA	Drug Enforcement Agency
DD	disabling disorder
DHEA	dehydroepiandrosterone, a steroid hormone manufactured by the adrenal glands
DPS	disturbed physician syndrome

EAP	Employee Assistance Program
EDR	electrodermal response
EDS	Ehlers-Danlos syndrome (joint hypermobility)
EEG	an electrical study of brain wave patterns, neuro-electrotherapy
E-Stim	electrical stimulation
EEOC	Equal Employment Opportunity Commission
EPA	Equal Pay Act
ERISA	Employee Retirement and Income Security Act
ETOIMS	electrical twitch-obtaining intramuscular stimulation
FM	fibromyalgia
FMily	fibromyalgia support group
FMLA	Family and Medical Leave Act
fMRI	functional magnetic resonance imaging, a type of specialized MRI scan
GH	growth hormone
GI	gastrointestinal
GWS	Gulf War syndrome
5-HT3	a serotonin receptor
5-HT	5-hydroxytryptamine, serotonin, a neurotransmitter manufactured by neurons within the central nervous system
5-HTT	serotonin transporters
5-HTP	5-hydroxytryptophan, an amino acid that is a serotonin precursor
HCP	health care provider
HGH	Human Growth Hormone
HIPAA	Health Insurance Portability and Accountability Act
HPA	hypothalamic-pituitary-adrenal axis
IBS	irritable bowel syndrome
IC	Interstitial cystitis
IgA	mucosal immunity antibody
IgE	immune mechanism, a type of antibody
IgM	immune mechanism, a type of antibody
IU	international units (metric)
IVIg	intravenous immunoglobulin
JAN	Job Accommodation Network

JCAHO	Joint Commission on Accreditation of Healthcare Organizations
LD	Lyme disease
LGS	leaky gut syndrome
MBHCO	Managed Behavioral Health Care Organization
MCS	multiple chemical sensitivity
MFR	myofascial release
MPS	myofascial pain syndrome
MRI	magnetic resonance imaging
MS	multiple sclerosis
MTP	myofascial trigger point
NADH	nicotinamide adenine dinucleotide
NAMTPT	National Association of Myofascial Trigger Point Therapists
NCPOA	National Chronic Pain Outreach Association
NIAMS	National Institute of Arthritis and Musculoskeletal and Skin Diseases
NK	natural killer cells—frontline of immune cells that respond immediately to attack
NMDA	N-methyl-D-aspartate
NMES	neuromuscular electrical simulation
NMH	Neurally mediated hypotension
NO	nitric oxide
NORD	National Organization for Rare Disorders
NS	nervous system
NSAIDS	non-steroidal anti-inflammatory medications
OA	osteoarthritis
OMT	osteopathic manipulative techniques
OT	occupational therapy
OTC	over-the-counter (medications)
PCOs	proanthocyanidins
PET	positron emission tomography
PLM	periodic limb movement
PMR	polymyalgia rheumatica
PMS	premenstrual syndrome
PN	peripheral neuropathy
POTS	postural orthostatic tachycardia syndrome

PT	physical therapy
PTSD	posttraumatic stress disorder
RA	rheumatoid arthritis
RHG	reactive hypoglycemia
RLS	restless leg syndrome
ROM	range of motion
RSDS	reflex sympathetic dystrophy syndrome
SAD	seasonal affective disorder
SAM-e	S-adenosyl-methionine
SEA	spontaneous electrical activity
SI	sacroiliac
SIBO	small intestinal bacterial overgrowth
SICCA	dryness of the cornea and conjuctiva
SLE	systemic lupus erythematosus
SO	significant other
SPECT	single photon emission computed tomography, a scan used to track blood
SSA	Social Security Administration
SSDI	Social Security Disability Insurance
SSRI	selective serotonin reuptake inhibitors
T4	thyroid hormone, thyroxine
T3	a thyroid hormone converted from T4
T-cells	white blood cells that are a critical part of the immune system
TAB	temporarily able-bodied
TANF	Temporary Assistance for Needy Families
TENS	transcutaneous electro-neuro stimulation units
THC	active ingredient in marijuana
TTT	things take time
THR	target heart rate
TMD/TMJ	temporomandibular dysfunction
TOS	thoracic outlet syndrome
TrP	myofascial trigger point
USDA	United States Department of Agriculture
USDL	U.S. Department of Labor

Notes

CHAPTER 1. FIBROMYALGIA PAIN, CHRONIC FATIGUE
IMMUNODYSFUNCTION, AND CHRONIC MYOFASCIAL PAIN
FROM TRIGGER POINTS

1. Centers for Disease Control and Prevention, www.cdc.gov/ (accessed April 24, 2008).

2. National Institute of Arthritis and Musculoskeletal and Skin Diseases, *NIAMS Information Package: Fibromyalgia,* AR-91 (Bethesda, Md.: National Institute of Arthritis and Musculoskeletal and Skin Diseases, 2000): 1–5.

3. R. B. Gremillion, "Fibromyalgia: recognizing and treating an elusive syndrome," *The Physician and Sportsmedicine* 16, no. 4 (1996): 55–56.

4. M. A. Dunkin, "Fibromyalgia—syndrome of the '90s," *Arthritis Today* (September–October 1997): 41–42.

5. Jenny. A. Fransen and I. Jon. Russell, *The Fibromyalgia Help Book: Practical Guide to Living Better with Fibromyalgia* (Saint Paul, Minn.: Smith House Press, 1996), 8.

6. Centers for Disease Control and Prevention, www.cdc.gov (accessed April 2008).

7. D. Buskila, L. Neumann, A. Alhoashle, and M. Abu-Shakra, "Fibromyalgia syndrome in men," *Seminars in Arthritis and Rheumatism* 30, no. 1 (2000): 47–51.

8. E. L. Peterson, "Fibromyalgia—management of a misunderstood disorder," *Journal of American Academy Nurse Practitioner* 19, no. 7 (2007): 341–48.

9. Centers for Disease Control and Prevention, www.cdc.gov (accessed April 2008).

10. F. Wolfe, H. Smythe, M. Yunus, R. M. Bennett, C. Bombardier, D. L. Goldenberg, P. Tugwell, S. M. Campbell, M. Abeles, P. Clark, et al, "The American college of rheumatology 1990 criteria for the classification of fibromyalgia," *Arthritis and Rheumatism* 33 (1990): 160–72.

11. Roland Staud, "Fibromyalgia pain: do we know the source?" *Current Opinion in Rheumatology* 16, no. 2 (2004): 157–63.

12. Devin. J. Starlanyl and Mary. E. Copeland, *Fibromyalgia & Chronic Myofascial Pain Syndrome: A Survival Manual* (Oakland, Calif.: New Harbinger Publications, Inc., 2001).

13. D. J. Starlanyl, personal correspondence to author (May 2008).

14. L. M. Arnold, J. I. Hudson, E. V. Hess, A. E. Ware, D. A. Fritz, M. B. Auchenbach, L. O. Starck, and P. E. Keck Jr., "Family study of fibromyalgia," *Arthritis & Rheumatism* 50, no. 3 (2004): 944–52.

15. D. Buskila, L. Neumann, and J. Press, "Genetic factors in neuromuscular pain," *CNS Spectrums* 10, no. 4 (2005): 281–84.

16. X. J. Caro, E. F. Winter, and A. J. Dumas, "A subset of fibromyalgia patients have findings suggestive of chronic inflammatory demyelinating polyneuropathy and appear to respond to IVIg," *Rheumatology* 47, no. 2 (2008): 208–11.

17. Gremillion, "Fibromyalgia: recognizing and treating an elusive syndrome."

18. E. Kasikcioglu, M. Dinler, and E. Berker, "Reduced tolerance of exercise in fibromyalgia may be a consequence of impaired microcirculation initiated by deficient action of nitric oxide," *Medical Hypotheses* 66, no. 5 (2006): 950–52.

19. R. M. Bennett, "Adult growth hormone deficiency in patients with fibromyalgia," *Currrent Rheumatology Reports* 4, no. 4 (2002): 306–12.

20. K. C. Yuen, R. M. Bennett, C. A. Hryciw, M. B. Cook, S. A. Rhoads, and D. M. Cook, "Is further evaluation for growth hormone (GH) deficiency necessary in fibromyalgia patients with low serum insulin-like growth factor (IGF)-I levels?" *Growth Hormone IGF Research* 17, no. 1 (2007): 82–88.

21. Bennett, "Adult growth hormone deficiency in patients with fibromyalgia."

22. Dunkin, "Fibromyalgia—syndrome of the '90s."

23. M. L. Mahowald and M. W. Mahowald, "Nighttime sleep and daytime functioning (sleepiness and fatigue) in less well-defined chronic rheumatic diseases with particular reference to the alpha-delta NREM sleep anomaly," *Sleep Medicine* 1, no. 3 (2000): 195–207.

24. J. C. Rains and D. B. Penzien, "Sleep and chronic pain: challenges to the alpha-EEG sleep pattern as a pain specific sleep anomaly," *Journal of Psychosomatic Research* 54, no. 1 (2003): 77–83.

25. H. Moldofsky, "The significance, assessment, and management of nonrestorative sleep in fibromyalgia syndrome," *CNS Spectrums* 13, no. 3 (2008): 22–26.

26. M. Calis, C. Gokce, F. Ates, S. Ulker, H. B. Izgi, H. Demir, M. Kirnap, S. Sofuoglu, A. C. Durak, A. Tutus, and F. Kelestimur, "Investigation of the hypothalamo-pituitary-adrenal axis (HPA) by 1 microg ACTH test and metyrapone test in patients with primary fibromyalgia syndrome," *Journal of Endocrinology Investment* 27, no. 1 (2004): 42–46.

27. K. Wingenfeld, C. Heim, I. Schmidt, D. Wagner, G. Meinlschmidt, and D. H. Hellhammer, "HPA Axis Reactivity and Lymphocyte Glucocorticoid Sensitivity in Fibromyalgia Syndrome and Chronic Pelvic Pain," *Psychosomatic Medicine* (December 2007).

28. R. Staud, J. G. Craggs, W. M. Perlstein, M. E. Robinson, and D. D. Price, "Brain activity associated with slow temporal summation of C-fiber evoked pain in fibromyalgia patients and healthy controls," *European Journal of Pain* (March 2008).

29. D. B. Cook, G. Lange, D. S. Ciccone, W. C. Liu, J. Steffener, and B. H. Natelson, "Functional imaging of pain in patients with primary fibromyalgia," *Journal of Rheumatology,* 31, no. 2 (2004): 364–78.

30. Z. Liu, M. Welin, B. Bragee, and F. Nyberg, "A high-recovery extraction procedure for quantitative analysis of substance P and opioid peptides in human cerebrospinal fluid," *Peptides* 21, no. 6 (2000): 853–60.

31. Adrienne Dellow, "Serotonin in Fibromyalgia and Chronic Fatigue Syndrome Serotonin Dysregulation: Symptoms & Treatment Options," http://chronicfatigue .about.com/od/treatingfmscfs/a/serotonin.htm (accessed July 28, 2009).

32. K. Riering, C. Rewerts, and W. Zieglgansberger, "Analgesic effects of 5–HT3 receptor antagonists," *Scandinavian Journal of Rheumatology,* Suppl. no. 119 (2004): 19–23.

33. M. Maes, R. Verkerk, L. Delmeir, A. Van Gastel, F. van Hunsel, and S. Scharpe, "Serotonergic markers and lowered plasma branched-chain-amino acid concentrations in fibromyalgia," *Journal of Psychiatric Research* 97, no. 1 (2000): 11–20.

34. R. Kwiatek, L. Barnden, R. Tedman, R. Jarrett, J. Chew, C. Rowe, and K. Pile, "Regional cerebral blood flow in fibromyalgia: single-photon-emission computed tomography evidence of reduction in the pontine tegmentum and thalami," *Arthritis & Rheumatism* 43, no. 12 (2000): 2823–33.

35. J. N. Baraniuk, G. Whalen, J. Cunningham, and D. J. Clauw, "Cerebrospinal fluid levels of opioid peptides in fibromyalgia and chronic low back pain," *BMC Musculoskeletal Disorders* 5, no. 1 (2004): 48.

36. L. A. Aaron and D. Buchwald, "Chronic diffuse musculoskeletal pain, fibromyalgia and co-morbid unexplained clinical conditions," *Best Practice & Research Clinical Rheumatology* 17, no. 4 (2003): 563–74.

37. R. Staud, "Evidence of involvement of central neural mechanisms in generating fibromyalgia pain," *Current Rheumatology Reports* 4, no. 4 (2002): 299–305.

38. R. Staud, D. D. Price, M. E. Robinson, A. P. Mauderli, and C. J. Vierck, "Maintenance of windup of second pain requires less frequent stimulation in fibromyalgia patients compared to normal controls," *Pain* 110, no. 3 (2004): 689–96.

39. D. J. Starlanyl, personal correspondence to author (April 2005).

40. S. B. McMahon, W. B. Cafferty, and F. Marchand, "Immune and glial cell factors as pain mediators and modulators," *Experimental Neurology* 192, no. 2 (2005): 444–62.

41. L. Bazzichi, A. Rossi, G. Massimetti, G. Giannaccini, T. Giuliano, F. De Feo, A. Ciapparelli, L. Dell'Osso, and Bombardieri, "Cytokine patterns in fibromyalgia and their correlation with clinical manifestations," *Clinical and Experimental Rheumatology* 25, no. 2 (2007): 225–30.

42. J. Wieseler-Frank, S. F. Maier, L. R. Watkins, "Glial activation and pathological pain," *Neurochemistry International* 45, no. 2–3 (2004): 389–95.

43. J. A. Macedo, J. Hesse, J. D. Turner, W. Ammerlaan, A. Gierens, D. H. Hell-manner, and C. P. Muller, "Adhesion molecules and cytokine expression in fibro-myalgia patients: increased L-selectin on monocytes and neutrophils," *Journal of Neuroimmunology* 188, no. 1–2 (2007): 159–66.

44. J. Wieseler-Frank, S. F. Maier, and L. R. Watkins, "Central proinflammatory cytokines and pain enhancement," *Neurosignals* 14, no. 4 (2005): 166–74.

45. M. Martinez-Lavin, "Biology and therapy of fibromyalgia. Stress, the stress response system, and fibromyalgia," *Arthritis Research & Therapy,* no. 4 (2007): 216.

46. "Automatic Dysfunction in FM," *Fibromyalgia Network Newsletter* (January 2002): 2–7.

47. H. C. Friederich, D. Schellberg, K. Mueller, C. Bieber, S. Zipfel, and W. Eich, "Stress and autonomic dysregulation in patients with fibromyalgia syndrome," *Schmerz* 2005 Jun., 19(3):185–88, 190–92, 194.

48. A. A. Larson, S. L. Giovengo, I. J. Russell, and J. E. Michalek, "Changes in the concentrations of amino acids in the cerebrospinal fluid that correlate with pain in patients with fibromyalgia: implications for nitric oxide pathways," *Pain* 87, no. 2 (2000): 201, 211.

49. R. L. Garrison and P. C. Breeding, "A metabolic basis for fibromyalgia and its related disorders: the possible role of resistance to thyroid hormone," *Medical Hypotheses* 61, no. 2 (2003): 182–89.

50. D. J. Wallace and D. S. Hallegua, "Fibromyalgia: the gastrointestinal link," *Current Pain and Headache Reports* 8, no. 5 (2004): 364–68.

51. R. Staud and M. Spaeth, "Psychophysical and neurochemical abnormalities of pain processing in fibromyalgia," *CNS Spectrums* 13, no. 3, suppl. no. 5 (2008): 12–17.

52. Centers for Disease Control and Prevention (accessed April 2008), www.cdc.gov/.

53. Ibid.

54. P. C. Rowe, "Neurally Mediated Hypotension and CFS." 1998 Clinical and Sci-entific Meeting, www.ahmf.org/98rowe.html (accessed August 2003).

55. The CFID Association of America, "Chronic Fatigue and Immune Dysfunction Syndrome (CFID) Fact Sheet" pamphlet (June 2001).

56. Centers for Disease Control and Prevention (accessed April 2008), www.cdc.gov/.

57. The CFID Association of America, "CFID and Youth" pamphlet (April 1999).

58. Ibid.

59. Centers for Disease Control and Prevention (accessed April 2008), www.cdc.gov/.

60. Ibid.

61. *About CFID: Symptoms*, The CFID Association of America, www.CFIDS.org (accessed March 2008).

62. Hal S. Blatman, M.D., Blatman Pain Clinic, www.blatmanpainclinic.com/blat_our_practice.htm (accessed September 1, 2009).

63. B. Evengard and N. Klimas, "Chronic fatigue syndrome: probable pathogenesis and possible treatments," *Drugs* 62, no. 17 (2002): 2433–46.

64. D. Racciatti, J. Vecchiet, A. Ceccomanncini, F. Ricci, E. Pizzigallo, "Chronic fatigue syndrome following toxic exposure," *Science of the Total Environment, Italy* 270, no. 1–3 (2001): 27–31.

65. E. Anyanwu, A. W. Campbell, J. Jones, J. E. Ehiri, and I. Akpan, "The neurological significance of abnormal natural killer cell activity in chronic toxigenic mold exposures," *Science World Journal* 3 (2003): 1128–37.

66. G. Kennedy, V. Spence, C. Underwood, J. J. Belch, "Increased neutrophil apoptosis in chronic fatigue syndrome," *Journal of Clinical Pathology* 57, no. 8 (2004): 891–93.

67. P. D. White, J. M. Thomas, P. F. Sullivan, and D. Buchwald, "The nosology of sub-acute and chronic fatigue syndromes that follow infectious mononucleosis," *Psychological Medicine* 34, no. 3 (2004): 499–507.

68. K. Gustaw, "Chronic fatigue syndrome following tick-borne diseases," *Neurologia i Neurochirurgia Polska* 37, no. 6 (2003): 1211–21.

69. J. Haier, M. Nasralla, and G. L. Nicholson, "Mycoplasmal Infections in Blood, Fibromyalgia Syndrome and Gulf War Illness," 1998 Clinical and Scientific Meeting, The Institute for Molecular Medicine, Huntington Beach, Calif., www.ahmf.org/98haier.html, (accessed December 28, 2001).

70. G. L. Nicholson, R. Gan, and J. Haier, "Multiple co-infections (mycoplasma, chlamydia, human herpes virus-6) in blood of chronic fatigue syndrome patients: association with signs and symptoms," *APMIS* 111, no. 5 (2003): 557–66.

71. L. M. Binder and K. A. Campbell, "Medically unexplained symptoms and neuropsychological assessment," *Journal of Clinical and Experimental Neuropsychology* 26, no. 3 (2004): 369–92.

72. Centers for Disease Control and Prevention, (accessed April 2008), www.cdc.gov.

73. V. Siemionow, Y. Fang, L. Calabrese, V. Sahgal, and G. H. Yue, "Altered central nervous system signal during motor performance in chronic fatigue syndrome," *Journal of Clinical Neurophysiology* 115, no. 10 (2004): 2372–81.

74. S. Yamamoto, Y. Ouch, I. H. Onoe, E. Yoshikawa, H. Tsukada, H. Takahashi, M. Iwase, K. Yamaguti, H. Kuratsune, and Y. Watanabe, "Reduction of serotonin transporters of patients with chronic fatigue syndrome," *Neuroreport* 15, no. 17 (2004): 2571–74.

75. A. Di Giorgio, M. Hudson, W. Jeres, and A. J. Cleare, "24–hour pituitary and adrenal hormone profiles in chronic fatigue syndrome," *Psychosomatic Medicine* 67, no. 3 (2005): 433–40.

76. A. J. Parker, S. Wessely, and A. J. Cleare, "The neuroendocrinology of chronic fatigue syndrome and fibromyalgia," *Psychological Medicine* 31, no. 8 (2001): 1331–45.

77. L. J. Crofford, E. A. Young, N. C. Engleberg, A. Korszun, C. B. Brucksch, L. A. McClure, M. B. Brown, and M. A. Demitrack, "Basal circadian and pulsatile ACTH and cortisol secretion in patients with fibromyalgia and/or chronic fatigue syndrome," *Brain, Behavior, and Immunity* 18, no. 4 (2004): 314–25.

78. A. J. Cleare, V. O'Keane, and J. P. Miell, "Levels of DHEA and DHEAS and responses to CRH stimulation and hydrocortisone treatment in chronic fatigue syndrome," *Psychoneuroendocrinology* 29, no. 6 (2004): 724–32.

79. K. J. Maher, N. G. Klimas, and M. A. Fletcher, "Chronic fatigue syndrome is associated with diminished intracellular perforin," *Clinical and Experimental Immunology* 142, no. 3 (2005): 505–11.

80. Kennedy, Spence, Underwood, Belch, "Increased neutrophil apoptosis in chronic fatigue syndrome."

81. J. Nijs, K. De Meirleir, M. Meeus, N. R. McGregor, and P. Englebienne, "Chronic fatigue syndrome: intracellular immune deregulations as a possible etiology for abnormal exercise response," *Medical Hypotheses* 62, no. 5 (2004): 759–65.

82. J. L. Newton, O. Okonkwo, K. Sutcliffe, A. Seth, J. Shin, and D. E. Jones, "Symptoms of autonomic dysfunction in chronic fatigue syndrome," *QJM* 100, no. 8 (2007): 519–26.

83. J. E. Naschitz, I. Rosner, M. Rozenbaum, S. Naschitz, R. Musafia-Priselac, N. Shaviv, M. Fileds, H. Isseroff, E. Zuckerman, D. Yeshurun, and E. Sabo, "The head-up tilt test with haemodynamic instability score in diagnosing chronic fatigue syndrome," *QJM* 96, no. 2 (2003): 133–42.

84. S. Fulle, S. Belia, J. Vecchiet, C. Morabito, L. Vecchiet, and G. Fano, "Modification of the functional capacity of sarcoplasmic reticulum membranes in patients suffering from chronic fatigue syndrome," *Neuromuscular Disorders* 13, no. 6 (2003): 479–84.

85. R. L. Garrison and P. C. Breeding, "A metabolic basis for fibromyalgia and its related disorders: the possible role of resistance to thyroid hormone," *Medical Hypotheses* 61, no. 2 (2003): 182–89.

86. AACFS Seventh International Clinical and Scientific Meeting, Madison, Wisconsin, October 2004, research overview prepared by A. Komaroff (Boston), www.iacfs.org (accessed May 5, 2005). Note: the proceedings of this meeting are no longer available at this website but to gain access to all the material offered at the conference go to: www.panda-clinic.com/pdf_word_docs/materialslist.pdf.

87. G. Moorkens, J. Berwaerts, H. Wyanants, and R. Abs, "Characterization of pituitary function with emphasis on GH secretion in the chronic fatigue syndrome," *Clinical Endocrinology* 53, no. 1 (2000): 99–106.

88. R. Glaser, D. A. Padgett, M. L. Litsky, R. A. Baiocchi, E. V. Yang, M. Chen, E. Yeh, N. G. Klimas, G. D. Marshall, T. Whiteside, R. Herberman, J. Kiecolt-

Glaser, and M. V. Williams, "Stress-associated changes in the steady-state expression of latent Epstein-Barr virus: implications for chronic fatigue syndrome and cancer," *Brain, Behavior, and Immunity* 19, no. 2 (2005): 91–103.

89. A. M. Lerner, S. H. Beqaj, R. G. Deeter, and J. T. Fitzgerald, "IgM serum antibodies to Epstein-Barr virus are uniquely present in a subset of patients with chronic fatigue syndrome," *In Vivo* 18, no. 2 (2004): 101–6.

90. A. Cocchetto, "The Ciguatera Epitope: So What Do We Really Know thus Far?" *The National Forum* 6, no. 4 (2003): 1, 4–5.

91. M. M. Brown and L. A. Jason, "Functioning in individuals with chronic fatigue syndrome: increased impairment with co-occurring multiple chemical sensitivity and fibromyalgia," *Dynamic Medicine* 6, no. 1 (2007): 6.

92. David Simons, Janet Travell, and Lois S. Simons, *Myofascial Pain and Dysfunction: The Trigger Point Manual*, 2nd ed. (Baltimore: Williams and Wilkins, 1999).

93. D. G. Simons, "Myofascial pain syndrome: One term but two concepts; a new understanding," *Journal of Musculoskeletal Medicine* 3, no. 1 (1995): 7–14.

94. C. Fernandez-de-las-Penas, M. L. Cuadrado, L. Arendt-Nielsen, D. G. Simons, and J. A. Pareja, "Myofascial trigger points and sensitization: an updated pain model for tension-type headache," *Cephalalgia* 27, no. 5 (2007): 383–93.

95. S. Mense, "Neurobiological basis of muscle pain," *Schmerz* 13, no. 1 (1999): 3–17.

96. Clair Davies, *The Trigger Pont Therapy Workbook: Your Self-Treatment Guide for Pain Relief,* 2nd ed. (Oakland, Calif.: New Harbinger Publications, 2004), 36–37.

97. Starlanyl, personal correspondence to author (May 2008).

98. Simons, et al., *Myofascial Pain and Dysfunction: The Trigger Point Manual.*

99. Starlanyl and Copeland, *Fibromyalgia & Chronic Myofascial Pain Syndrome: A Survival Manual*, 25.

100. Ibid.

101. Starlanyl, personal correspondence to author (March 2005).

102. John Whiteside, MBBS, BSc, "Myofascial Medicine," www.myomed.com.au (accessed September 2009).

103. Ibid.

104. Ibid.

105. "Natural Course of Myofascial Trigger Points," www.pain-education.com/100256 .php (accessed August, 2009).

106. John Whiteside, MBBS, BSc, "Myofascial Pain Syndromes and Trigger Point Injection Therapy," www.pain-education.com/100134.php (accessed September 2009).

107. Starlanyl, personal correspondence to author (April 1, 2005).

108. Simons, et al., *Myofascial Pain and Dysfunction: The Trigger Point Manual.*

109. Starlanyl and Copeland, *Fibromyalgia & Chronic Myofascial Pain Syndrome: A Survival Manual.*

110. R. D. Gerwin, "Classification, epidemiology, and natural history of myofascial pain syndrome," *Current Pain and Headache Reports,* no. 5 (2001): 412–20.

111. J. G. Travell and D. G. Simons, *Myofascial Pain and Dysfunction: The Trigger Point Manual*, Vol. 2, 2nd ed. (Baltimore: Lippincott, Williams and Wilkins, 1992), 110–29.

112. D. Simons, et al., *Myofascial Pain and Dysfunction: The Trigger Point Manual.*

113. C. Z. Hong and D. G. Simons, "Pathophysiologic and electrophysiologic mechanisms of myofascial trigger points," *Archives of Physical Medicine and Rehabilitation* 79, no. 7 (1998): 863–72.

114. D. M. Niddam, R. C. Chan, S. H. Lee, T. C. Yeh, and J. C. Hsieh, "Central representation of hyperalgesia from myofascial trigger point," *NeuroImage* 39 (2008): 1299–1306.

115. D. G. Simons and S. Mense, "Diagnosis and therapy of myofascial trigger points," *Schmerz* 17, no. 6 (2003): 419–24.

116. C. Z. Hong, "New Trends in myofascial pain syndrome," *Zhonghua Yi Xue Za Zhi* (Taipei) 65, no. 11 (2002): 501–12.

117. Simons, et al., *Myofascial Pain and Dysfunction: The Trigger Point Manual.*

118. R. Gerwin, "Trigger points: a comprehensive hypothesis of trigger point formation," *Journal of Musculoskeletal Pain* 15, no. 13 (2007): 12.

119. Wieseler-Frank, Maier, and Watkins, "Central proinflammatory cytokines and pain enhancement."

120. A. Gur, R. Cevik, K. Nas, L. Colpan, and S. Sarac, "Cortisol and hypothalamic–pituitary–gonadal axis hormones in follicular-phase women with fibromyalgia and chronic fatigue syndrome and effect of depressive symptoms on these hormones," *Arthritis Research & Therapy* 6, no. 3 (2004): R232–R238.

121. J. E. Naschitz, M. Rozenbaum, I. Rosner, E. Sabo, R. M. Priselac, N. Shaviv, A. Ahdoot, M. Ahdoot, L. Gaitin, S. Eldar, and D. Yeshurun, "Cardiovascular response to upright tilt in fibromyalgia differs from that in chronic fatigue syndrome," *Journal of Rheumatology* 28, no. 6 (2001): 1356–60.

122. J. E. Naschitz, G. Slobodin, D. Sharif, M. Fields, H. Isseroff, E. Sabo, and I. Rosner, "Electrocardiographic QT interval and cardiovascular reactivity in fibromyalgia differ from chronic fatigue syndrome," *European Journal of Internal Medicine* 19, no. 3 (2008): 187–91.

123. Gremillion, "Fibromyalgia: recognizing and treating an elusive syndrome": 55–56.

124. M. N. Baliki, P. Y. Geha, and A. V. Apkarian, "Spontaneous pain and brain activity in neuropathic pain: functional MRI and pharmacologic functional MRI studies," *Current Pain and Headache Reports* 11, no. 3 (2007): 171–77.

125. B. H. Natelson, Contempo Updates: "Linking Evidence and Experience: Chronic Fatigue Syndrome," *JAMA* 285, no. 20 (2001).

126. "Fibro Forum," *The National Forum* 6, no. 4 (2003): 21–22.

127. D. J. Clauw, "Potential mechanisms in chemical intolerance and related conditions," *Annals of the New York Academy of Sciences* 933 (2001): 235–53.

CHAPTER 2. COMMUNICATING YOUR HEALTH CARE NEEDS

1. R. Staud, D. D. Price, M. E. Robinson, and C. J. Vierck Jr., "Body pain area and pain-related negative effect predict clinical pain intensity in patients with fibromyalgia," *Journal of Pain* 5, no. 6 (2004): 338–43.

2. Fransen and Russell, *The Fibromyalgia Help Book: Practical Guide to Living Better with Fibromyalgia.*

3. S. Pay, M. Calguneri, Z. Caliskaner, A. Dinc, S. Apras, I. Ertenli, S. Kiraz, and V. Cobankara, "Evaluation of vascular injury with proinflammatory cytokines, thrombomodulin and fibronectin in patients with primary fibromyalgia," *Nagoya Journal of Medical Science* 63, no. 3–4 (2000): 115–22.

4. Devin J. Starlanyl and Mary E. Copeland, *Fibromyalgia & Chronic Myofascial Pain: A Survival Manual,* 2nd ed. (Oakland, Calif.: New Harbinger Publications, Inc., 2001), 51.

5. Ibid., 41–50.

6. Ibid., 168–70.

7. Ibid., 41–50.

8. Ibid.

9. Clair Davies, *The Trigger Point Therapy Workbook: Your Self-treatment Guide for Pain Relief* (Oakland, Calif.: New Harbinger Publications, Inc., 2004).

10. D. R. Hubbard, "Persistent muscular pain: Approaches to relieving trigger points," *Journal of Musculoskeletal Medicine* 15, no. 5 (1998): 16–20, 23–26.

11. L. A. Aaron, R. Herrell, S. Ashton, M. Belcourt, K. Schmaling, J. Goldberg, and D. Buchwald, "Comorbid clinical conditions in chronic fatigue: a co-twin control study," *Journal of General Internal Medicine* 16, no. 1 (2001): 24–31.

12. Starlanyl and Copeland, *Fibromyalgia & Chronic Myofascial Pain: A Survival Manual,* 2nd ed., 43.

13. G. L. Nicolson, R. Gan, and J. Haier, "Multiple co-infections (Mycoplasma, Chlamydia, and human herpes virus 6) in blood of chronic fatigue syndrome patients: associated with signs and symptoms," *APMIS* 111 (2003): 557–66 [Denmark].

14. National ME/FM Action Network, *Myalgic Encephalomyelitis/Chronic Fatigue Syndrome: A Clinical Case Definition for Medical Practitioners—An Overview of Canadian Consensus Document.* www.CFID-me.org (accessed March 2008).

15. S. Reid, M. Hotopf, L. Hull, K. Ismail, C. Unwin, and S. Wessely, "Multiple chemical sensitivity and chronic fatigue syndrome in British Gulf War veterans," *American Journal of Epidemiology* 153, no. 6 (2001): 604–9.

16. Centers for Disease Control and Prevention, "Chronic Fatigue Syndrome: What is CFS?" www.cdc.gov/ncidod/diseases/cfs/info.htm (accessed April 4, 2005).

17. J. A. Bellanti, A. Sabra, H. J. Castro, J. R. Chavez, J. Malka-Rais, and J. M. de Inocencio, "Are attention deficit, hyperactivity disorder, and chronic fatigue syndrome allergy related? What is fibromyalgia?" *Allergy and Asthma Proceedings* 26, no. 1 (2005): 19–28.

18. Starlanyl and Copeland, *Fibromyalgia & Chronic Myofascial Pain: A Survival Manual,* 72–73.

19. T. Kato, J. Y. Montplaisir, F. Guitard, B. J. Sessle, J. P. Lund, and G. J. Lavigne, "Evidence that experimentally induced sleep bruxism is a consequence of transient arousal," *Journal of Dental Research* 82, no. 4 (2003): 284–88.

20. Starlanyl and Copeland, *Fibromyalgia & Chronic Myofascial Pain: A Survival Manual,* 82.

21. GI Problems—Is Bacteria to Blame? *Fibromyalgia Network Newsletter* (July 2000): 3.

22. Starlanyl and Copeland, *Fibromyalgia & Chronic Myofascial Pain: A Survival Manual,* 48.

23. R. E. Cater, 2nd, "Chronic intestinal candidiasis as a possible etiological factor in the chronic fatigue syndrome," *Medical Hypotheses* 44, no. 6 (June 1995): 507–15.

24. Starlanyl and Copeland, *Fibromyalgia & Chronic Myofascial Pain: A Survival Manual,* 296.

25. R. Baron and G. Wasner, "Complex Regional Pain Syndromes," *Current Pain and Headache Reports* 5 (2001), 114–23.

26. S. Bruehl, R. N. Harden, B. S. Galer, S. Saltz, M. Backonja, and M. Stanton-Hicks, "Complex regional pain syndrome: are there distinct subtypes and sequential stages of the syndrome?" *Pain* 95 (2002): 119–24.

27. Starlanyl and Copeland, *Fibromyalgia & Chronic Myofascial Pain Syndrome: A Survival Manual,* 43.

28. Gulf War Syndrome: The Case for Multiple Origin Mixed Chemical/Biotoxin Warfare Related Disorder. Staff Report to U.S. Senator Donald W. Riegle Jr. (the "Riegle report," S.R. 103-900) Chronicillnet.org: PGWS, www.gulfweb.org (accessed August 31, 2009).

29. G. Nicolson, M. Y. Nasralla, J. Haier, R. Erwin, N. L. Nicolson, and R. Ngwenya, "Mycoplasmal Infections in Chronic Illnesses: Fibromyalgia & Chronic Fatigue Syndromes, Gulf War Illness, HIV-AIDS, and Rheumatoid Arthritis," Gulfwarvets.com (accessed August 2003).

30. Starlanyl and Copeland, *Fibromyalgia & Chronic Myofascial Pain Syndrome: A Survival Manual,* 44.

31. M. F. Peres, E. Zukerman, C. A. Senne Soares, E. O. Alonso, B. F. Santos, and M. H. Faulhaber, "Cerebrospinal fluid glutamate levels in chronic migraine," *Cephalalgia* 24, no. 9 (2004): 735–39.

32. Starlanyl and Copeland, *Fibromyalgia & Chronic Myofascial Pain Syndrome: A Survival Manual,* 44.

33. D. F. Barron, B. A. Cohen, M. T. Geraghty, R. Violand, and P. C. Rowe, "Joint hypermobility is more common in children with chronic fatigue syndrome than in healthy controls," *Journal of Pediatrics* 141, no. 3 (2002): 421–25.

34. D. G. Simons, J. G. Travell, and L. S. Simons, *Myofascial Pain and Dysfuntion:*

The Trigger Point Manual, vol. 1, 2nd ed. (Baltimore: Lippincott, Williams and Wilkins, 1999), 179–84.

35. J. F. Brun, C. Fedou, and J. Mercier, "Postprandial reactive hypoglycemia," *Diabetes/Metabolism Research and Reviews* 26, no. 5 (2000): 337–51.

36. Starlanyl and Copeland, *Fibromyalgia & Chronic Myofascial Pain Syndrome: A Survival Manual,* 65.

37. L. Bazzichi, A. Rossi, T. Giuliano, F. De Feo, C. Giacomelli, A. Consensi, A. Ciapparelli, G. Consoli, L. Dell'osso, and S. Bombardieri, "Association between thyroid autoimmunity and fibromyalgic disease severity," *Clinical Rheumatology* 26, no. 12 (2007): 2115–20.

38. Starlanyl and Copeland, *Fibromyalgia & Chronic Myofascial Pain Syndrome: A Survival Manual,* 44.

39. Simons, and Simons, *Myofascial Pain and Dysfuntion: The Trigger Point Manual,* 308–16.

40. D. J. Clauw, M. Schmidt, D. Radulovic, A. Singer, P. Katz, and J. Bresette, "The relationship between fibromyalgia and interstitial cystitis," *Journal of Psychiatric Research* 31, no. 1 (1997): 125–31.

41. Starlanyl and Copeland, *Fibromyalgia & Chronic Myofascial Pain Syndrome: A Survival Manual,* 44.

42. D. J. Starlanyl, "What Your Urologist Should Know," www.sover.net/~devstar/urol.pdf (accessed May 3, 2001).

43. D. W. Acheson and S. Luccioli, "Microbial-gut interactions in health and disease. Mucosal immune responses," *Best Practice & Research Clinical Gastroenterology* 18, no. 2 (2004): 387–404.

44. Starlanyl and Copeland, *Fibromyalgia & Chronic Myofascial Pain Syndrome: A Survival Manual,* 296.

45. R. Staud, "Are patients with systemic lupus erythematosus at increased risk for fibromyalgia?" *Current Rheumatology Reports* 8, no. 6 (2006): 430–35.

46. Pay, et al., "Evaluation of vascular injury with proinflammatory cytokines, thrombomodulin and fibronectin in patients with primary fibromyalgia."

47. Ibid., 46.

48. Ibid., 46.

49. J. E. Naschltz, I. Rosner, M. Rozenbaum, S. Naschitz, R. Musafia-Priselac, N. Shaviv, M. Fields, H. Isseroff, E. Zuckerman, D. Yeshurun, and E. Sabo, "The head-up tilt test with haemodynamic instability score in diagnosing chronic fatigue syndrome," *QJM* 96, no. 2 (2003): 133–42.

50. R. L. Swezey and J. Adams, "Fibromyalgia: a risk factor for osteoporosis," *Journal of Rheumatology* 26, no. 120 (1999): 2642–44.

51. R. L. Bruno, S. J. Creange, and N. M. Frick, "Parallels between post-polio fatigue and chronic fatigue syndrome: a common pathophysiology?" *The American Journal of Medicine* 105, no. 3A (1998): 66S–73S.

52. M. L. Pall, "Common etiology of posttraumatic stress disorder, fibromyalgia,

chronic fatigue syndrome and multiple chemical sensitivity via elevated nitric oxide/peroxynitrite," *Medical Hypotheses* 57, no. 2 (2001): 139–45.

53. M. J. Pellegrino, D. Van Fossen, C. Gordon, J. M. Ryan, and G. W. Waylonis, "Prevalence of mitral valve prolapse in primary fibromyalgia: a pilot investigation," *Archives of Physical Medicine and Rehabilitation* 70, no. 7 (1989): 541–43.

54. R. M. Bennett, S. R. Clark, S. M. Campbell, S. B. Ingram, C. S. Burckhardt, D. L. Nelson, and J. M. Porter, "Symptoms of Raynaud's syndrome in patients with fibromyalgia. A study utilizing the Nielsen test, digital photoplethysmography, and measurements of platelet alpha 2–adrenergic receptors," *Arthritis & Rheumatism* 34, no. 3 (1991): 264–69.

55. D. J. Starlanyl, personal correspondence to author (March 31, 2005).

56. E. J. Price and P. J. Venables, "Dry eyes and mouth syndrome—a subgroup of patients presenting with sicca symptoms," *Rheumatology* 41, no. 4 (2002): 416–22.

57. D. J. Starlanyl, personal correspondence to author (April 1, 2005).

58. Starlanyl and Copeland, *Fibromyalgia & Chronic Myofascial Pain Syndrome: A Survival Manual,* 48.

59. Ibid., 125–42.

60. Psychological Status in Fibromyalgia and Associated Syndromes based on based on an interview with Muhammad B. Yunus, M.D. http://sh1.webring.com/people/fc/cfsdays/yunus.htm. Accessed September 1, 2009. Original interview, L. Lorden, "It's not all in your head," National Fibromyalgia Association, www.Fmaware.org/patient/research/inyourheadFP.htm (accessed March 17, 2005).

61. I. Mori, "Chronic Pain and the Doctor-Client Relationship—An Action Research Project" (a report of the project up to April 1997), www.moritherapy.org/chronic-pain/chronic-pain-and-the-doctor-patient-relationship/comment-page-1 (accessed August 31, 2009).

62. A. Deale and S. Wessely, "Patients' perceptions of medical care in chronic fatigue syndrome," *Social Science & Medicine* 52, no. 12 (2001): 1859–64.

63. Bernie. Siegel, *Peace, Love and Healing: Bodymind Communication and the Path to Self-healing and Exploration,* 1st ed. (New York: Harper & Row Publishers, 1990), 118.

CHAPTER 3. DIALOGUES WITHIN AND WITHOUT

1. Jenny Fransen and I. Jon. Russell, *The Fibromyalgia Help Book: Practical Guide to Living Better with Fibromyalgia* (St. Paul, Minn.: Smith House Press, 1996), 174.

2. P. McGraw, *O, The Oprah Magazine* (September 2001): 60.

3. Bernie Siegel, *Love, Medicine & Miracles: Lessons Learned about Self-healing from a Surgeon's Experience with Exceptional Patients* (New York: Harper and Row, 1988), 112–24.

4. Lynn Vanderzalm, *Finding Strength in Weakness: Help and Hope for Families Battling Chronic Fatigue Syndrome* (Grand Rapids, Mich.: Zondervan, 1995).

5. C. Eustice and R. Eustice, "Arthritis and Sexuality: pain, fatigue and limitation can interfere," *About.com*, www.arthritis.about.com/cs/sex/a/sexualityarth.htm (accessed December 28, 2004).

6. William Elliott, *Tying Rocks to Clouds: Meetings and Conversations with Wise and Spiritual People* (New York: Doubleday, 1995), 162–75.

7. L. Buscaglia, *The Disabled and Their Parents: A Counseling Challenge* (Thorofare, N.J.: Slack, Inc., 1983).

8. Ibid.

9. M. E. Bedard, "Bankruptcies of the Heart: Secondary Losses from Disabling Chronic Pain," Women's Studies Program, California State University at Fresno, a paper presented by the author at the 1998 Society for Disability Studies Annual Meeting.

10. Dealing with the Temporarily Able Bodied (TABs) [handout], Michigan Handicapper Alliance (1978).

CHAPTER 4. MY BODY IS MATTER AND IT MATTERS

1. C. R. Chapman and M. Stillman, "Pathological Pain," in *Pain and Touch.* Edited by Lawrence Krueger, Morton Friedman, and Edward Carterette (Burlington, Mass.: Elsevier 1996), 315–40.

2. M. Irwin, J. McClintick, C. Costlow, M. Fortner, J. White, and J. C. Gillin, "Partial night sleep deprivation reduces natural killer and cellular immune responses in humans," *Federation of American Societies for Experimental Biology* 10, no. 5 (1996): 643–53.

3. H. Moldofsky, "The assessment and significance of the sleep/waking brain in patients with chronic widespread musculoskeletal pain and fatigue syndromes," *Journal of Musculoskeletal Pain* 15 Suppl. no. 13 (2007): 4 [Myopain 2007 poster].

4. B. Kundermann, J. C. Krieg, W. Schreiber, and S. Lautenbacher, "The effect of sleep deprivation on pain," *Pain Research & Management* 9, no. 1 (2004): 25–32.

5. M. Irwin, et al., "Partial night sleep deprivation reduces natural killer and cellular immune responses in humans."

6. A. R. Gold, F. Dipalo, M. S. Gold, and J. Broderick, "Inspiratory airflow dynamics during sleep in women with fibromyalgia," *Sleep* 27, no. 3 (2004): 459–66.

7. E. R. Unger, R. Nisenbaum, H. Moldofsk, A. Cesta, C. Sammut M. Reyes, and W. C. Reeves, "Sleep assessment in a population-based study of chronic fatigue syndrome," *BMC Neurology* 4, no. 1 (2004): 6.

8. M. L. Mahowald and M. W. Mahowald, "Nighttime sleep and daytime functioning, sleepiness and fatigue, in well-defined chronic rheumatic diseases," *Journal of Clinical Sleep Medicine* 1, no. 3 (2000): 179–93.

9. H. K. Moldofsky, "Disordered sleep in fibromyalgia and related myofascial pain condition," *Journal of Clinical Dentistry, North America* 45, no. 4 (2001): 701–13.

10. E. Vazquez-Delgado, J. Schmidt, C. Carlson, R. DeLeeuw, and J. Okeson, "Psychological and sleep quality differences between chronic daily headache and temporomandibular disorders patients," *Cephalgia* 24, no. 6 (2004): 446–54.

11. M. K. Millott and R. M. Berlin, "Treating sleep disorders in patients with fibromyalgia: exercise, behavior, and drug therapy may all help," *Journal of Musculoskeletal Medicine* 14 (1993): 25–28.

12. N. Ishii, T. Iwata, M. Dakeishi, and K. Murata, "Effects of shift work on autonomic and neuromotor function in female nurses," *Journal of Occupational Health* 46, no. 5 (2004): 352–58.

13. J. C. Rains and D. B. Penzien, "Sleep and chronic pain: challenges to the alpha-EEG sleep pattern as a pain specific sleep anomaly," *Journal of Psychosomatic Research* 54, no. 1 (2003): 77–83.

14. A. Korszun, L. Sackett, Lundeen, E. Papadopoulos, C. Brucksch, L. Masterson, N. C. Engelberg, E. Hause, M. A. Demitrack, and L. Crofford, "Melatonin levels in women with fibromyalgia and chronic fatigue syndrome," *Journal of Rheumatology* 26, no. 12 (1999): 2675–80.

15. Joint Commission on Accreditation of Health Care Organizations (JCAHO), Pain Mangement, www.jointcommission.org/NewsRoom/health_care_issues.htm#9 (accessed September 1, 2009)

16. C. S. Hill Jr., "Government regulatory influences on opiod prescribing and their impact on the treatment of pain of nonmalignant origin," *Journal of Pain Symptom Management* 11, no. 5 (1996): 287.

17. S. D. Passik and H. J. Weinreb, "Managing chronic non-malignant pain: overcoming obstacles to the use of opiods," *Advances in Therapy* 17, no. 2 (2000): 70–83.

18. G. Kansky, "The Illegal Creation of Neurontin," *The National Forum* 6, no. 4 (2003): 14.

19. L. J. Crofford, P. J. Mease, S. L. Simpson, J. P. Young Jr., S. A. Martin, G. M. Haig, and U. Sharma, "Fibromyalgia relapse evaluation and efficacy for durability of meaningful relief (FREEDOM)," *Pain* 136, no. 3 (2008) 419–31 (e-publication ahead of print April 8, 2008).

20. D. R. Grothe, B. Scheckner, and D. Albano, "Treatment of pain syndromes with venlafaxine," *Journal of Clinical Pharmacology, Therapy and Toxicology* 24, no. 5 (2004): 621–29.

21. S. R. Savage, "Assessment for addiction in pain-treatment setting," *Clinical Journal of Pain* 18, Suppl. no. 4 (2002): S28–S38.

22. Ibid.

23. B. H. McCarberg and R. L. Barkin, "Long-acting opiods for chronic pain: pharmacolacotherapeutic opportunities to enhance compliance, quality of life and analgesia," *American Journal of Therapeutics* 8, no. 3 (2001): 181–86.

24. H. A. Heit, "The truth about pain management: the difference between a pain patient and an addicted patient," *European Journal of Pain* 5, Suppl. no. A (2001): 27–29.

25. P. Comptom, P. Athanasos, "Chronic pain, substance abuse and addiction," *Nursing Clinics of North America* 38, no. 3 (2003): 525–37.

26. J. Devulder, U. Richarz, S. H. Nataraja, "Impact of long-term use of opioids on quality of life in patients with chronic, non-malignant pain," *Current Medical Research and Opinion* 21, no. 10 (2005): 1555–68.

27. D. S. Ciccone, N. Just, E. B. Bandilla, E. Reimer, M. S. Ilbeigi, and W. Wu, "Psychological correlates of opiods use in patients with chronic non-malignant pain: a preliminary test of the downhill spiral hypothese," *Journal of Pain Symptom Management* 29, no. 3 (2000): 180–92.

28. R. Galski, J. B. Williams, and H. T. Ehle, "Effects of opiods on driving ability," *Journal of Pain Symptom Management* 19, no. 3 (2000): 200–08.

29. M. L. Mahowald, J. A. Singh, and P. Majeski, "Opioid use by patients in an orthopedics spine clinic," *Arthritis & Rheumatism* 52, no. 1 (2005): 312–21.

30. G. W. Pasternak, "The pharmacology of mu analgesics: from patients to genes," *Neuroscientist* 7, no. 3 (2001): 220–31.

31. R. E. Harris, D. J. Clauw, D. J. Scott, S. A. McLean, R. H. Graceley, and J. K. Zubieta, "Decreased central mu-opioid receptor availability in fibromyalgia," *Journal of Neuroscience* 27, no. 37 (2007): 10000–06.

32. Savage, "Assessment for addiction in pain-treatment setting."

33. D. T. Cowan, L. Allan, and S. P. Griffith, "A pilot study into the problematic use of opiod analgesics in chronic non-cancer pain patients," *International Journal of Nursing Studies* 39, no. 1 (2002): 59–69.

34. C. B. Willmore, K. L. LaVecchia, and J. L. Wiley, "NMDA antagonists produce site-selective impairment of accuracy in delayed nonmatch-to-sample task in rats," *NeuroPharmacology* 41, no. 8 (2001): 916–27.

35. P. M. McConaghy, P. McSorley, W. McCaughey, and W. I. Campbell, "Dextromethorphan and pain after total abdominal hysterectomy," *British Journal of Anaesthesia* 81, no. 5 (1998): 731–36.

36. Ibid.

37. G. J. Bennett, "Update on the neurophysiology of pain transmission and modulation: focus on the NMDA-receptor," *Journal of Pain and Symptom Management* 19, Suppl. no. 1 (2000): S2–S6.

38. E. B. Russo, "Clinical endocannabinoid deficiency (CECD): Can this concept explain therapeutic benefits of cannabis in migraine, fibromyalgia, irritable bowel syndrome and other treatment-resistant conditions?" *Neuroendocrinol Letter* 2, no. 2 (2008): 192–200.

39. Adapted from materials provided by the American Pain Society, "Marijuana-based drug reduces fibromyalgia pain, study suggests," *Science Daily* (February 18, 2008), retrieved from www.sciencedaily.com/releases/2008/02/080217214547 .htm (accessed September 2009).

40. R. W. Foltin, M. W. Fischman, and M. F. Byrne, "Effects of smoked marijuana on food intake and body weight of humans living in a residential laboratory," *Appetite* 11 (1988): 1–14.

41. M. S. Rosenthal and H. D. Kleber, "Making sense of medical marijuana," *Proceedings of the Association of American Physicians,* 111, no. 2 (1999): 159–65.

42. G. D. Carlo and A. A. Izzo, "Cannabinoids for gastrointestinal diseases: potential therapeutic applications," *Expert Opinion on Investigational Drugs* 12, no. 1 (2003): 39–49.

43. Cannabis drug cuts arthritis pain, BBC News, http://news.bbc.co.uk/2/hi/health/3790227.stm (June 9, 2004).

44. J. L. Croxford, "Therapeutic potential of cannabinoids in CNS disease," *CNS Drugs* 17, no. 3 (2003): 179–202.

45. T. W. Klein, "Cannabinoid-based drugs as anti-inflammatory therapeutics," *Nature Reviews Immunology* 5, no. 5 (2005): 400–11.

46. I. Mainville, Y. Arcand, and E. R. Farnworth, "A dynamic model that simulates the human upper gastrointestinal tract for the study of probiotics," *International Journal of Food Microbiology* 99, no. 3 (2000): 2872–96.

47. J. L. Swerdlow, *Nature's Medicine: Plants That Heal* (Washington, D.C.: National Geographic Society, 2000), 302.

48. J. N. Hathcock, A. Azzi, J. Blumberg, T. Bray, A. Dickinson, B. Fre, I. Jialal, C. S. Johnston, F. J. Kelly, K. Kraemer, L. Packer, S. Parthasarathy, H. Sies, and M. G. Traber, "Vitamins E and C are safe across a broad range of intakes," *American Journal of Clinical Nutrition* 81, no. 4 (2005): 736–45.

49. Swerdlow, *Nature's Medicine: Plants That Heal*, 390.

50. M. F. McCarty, "Chromium picolinate may favorably influence the vascular risk associated with smoking by combating cortisol-induced insulin resistance," *Medical Hypotheses* 64, no. 6 (2005): 1220–24.

51. W. J. Kong, Y. C. Han, Y. Wang, Y. J. Hu, J. Liu, and Q. Wang, "Protective roles of vitamin E and coenzyme Q10 in the inner ear mitochondrial DNA 4834 bp deletion mutation of rats," *Zhonghua Er Bi Yan Hou Ke Za Zhi* 39, no. 12 (2004): 707–11 [Chinese].

52. R. Sahelian, S. Borken, "Dehydroepiandrosterone and cardiac arrhythmia," *Annals of Internal Medicine* 129, no. 7 (1998): 588.

53. O. Bruyere, K. Pavelka, L. C. Rovati, R. Deroisy, M. Olejarova, J. Gatterova, G. Giacovelli, and J. Y. Reginster, "Glucosamine sulfate reduces osteoarthritis progression in postmenopausal women with knee osteoarthritis: evidence from two 3-year studies," *Menopause* 11, no. 2 (2004): 138–43.

54. Devin J. Starlanyl and Mary E. Copeland, *Fibromyalgia & Chronic Myofascial Pain: A Survival Manual,* 2nd ed. (Oakland, Calif.: New Harbinger Publications, Inc., 2001), 170–71.

55. D. J. Starlanyl, J. L. Jeffrey, G. Roentsch, and C. Taylor-Olson, "The effect of transdermal T3 (3, 3', 5–triiodothyronine) on geloid masses found in patients

with both fibromyalgia and myofascial pain: double-blinded, N of 1 clinical study," *Myalgies International* 2, no. 2: 8–18.

56. D. Bagchi, C. K. Sen, S. D. Ray, D. K. Das, M. Bagchi, H. G. Preuss, and J. A. Vinson, "Molecular mechanisms of cardio-protection by novel grape seed proanthocyanidins extract," *Mutation Research* 523–524 (2003): 87–97.

57. R. M. Bennett, "Adult growth hormone deficiency in patients with fibromyalgia." *Current Rheumatology Reports* 4, no. 4 (2002): 306–12.

58. M. Nicolodi and F. Sicuteri, "Fibromyalgia and migraine, two faces of the same mechanism: serotonin as the common clue for pathogenesis and therapy," *Advances in Experimental Medicine and Biology* 398 (1996): 373–79.

59. Caruso, et al., "Double blind study of 5–hydroytryptophan versus placebo in the treatment of primary fibromyalgia syndrome," *Journal of International Medical Research* 18 (1990): 201–9.

60. P. S. Puttine and I. Caruso, "Primary fibromyalgia syndrome and 5–hydroxy-L-tryptophan, a 90-day open study," *Journal of International Medical Research* 20 (1992): 182–89.

61. K. Shinomiya, T. Inoue, Y. Utsu, S. Tokunaga, T. Masuoka, A. Ohmori, and C. Kamei, "Effects of kava-kava extract on the sleep-wake cycle in sleep-disturbed rats," *PsychoPharmacology* 180, no.3 (2005) 564–69.

62. T. J. Romano and J. W. Stiller, "Magnesium deficiency in fibromyalgia syndrome," *Journal of Nutritional Medicine* 4 (1994): 165–67.

63. B. M. Altura and B. T. Altura, "Tension headaches and muscle tension: is there a role for magnesium?" *Medical Hypotheses* 57, no. 6 (2001): 705–13.

64. Ibid.

65. G. Abraham, "Management of fibromyalgia: rationale for the use of magnesium and malic acid," *Journal of Nutritional Medicine* 3 (1992): 49–59.

66. J. Sonsiadek (chiropractic physician, biochemist), personal correspondence to author (June 2008).

67. I. J. Russell, J. E. Michalek, J. D. Flechas, and G. E. Abraham, "Treatment of fibromyalgia syndrome with Super Malic: a randomized, double blind, placebo controlled, crossover pilot study," *Journal of Rheumatology* 22, no. 5 (1995): 953–58.

68. D. E. Moulin, "Systemic drug treatment for chronic musculoskeletal pain," *Clinical Journal of Pain* 17, Suppl. no. 4 (2001): S86–93.

69. U. D. Rohr and J. Herold, "Melatonin deficiencies in women," *Maturitas* 41, Suppl. no. 1 (2002): S85–S104 [German].

70. G. Williams, J. Waterhouse, J. Mugarza, D. Minors, and K. Hayden, "Therapy of circadian rhythm disorders in chronic fatigue syndrome: no symptomatic improvement with melatonin or phototherapy," *European Journal of Clinical Investigation* 32, no. 11 (2002): 831–37.

71. S. Naylor and G. J. Gleich, "Over-the-counter melatonin products and contamination," *American Family Physician* 59, no. 2 (1999): 284, 287–88.

72. F. W. Turek and M. U. Gillette, "Melatonin, sleep, and circadian rhythms: rationale for development of specific melatonin agonists," *Journal of Clinical Sleep Medicine* 5, no. 6 (2004): 523–32.

73. G. D. Birkmayer, G. G. Kay, and E. Vurre, "Stabilized NADH (ENADA) improves jet lag-induced cognitive performance deficit," *Wien Med Wochenschr* 152, no. 17–18 (2002): 450–54.

74. L. M. Forsyth, H. G. Preuss, A. L. MacDowell, L. Chiazze, Jr., G. D. Birkmayer, J. A. Bellanti, "Therapeutic effects of oral NADH on the symptoms of patients with chronic fatigue syndrome," *Ann Aller Asthma Immunol* 82, no. 2 (1999): 185–91.

75. S. Ozgocmen, S. A. Catal, O. Ardicoglu, and A. Kamanli, "Effect of omega-3 fatty acids in the management of fibromyalgia syndrome," *International Journal of Clinical Pharmacology and Therapeutics* 38, no. 7 (2000): 362–63.

76. B. K. Puri, J. Holmes, and G. Hamilton, "Eicosapentaenoic acid-rich essential fatty acid supplementation in chronic fatigue syndrome associated with symptom remission and structural brain changes," *International Journal of Clinical Practice* 58, no. 3 (2004): 297–99.

77. R. Staud, "Fibromyalgia pain: do we know the source?" *Current Opinion in Rheumatology* 16, no. 2 (2004): 157–63.

78. R. A. Shippy, D. Mendez, K. Jones, I. Cergnul, and S. E. Karpiak, "S-adenosylmethionine (SAM-e) for the treatment of depression in people living with HIV/AIDS," *BMC Psychiatry* 4, no. 38.

79. *Arthritis Today* on-line supplement guide, www.arthritistoday.org/treatments/supplement-guide/supplements/sam-e.php (accessed August 2009).

80. www.nlm.nih.gov/medlineplus/druginfo/natural/patient-stjohnswort.html (accessed August 25, 2009).

81. D. V. Awang and A. Fugh-Berman, "Herbal interactions with cardiovascular drugs," *Journal of Cardiovascular Nursing* 16, no. 4 (2002): 64–70.

82. J. S. Markowitz and C. L. DeVane, "The emerging recognition of herb-drug interactions with a focus on St. John's wort (Hypercium perforatum)," *Psychopharmacology Bulletin* 35, no. 1 (2001): 53–64.

83. K. P. White and M. Harth, "An Analytical Review of 24 Controlled Clinical Trials for Fibromyalgia Syndrome (FMS)," *Pain* 64 (1996): 211–19.

84. J. A. Wilken, R. L. Kane, A. K. Ellis, E. Rafeiro, M. P. Briscoe, C. L. Sullivan, and J. H. Day, "A comparison of the effect of diphenhydramine and desloratadine on vigilance and cognitive function during treatment of ragweed-induced allergic rhinitis," *Annals of Allergy, Asthma and Immunology* 91, no. 4 (2003): 375–385.

85. Starlanyl and Copeland, *Fibromyalgia and Chronic Myofascial Pain Syndrome: A Survival Manual,* 263.

86. Z. H. Cho, S. C. Chung, J. P. Jones, H. J. Park, H. J. Lee, E. K. Wong, and B. I. Min, "Corresponding brain cortices using functional MRI," *Proceedings of the National Academy of Sciences* 95, no. 5 (1998): 2670–73.

87. G. Goddard, H. Karibe, C. McNeil, and E. Villafuerte, "Acupuncture and sham acupuncture reduce muscle pain in myofascial pain patients," *Journal of Orofacial Pain* 16, no. 1 (2002): 71–76.

88. National Institutes of Health, Overview of NIH Consensus Conference: Acupuncture, [no authors listed], *JAMA* 280, no. 17 (1998): 1518–24.

89. B. Duncan, A. White, and A. Rahman, "Acupuncture in the treatment of fibromyalgia in tertiary care—a case series," *Acupuncture in Medicine* 25, no. 4 (2007): 137–47.

90. A. B. Newberg, P. J. Lariccia, B. Y. Lee, J. T. Farrar, L. Lee, and A. Alavi, "Cerebral blood flow effects of pain and acupuncture: a preliminary single-photon emission computed tomography imaging study," *Journal of Neuroimaging* 15, no. 1 (2005): 43–49.

91. D. Munguía-Izquierdo and A. Legaz-Arrese, "Exercise in warm water decreases pain and improves cognitive function in middle-aged women with fibromyalgia," *Clinical and Experimental Rheumatology* 25, no. 6 (2007): 823–30.

92. R. Neblett, R. J. Gatchel, and T. G. Mayer, "A clinical guide to surface-EMG-assisted stretching as an adjunct to chronic musculoskeletal pain rehabilitation," *Applied Psychophysiology and Biofeedback* 28, no. 2 (2003): 147–60.

93. A. S. Babu, E. Mathew, D. Danda, et al., "Management of patients with fibromyalgia using biofeedback: a randomized control trial," *Indian Journal of Medical Sciences* 61, no. 8 (2007): 455–61.

94. D. C. Hammond, "Treatment of chronic fatigue with neurofeedback and self hypnosis," *NeuroRehabilitation* 16, no. 4 (2001): 295–300.

95. American Dietetic Association, Position of the American Dietetic Association: Food fortification and dietary supplements, *Journal of the American Dietetic Association* 101, no. 1 (2001): 115–25.

96. R. S. Ivker and T. Nelson, *Arthritis Survival: The Holistic Medical Treatment Program for Osteoarthritis* (New York: Jeremy P. Tarcher, an imprint of Penguin Group, Inc., 2001).

97. I. R. Bell, C. M. Baldwin, E. Stoltz, B. T. Walsh, and G. E. Schwartz, "EEG Beta 1 oscillation and sucrose sensitization in fibromyalgia with chemical intolerance," *International Journal of Neuroscience,* 180, no. 102 (2001): 31–42.

98. T. Hung, J. L. Sievenpiper, A. Marchie, C. W. Kendall, and D. J. Jenkins, "Fat versus carbohydrates in insulin resistance, obesity, diabetes and cardiovascular disease," *Current Opinion in Clinical Nutrition & Metabolic Care* 6, no. 2 (2003): 165–76.

99. Starlanyl and Copeland, *Fibromyalgia and Chronic Myofascial Pain Syndrome: A Survival Manual,* 297–99.

100. P. E. Cryer, "Symptoms of hypoglycemia, thresholds for their occurrence and hypoglycemia unawareness," *Endocrinology and Metabolism Clinics of North America* 28, no. 3 (1999): 495–500, v-vi.

101. Starlanyl and Copeland, *Fibromyalgia and Chronic Myofascial Pain Syndrome: A Survival Manual,* 298.

102. Ibid., 47, 297.

103. J. F. Brun, C. Fedou, and J. Mercier, "Postprandial reactive hypoglycemia," *Diabetes/Metabolism Research and Reviews* 26, no. 5 (2000): 337–51.

104. D. G. Simons and J. Goodgold, eds., *Rehabilitation Medicine,* "Myofascial pain syndrome due to trigger points," (St. Louis: Mosby, 1988), 686–732.

105. R. D. Oles, "Glucose intolerance associated with temporomandibular joint pain-dysfunction syndrome," *Oral Surgery, Oral Medicine, Oral Pathology, Oral Radiology and Endodontology* 43, no. 4 (1977): 546–53.

106. Starlanyl and Copeland, *Fibromyalgia and Chronic Myofascial Pain Syndrome: A Survival Manual,* 298.

107. B. Sears, *Zone-Perfect Meals in Minutes* (New York: Harper Collins, 1997).

108. Food pyramid, http://encyclopedia2.thefreedictionary.com/food+pyramid (accessed September, 2009).

109. Dietary Guidelines for Americans 2005, www.health.gov/DietaryGuidelines/ (accessed September, 2009).

110. World Health Organization, www.who.int/dietphysicalactivity/diet/en/index .html (accessed August 26, 2009).

111. David Simons, Janet Travell, and Lois. S. Simons, *Myofascial Pain and Dysfunction: The Trigger Point Manual,* Vol. I, 2nd ed. (Baltimore: Williams and Wilkins, 1999), 149.

112. R. L. Swezey, A. Swezey, and J. Adams, "Isometric progressive resistive exercise for osteoporosis," *Journal of Rheumatology* 27, no. 5 (2000): 1260–64.

113. E. Bourne, *The Anxiety & Phobia Workbook,* 4th ed. (Oakland, Calif.: New Harbinger Publications, 2005).

114. K. Lewit and D. G. Simons, "Myofascial pain: relief by post-isometric relaxation," *Archives of Physical Medicine and Rehabilitation* 65, no. 8 (1984): 452–56.

115. D. S. Rooks, C. B. Silverman, and F. G. Kantrowitz, "The effects of progressive strength training and aerobic exercise on muscle strength and cardiovascular fitness in women with fibromyalgia: a pilot study," *Arthritis & Rheumatism* 47, no. 1 (2002): 22–28.

116. C. R. Snell, J. M. Vanness, D. R. Strayer, and S. R. Stevens, "Exercise capacity and immune function in male and female patients with chronic fatigue syndrome (CFS)," *In Vivo* 19, no. 2 (2005): 387–90.

117. C. D. Black, P. J. O'Connor, and K. K. McCully, "Increased daily physical activity and fatigue symptoms in chronic fatigue syndrome," *Dynamic Medicine* 4, no. 1 (2005): 3.

118. Starlanyl and Copeland, *Fibromyalgia and Chronic Myofascial Pain: A Survival Manual,* 222.

119. M. van Santen, P. Bolin, R. Landewe, F. Verstappen, C. Bakker, A. Hidding, D. van Der Kemp, H. Houben, and S. van Der Linden, "High or low intensity aerobic fitness training in fibromyalgia: does it matter?" *Journal of Rheumatology* 3 (March 2002): 582–87.

120. C. Sieverling, "Dr. Cheney's Basic Treatment Plan for Chronic Fatigue Syndrome," Prohealth.com/library (accessed September, 2009).

121. R. Jahnke, "The Most Profound Medicine, II," *Townsend Letter for Doctors* 91/92 (1991): 124.

122. B. Douglas, *The Complete Idiot's Guide to T'ai Chi & QiGong* (New York: Alpha Books, 1999).

123. K. W. Chen, A. L. Hassett, F. Hou, J. Staller, and A. S. Lichtbroun, "A pilot study of external qigong therapy for patients with fibromyalgia," *Journal of Alternative and Complementary Medicine* 12, no. 9 (2006): 851–56.

124. Y. I. Shin and M. S. Lee, "Qi therapy (external qigong) for chronic fatigue syndrome: case studies," *American Journal of Chinese Medicine* 33, no. 1 (2005): 139–41.

125. G. D. Silva, G. Lorenzi-Filho, and L. V. Lage, "Effects of yoga and the addition of tui na in patients with fibromyalgia," *Journal of Alternative and Complementary Medicine* 13, no. 10 (2007): 1107–14.

126. S. E. Bentler, A. J. Hartz, and E. M. Kuhn, "Prospective observational study of treatments for unexplained chronic fatigue," *Journal of Clinical Psychiatry* 66, no. 5 (2005): 625–32.

127. Ibid.

128. C. Hassed, "How humor keeps you well," *Australian Family Physician* 30, no. 1 (2001): 25–28.

129. I. H. Jonsdottir, "Exercise immunology: neuroendocrine regulation of NK-cells," *International Journal of Sports Medicine* 21, Suppl. no. 1 (2000): S20–S30.

130. Starlanyl and Copeland, *Fibromyalgia and Chronic Myofascial Pain Syndrome: A Survival Manual,* 237.

131. B. Denison, "Touch the pain away: new research on therapeutic touch and persons with fibromyalgia syndrome," *Holistic Nursing Practice* 18, no. 3 (2004): 142–51.

132. Clair Davies, personal correspondence to author (April 13, 2005).

133. A. A. Deodhar, R. A. Fisher, C. V. Blacker, and A. D. Woolf, "Fluid retention syndrome and fibromyalgia," *British Journal of Rheumatology* 33, no. 6 (1994): 576–82.

134. D. J. Starlanyl, personal correspondence to author (April 11, 2005).

135. S. M. Johnson, M. E. Kurtz, "Perceptions of philosophic and practice differences between U.S. osteopathic physicians and their allopathic counterparts," *Social Science & Medicine* 55, no. 12 (2002): 2141–48.

136. B. Williams, D.O., personal communication (August 8, 2003).

137. W. R. Nielson and R. Weir, "Biopsychosocial approaches to the treatment of chronic pain," *The Clinical Journal of Pain* 17, Suppl. no. 4 (2001): S114–S127.

138. W. P. Hanten, S. L. Olson, N. L. Butts, and A. L. Nowicki, "Effectiveness of a home program of ischemic pressure followed by sustained stretch for treatment of myofascial trigger points," *Physical Therapy* 80, no. 10 (2000): 997–1003.

139. Janet G. Travell and David G. Simons, *Myofascial Pain and Dysfunction: The Trigger Point Manual* (Baltimore: Lippincott, Williams & Wilkins, 1983), 126–47.

140. Ibid.

141. Starlanyl and Copeland, *Fibromyalgia and Chronic Myofascial Pain Syndrome: A Survival Manual,* 227–28.

142. Ibid.

143. J. Borg-Stein and D. G. Simons, "Focused review: Myofascial pain," *Archives of Physical Medicine and Rehabilitation* 83, no. 3, Suppl. no. 1 (2002): 540–47, S48–49.

144. C. Z. Hong, "Lidocaine injection versus dry needling to myofascial trigger point: The importance of the local twitch response," *American Journal of Physical Medicine & Rehabilitation* 73 (1994): 256–63.

145. Starlanyl and Copeland, *Fibromyalgia and Chronic Myofascial Pain Syndrome: A Survival Manual,* 288–89.

146. Ibid., 288–89.

147. Ibid., 288.

148. John Whiteside, "Myofascial Pain Syndromes and Trigger Point Injection Therapy," www.pain-education.com/100134.php (accessed September 2009).

149. G. Sheean, "Botulinum toxin for the treatment of musculoskeletal pain and spasm," *Current Pain and Headache Reports* 6, no. 6 (2002): 460–69.

150. J. De Andres, G. Cerda-Olmedo, J. C. Valia, V. Monsalve, D. Lopez-Alarcón, and A. Minguez, "Use of botulinum toxin in the treatment of chronicmyofascial pain," *Clinical Journal of Pain* 19, no. 4 (2003): 269–75.

151. C. K. Hou, L. C. Tsai, K. F. Cheng, K. C. Chung, and C. Z. Hong, "Immediate effects of various physical therapeutic modalities on cervical myofascial pain and trigger point sensitivity," *Archives of Physical Medicine and Rehabilitation* 83, no. 10 (2002): 1406–14.

152. D. A. Lake, "Neuromuscular electrical stimulation: an overview and its application in the treatment of sports injuries," *Sports Medicine* 13, no. 5 (1992): 320–36.

153. F. L. Cramp, G. Noble, A. J. Lowe, D. M. Walsh, and J. C. Willer, "A controlled study on the effects of transcutaneous electrical neuro stimulation and interferential therapy upon the RIII nociceptive and H-reflexes in humans," *Archives of Physical Medicine and Rehabilitation* 81, no. 3 (2000): 324–33.

154. "What Is CAM?" National Center for Complementary and Alternative Medicine Health Info, www.nccam.nih.gov/health/whatiscam/ (accessed September, 2009).

155. Ibid.

156. M. Ebell and E. Beck, "How effective are complementary/alternative medicine (CAM) therapies for fibromyalgia?" *Journal of Family Practice* 50, no. 5 (2001): 400.

157. N. Afari, D. M. Eisenberg, R. Herrell, J. Goldberg, E. Kleyman, S. Ashton, and D. Buchwald, "Use of alternative treatments by chronic fatigue syndrome discordant twins," *Integrative Medicine* 2, no. 2 (2000): 97–103.

158. C. Barbour, "Use of complementary and alternative treatments by individuals with fibromyalgia syndrome," *Journal of the American Academy of Nurse Practitioners* 12, no. 8 (2000): 311–16.

159. D. L. Goldenberg, C. Burckhardt, and L. Crofford, "Management of Fibromyalgia Syndrome," *JAMA* 292, no. 19 (2004): 2388–95.

160. R. H. Gracely, F. Petske, J. M. Wolf, and D. J. Clauw, "Functional magnetic resonance imaging evidence of augmented pain processing in fibromyalgia," *Arthritis & Rheumatism* 46, no. 5 (2002): 1333–43.

161. P. Schweinhardt, K. M. Sauro, and M. C. Bushnell, "Fibromyalgia: a disorder of the brain?" *Neuroscientist* 14, no. 5, (2008): 415–21.

162. A. J. Cleare, "The HPA axis and the genesis of chronic fatigue syndrome," *Trends in Endocrinology and Metabolism* 15, no. 2 (2004): 55–59.

CHAPTER 5. THE POWER OF MIND, BODY, AND SPIRIT

1. M. Gustafsson, J. Ekholm, and A. Ohman, "From shame to respect: musculoskeletal pain patients experience of rehabilitation programme, a qualitative study," *Journal of Rehabilitation Medicine* 36, no. 3 (2004): 97–103.

2. Viane, et al., "Acceptance of pain is an independent predictor of mental well-being in patients with chronic pain: empirical evidence and reappraisal."

3. P. Arnstein, C. Wells-Federman, and M. Caudill, "The effect of an integrated cognitive-behavioral pain management program on pain intensity, self-efficacy beliefs and depression in chronic pain patients on completion and one year later," *Pain Medicine* 2, no. 3 (2001): 238–39.

4. William Elliott, *Tying Rocks to Clouds: Meetings and Conversations with Wise and Spiritual People* (New York: Doubleday, 1995), 215–22.

5. Ibid., 216.

6. Ibid.

7. *Spirituality and Medicine*, Med CEU. www.medceu.com/course.cfm?CID=563 (accessed September 20, 2002).

8. L. Dossey, *Prayer Is Good Medicine: How to Reap the Healing Benefits of Prayer* (San Francisco: HarperCollins, 1996).

9. R. Walsh, *Essential Spirituality: The 7 Central Practices to Awaken Heart and Mind* (New York: John Wiley & Sons, Inc., 1999).

10. E. A. Dedert, J. L. Studts, I. Weissbecker, P. G. Salmon, P. L. Banis, and S. E. Sephton, "Religiosity may help preserve the cortisol rhythm in women with stress-related illness," *International Journal of Psychiatry in Medicine* 34, no. 1 (2004): 61–77.

11. Elliott, *Tying Rocks to Clouds,* 76–98.

12. Ibid.

13. Ibid.

14. I. Viane, G. Crombez, C. Eccleston, C. Poppe, J. Devulder, B. Van Houdenhove, and W. De Corte, "Acceptance of pain is an independent predictor of mental well-being in patients with chronic pain: empirical evidence and reappraisal," *Pain* 106, no. 1–2 (2003): 65–72.

15. Elliot, *Tying Rocks to Clouds,* 26–44.

16. Ibid., 52–60.

17. J. Kabat-Zinn, *Full Catastrophe Living: Using the Wisdom of Your Body and Mind to Face Stress, Pain and Illness* (New York: Delta, 1990).

18. Elliot, *Tying Rocks to Clouds,* 61–75.

19. Ibid., 120–32.

20. Ibid., 144–48.

21. Ibid.

22. Ibid., 149–61.

23. Ibid.

24. Ibid., 162–75.

25. Ibid.

26. Ibid.

27. Ibid.

28. Ibid., 223–35.

29. Ibid.

30. Ibid.

31. Ibid.

32. K. E. Ferner, "Mind-body-spirit, treating the whole person," *Paradigm* 7, no. 1 (2003): 8–9.

33. Ibid.

34. W. Elliot, *Tying Rocks to Clouds,* 76–98

35. Bernie Siegel, *Peace, Love and Healing: Body-mind Communication and the Path to Self-healing and Exploration,* 1st ed. (NY: Harper & Row Publishers, 1990).

36. D. Cheek, "Fibromyalgia, Creative Imagery and Healing," reprinted from Suite 101.com, www.healingwell.com/library/fibro/cheek3.asp (accessed September, 2009).

37. E. A. Fors, H. Sexton, and K. G. Gotestam, "The effect of guided imagery and amitriptyline on daily fibromyalgia pain: a prospective, randomized, controlled trial," *Journal of Psychiatric Research* 36, no. 3 (2002): 179–87.

38. *Science, Spirit and Soul: Toward a New Model of Healing* with Larry Dossey, M.D. at the Conference: Expanding the Spectrum of Medicine, Sounds True Series, audio recording available from http://shop.soundstrue.com/authors.soundstrue.com/author.

39. R. C. Byrd, "Positive therapeutic effects of intercessory prayer in a coronary care unit population," *Southern Medical Journal* 81, no. 7 (1988): 826–29.

40. Jon Kabat-Zinn, *Mindfulness Meditation, Cultivating the Wisdom of Your Body and Mind.* Audio recording by Simon & Schuster Sound Ideas, 1988.

41. Elliott, *Tying Rocks to Clouds,* 159.

42. Ibid.*,* 125.

43. J. Donovan, *Handbook to a Happier Life: A Simple Guide to Creating the Life You've Always Wanted* (Buckingham, Pa.: Bovan Publishing Group, Inc., 1996).

CHAPTER 6. DEALING WITH CIRCUIT OVERLOAD

1. K. Campbell and D. G. Cowan, *Neuropsychological Deficits Associated with Chronic Fatigue Syndrome.* Unpublished master's thesis, University of Missouri–Kansas City (2002).

2. D. C. Park, J. M. Glass, M. Minear, and L. J. Crofford, "Cognitive function in fibromyalgia patients," *Arthritis & Rheumatism* 44, no. 9 (2001): 2125–33.

3. Starlanyl and Copeland, *Fibromyalgia & Chronic Myofascial Pain Syndrome: A Survival Manual,* 16–17, 140.

4. Ibid., 297.

5. B. D. Dick and S. Rashiq, "Disruption of attention and working memory traces in individuals with chronic pain," *Anesthesia & Analgesia* 104, no. 5 (2007): 1223–29.

6. A. V. Apkarian, Y. Sosa, B. R. Krauss, P. S. Thomas, B. E. Fredrickson, R. E. Levy, R. N. Harden, and D. R. Chialvo, "Chronic pain patients are impaired on an emotional decision-making task," *Pain* 108, no. 1–2 (2004): 129–36.

7. Swami Beyondananda (Steve Bhaerman), *Driving Your Own Karma: Swami Beyondananda's Tour Guide to Enlightenment* (Rochester, Vt.: Inner Traditions, 1989).

8. Ibid.

CHAPTER 7. APPROACHING THE SYSTEM SYSTEMATICALLY

1. ADA, Americans with Disabilities Act homepage, www.ncd.gov/newsroom/publications/2006/ada16years.htm/ (accessed September 2009).

2. Job Accommodation Network, ADA: A Brief Overview, www.jan.wvu.edu/links/adasummary.htm (accessed September 2009).

3. The ADA questions and answers, www.eeoc.gov/facts/adaqa1.html (accessed September 2009).

4. S. Cooper, human resource specialist, personal correspondence with author (April 20, 2005).

5. F. Kavaler and A. D. Spiegel, *Risk Management in Health Care Institutions: A Strategic Approach* (Sudbury, Mass.: Jones and Bartlett Publishers, 1997), 63–64.

6. Cooper, personal correspondence with author.

7. Ibid.

8. Technical Assistance Manual: Title I of the ADA, www.jan.wvu.edu/links/adatam1.html (accessed, September, 2009).

9. Americans with Disabilities Act, Tax Incentives, www.ada.gov/taxpack.htm (accessed September 2009).

10. U.S. Department of Labor website, Equal Employment Opportunity, www.dol
   .gov/dol/topic/discrimination/disabilitydisc.htm (accessed September 2009).

11. Cooper, personal correspondence.

12. Ibid.

13. Disability.gov, "Tax Information," www.disability.gov/employment/employer_
   resources/tax_information (accessed September 2009).

14. EEOC, Equal Employment Opportunity Commission, www.eeoc.gov (accessed
   September 2009).

15. Ibid.

16. Ibid.

17. Job Accommodation Network, "ADA: A Brief Overview," www.jan.edu/links/
   adasummary.htm (accessed September 2009).

18. Kavaler and Spiegel, *Risk Management in Health Care Institutions: A Strategic
   Approach*, 62.

19. Social Security Administration, www.ssa.gov (accessed April 2008).

20. Ibid.

21. F. Wolfe and J. Potter, "Fibromylagia and work disability: is fibromylagia a disabling disorder?" *Rheumatology Disability Clinics of North America* 22 (1996):
   369–91.

22. Social Security Administation, "Disability Evaluation under Social Security" ("Blue
   Book"), www.ssa.gov/disability/professionals/bluebook/listing-impairments
   .htm, SSA Publication No. 64–039 (accessed August 2009).

23. World Health Organization, www.who.int/topics/disabilities (accessed September 2009).

24. Social Security Administration, "Retirement Planner," www.socialsecurity.gov/
   retire2/credits3.htm (accessed April 22, 2008). [To access this information,
   search for "work credit" at SSA.gov. You will be directed to the htm link.]

25. Ibid.

26. Social Security Administration, "Code of Regulations," www.ssa.gov/OP_Home/
   cfr20/404/404-1520.htm (accessed September 2009).

27. Social Security Administration, "Code of Regulations," www.ssa.gov/OP_Home/
   cfr20/404/404-1563.htm (accessed September 2009).

28. Social Security Administration, "Code of Regulations," www.ssa.gov/OP_Home/
   cfr20/404/404-1564.htm (accessed September, 2009).

29. Social Security Administration, "Code of Regulations," www.ssa.gov/OP_Home/
   cfr20/404/404-1545.htm (accessed September 2009).

30. Social Security, Code of Federal Regulations, Appendix 2 to Subpart P of Part
   404—"Medical-Vocational Guidelines," www.ssa.gov/OP_Home/cfr20/404/
   404-ap11.htm (accessed September 2009).

31. Social Security Administration, "Code of Regulations," www.ssa.gov/OP_Home/
   cfr20/404/404-1572.htm (accessed September 2009).

32. Office of Retirement and Disability Policy: Annual Statistical report on the

Social Security Disability Insurance Program 2008, www.ssa.gov/policy/docs/statcomps/di_asr/2008/sect04.html#table59 (accessed September 2009).

33. Social Security Administration, "Appeals Process," www.socialsecurity.gov/pubs/10041.html (accessed September 2009).

34. Ibid.

35. Ibid.

36. Ibid.

37. Social Security Administration, *Social Security Handbook,* www.socialsecurity.gov/OP_Home/handbook/handbook.html (accessed September 2009).

38. Ibid.

39. The American Academy of Pain Management, www.aapainmanage.org/info/BillOfRights.php (accessed September 2009).

40. The Library of Congress, www.thomas.loc.gov.

41. Missouri Revised Statutes, Chap. 334—Physicians and Surgeons-Therapists-Athletic Trainers-Health, www.moga.mo.gov/STATUTES/C334.HTM (accessed September 2009).

42. California Pain Patient's Bill of Rights, S. B. 402, The National Foundation for the Treatment of Pain, www.paincare.org/pain_management/advocacy/ca_bill.html (accessed September 2009).

43. B. J. Bogart, *Legal Nurse Consultants: Principles and Practices* (New York: CRC Press, 1998), 717.

44. Ibid., 724

45. U.S. Department of Labor, Employee Benefits Security Administration, FAQs For Employees About COBRA Continuation Health Coverage, www.dol.gov/ebsa/faqs/faq_consumer_cobra.HTML (accessed September 2009).

46. COBRA Small Employer Exemption, www.wpsic.com/pdf/faq_groups_cobra.pdf (accessed September 2009).

47. U.S. Department of Labor, Employee Benefits Security Administration. FAQs For Employees About COBRA Continuation Health Coverage, www.dol.gov/ebsa/faqs/faq_consumer_cobra.HTML (accessed September 2009).

48. U.S. Department of Labor, Employee Benefits Security Administration, FAQs About Portability Of Health Coverage And HIPAA, www.dol.gov/ebsa/faqs/faq_consumer_hipaa.html. (accessed September 2009).

49. Bogart, *Legal Nurse Consultants: Principles and Practices,* 718–19.

50. U.S. Department of Labor website, www.dol.gov/dol/topic/health-plans/erisa.htm (accessed September 2009).

51. M. A. McKuin, "ERISA-Governed Claim Denials," www.mckuinlaw.com/FAQs-Page-2.html (accessed September 2009).

52. *The Family and Medical Leave Act of 1993,* U.S. Department of Labor website, www.dol.gov/compliance/laws/comp-fmla.htm (accessed September 2009).

53. *The Family and Medical Leave Act, Fact Sheet,* U.S. Department of Labor website, www.dol.gov/esa/whd/regs/compliance/whdfs28.pdf (accessed September, 2009).

54. S. Cooper, personal correspondence with author.

55. Ibid.

56. *The Family and Medical Leave Act, Fact Sheet,* U.S. Department of Labor website, www.dol.gov/esa/whd/regs/compliance/whdfs28.pdf (accessed September 2009).

57. Ibid.

58. U.S. Department of Labor website, "Rights of Key Employees," www.dol.gov/dol/allcfr/esa/Title_29/Part_825/29CFR825.219.htm (accessed September 2009).

59. *The Family and Medical Leave Act, Fact Sheet,* U.S. Department of Labor website, www.dol.gov/esa/whd/regs/compliance/whdfs28.pdf (accessed September 2009).

60. M. Skelly and S. Helm, *Alternative Treatments for Fibromyalgia and Chronic Fatigue Syndrome: Insights from Practitioners and Patients,* 1st ed. (Alameda, Calif.: Hunter House, Inc., 1999), chap. 7.

About the Authors

Celeste Cooper, R.N.

As a registered nurse for more than twenty years, Celeste's experience includes board-certified emergency nursing, critical care nursing, trauma nursing certification, and working as a nurse educator with agencies such as the American Heart Association and the Missouri State Board of Nursing. She has also been an expert witness as a nurse paralegal. She views this book as a vessel for sharing the trials, setbacks, and successes brought about by learning to cope with fibromyalgia, chronic fatigue immunodysfunction, and the chronic myofascial pain caused by persistent, restricting, and painful trigger points

Believing that knowledge is a necessary step to achieving wellness, Celeste's understanding of wellness is not limited to physical being, but includes intellectual, emotional, and spiritual balance. Any one of the disorders featured in this book has the ability to immobilize a life, but she believes one should view this "deer caught in the headlights" effect as a temporary setback. Her goal is to share ways to overcome obstacles and turn roadblocks into a road trip full of opportunities.

In addition to being an author, Celeste is an amateur photographer who enjoys life with her friends, husband, four children, three children-in-law, three grandchildren, and the many people she has had the pleasure of knowing because of these disorders.

For more information about Celeste Cooper, as well as continually updated information about fibromyalgia, chronic fatigue immunodysfunction, and chronic myofascial pain, visit Celeste's website at:

www.TheseThree.com

Jeffrey Miller, Ph.D.

A psychologist in private practice in suburban Kansas City, Missouri, Jeffrey Miller, Ph.D., was trained at Macalester College, Western Michigan University, and the University of Missouri-Kansas City. He has extensive post-graduate training through the Milton H. Erickson Institute in hypnotherapy and utilization approaches to behavior change. Jeff sees a broad range of clients but has emphases in medical issues, family systems, dissociative disorders, and existential questions. His work is informed and influenced by Dr. Erickson, psychologist Dr. Roger Ulrich, psychotherapist Jay Haley, family therapist Dr. Carl Whittaker, Tibetan Buddhist Lama Surya Das, filmmaker Robert Altman, spiritual master Shanti Mayi, humorist and political philosopher Steve Bhaerman, and spiritual devotee Baba Ram Das.

Jeff grew up between Kingston, Jamaica, and Sault Saint Marie, Michigan, before settling in central Arkansas. He moved to Kansas City in 1979, married Marji Datwyler in 1993, and now learns life's most worthwhile lessons from their children, Corina and Wilson. He has been blessed by the interdiction of fate improbable at every turn, which has prompted him to listen for guidance from dreams, song lyrics, wise folk, and fools. Jeff believes that if we do not learn to laugh at ourselves, we leave that job to others. He is currently finishing a primer on Stand-Up Therapy called "Your Second Wish."

For more information about Jeff Miller visit his website at:

www.jeffmiller.org

Index

Page numbers in *italics* refer to illustrations.

Books of Related Interest

Trigger Point Therapy for Myofascial Pain
The Practice of Informed Touch
by Donna Finando, L.Ac., L.M.T., and Steven Finando, Ph.D., L.Ac.

The New Rules of Posture
How to Sit, Stand, and Move in the Modern World
by Mary Bond

Preventing and Reversing Arthritis Naturally
The Untold Story
by Raquel Martin and Karen J. Romano, R.N., D.C.

Adaptogens
Herbs for Strength, Stamina, and Stress Relief
by David Winston and Steven Maimes

The Healing Power of Neurofeedback
The Revolutionary LENS Technique for Restoring Optimal Brain Function
by Stephen Larsen, Ph.D.

Traditional Foods Are Your Best Medicine
Improving Health and Longevity with Native Nutrition
by Ronald F. Schmid, N.D.

The Acid–Alkaline Diet for Optimum Health
Restore Your Health by Creating pH Balance in Your Diet
by Christopher Vasey, N.D.

Decoding the Human Body-Field
The New Science of Information as Medicine
by Peter H. Fraser and Harry Massey with Joan Parisi Wilcox

INNER TRADITIONS • BEAR & COMPANY
P.O. Box 388
Rochester, VT 05767
1-800-246-8648
www.InnerTraditions.com

Or contact your local bookseller